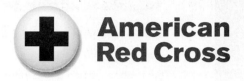

Responding to Emergencies:
Comprehensive First Aid/CPR/AED

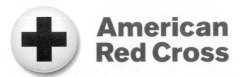

American Red Cross

This textbook is part of the American Red Cross Responding to Emergencies: Comprehensive First Aid/CPR/AED program. Visit redcross.org to learn more about this program.

The emergency care procedures outlined in this textbook reflect the standard of knowledge and accepted emergency practices in the United States at the time this textbook was published. It is the reader's responsibility to stay informed of changes in emergency care procedures.

Published by The StayWell Company, LLC

Printed in the United States of America

ISBN: 978-1-58480-684-4

Acknowledgments

The *Responding to Emergencies: Comprehensive First Aid/CPR/AED* textbook was developed through the dedication of both employees and volunteers. Their commitment to excellence made this textbook possible.

The emergency care steps outlined in this textbook are consistent with the 2015 International Consensus on CPR and Emergency Cardiovascular Care (ECC) Science With Treatment Recommendations and the 2015 American Heart Association and American Red Cross Guidelines Update for First Aid.

American Red Cross Scientific Advisory Council

Guidance for the Responding to Emergencies: Comprehensive First Aid/CPR/AED program was provided by members of the American Red Cross Scientific Advisory Council.

The Council is a panel of nationally recognized experts drawn from a wide variety of scientific, medical and academic disciplines. The Council provides authoritative guidance on first aid, CPR, emergency treatments, rescue practices, emergency preparedness, aquatics, disaster health, nursing, education and training.

For more information on the Scientific Advisory Council, visit redcross.org/science.

Dedication

This textbook is dedicated to the thousands of employees and volunteers of the American Red Cross who contribute their time and talent to supporting and teaching lifesaving skills worldwide, and to the thousands of course participants who have decided to be prepared to take action when an emergency strikes.

Table of Contents

Detailed Table of Contents

PART ONE
Introduction / 1

PART TWO
Assessment / 40

PART THREE
Life-Threatening Emergencies / 78

PART FOUR
Injuries / 158

PART FIVE
Medical Emergencies / 254

ABOUT THIS COURSE

People need to know what to do in an emergency before medical help arrives. It is, after all, trained lay responders such as yourself who are most likely to be on the scene of an emergency first. This course will prepare you to make appropriate decisions regarding first aid care, and equip you to act on your decisions, whether at home, at your workplace or in the community.

The first critical step in any emergency depends on the presence of someone who is willing to act and take appropriate action. After completing this course, you should be able to:

- Recognize when an emergency has occurred.

- Follow the emergency action steps:
  CHECK—CALL—CARE.

- Give care for an injury or sudden illness until emergency medical services (EMS) personnel arrive.

How You Will Learn

Course content is presented in various ways. The textbook, which will be assigned reading, contains the information that will be discussed in class, as well as visual support to illustrate the key skills and concepts you will be learning. In addition, you will view videos demonstrating how to correctly perform specific skills in preparation for skill practice sessions. Participating in all class activities will increase your confidence in your ability to respond to a variety of emergencies.

The course design allows you to frequently evaluate your progress in terms of skills competency, knowledge and decision making. Certain chapters in the textbook include directions for skill practice sessions that are designed to help you learn specific first aid skills. Some of the practice sessions require practice on a manikin. Others give you the opportunity to practice with another person. This will give you a sense of what it would be like to care for a real person in an emergency situation and help reduce any concerns or fears you may have about giving care. Your ability to perform specific skills competently will be checked by your instructor during the practice sessions.

Your ability to make appropriate decisions when faced with an emergency will be enhanced as you participate in the class activities. Periodically, you will be given situations in the form of scenarios that provide you the opportunity to apply the knowledge and skills you have learned. These scenarios also provide an opportunity to discuss with your instructor the many different situations that you may encounter in any emergency.

Requirements for American Red Cross Certification

By taking this course, you will be eligible for American Red Cross certification in Responding to Emergencies: Comprehensive First Aid/CPR/AED.

Red Cross certification means that on a particular date an instructor verified that a participant demonstrated competency in all required skills taught in the course. Competency is defined as being able to demonstrate correct decision making, sequence care steps properly, and proficiently complete all required skills without any coaching or assistance from the instructor or another participant.

To obtain certification, you must:

- Attend and participate in all class sessions.

  ○ *Note: If a participant must miss a session, the instructor should assign the appropriate make-up work to cover the course material missed during the participant's absence.*

- Participate in all skill sessions.

- Demonstrate competency in all required skills and scenarios.

- Pass each section of the written exam with a score of 80 percent or better.

If this course is taught at a college or university, there may be additional academic requirements, such as graded quizzes and other assignments, in order to pass this course. Your instructor will explain these requirements to you.

How to Use This Textbook

This textbook has been designed to facilitate your learning and understanding of the knowledge and skills required to effectively respond to emergency situations. The following pages graphically point out the features of this textbook so that you may use them to your best advantage.

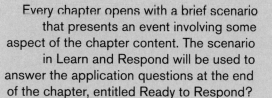

Learn and Respond ▶

Every chapter opens with a brief scenario that presents an event involving some aspect of the chapter content. The scenario in Learn and Respond will be used to answer the application questions at the end of the chapter, entitled Ready to Respond?

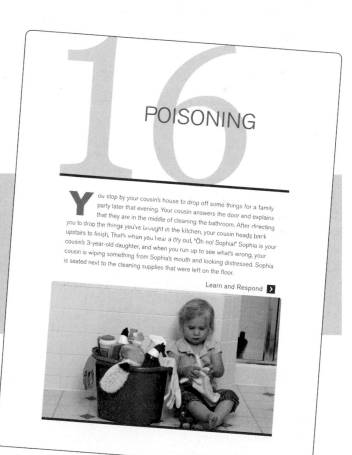

16

POISONING

You stop by your cousin's house to drop off some things for a family party later that evening. Your cousin answers the door and explains that they are in the middle of cleaning the bathroom. After directing you to drop the things you've brought in the kitchen, your cousin heads back upstairs to finish. That's when you hear a cry out, "Oh no! Sophia!" Sophia is your cousin's 3-year-old daughter, and when you run up to see what's wrong, your cousin is wiping something from Sophia's mouth and looking distressed. Sophia is seated next to the cleaning supplies that were left on the floor.

Learn and Respond ▶

Objectives ▶

At the beginning of each chapter is a bulleted list of objectives. Each item describes something you should know or be able to do after reading the chapter and participating in class activities. Read this list carefully, and refer back to it as you read the chapter. These objectives form the basis for the testing and assessment that will determine your mastery of the material.

OBJECTIVES

After reading this chapter, you should be able to:

- List four conditions that must be present for disease transmission to occur.
- Identify two ways in which a pathogen can enter the body.
- Describe how to minimize the risk of disease transmission when giving care in a situation that involves visible blood.
- Describe the difference between consent and implied consent.
- Describe the purpose of Good Samaritan laws.
- List three situations in which moving a person is necessary.
- List seven limitations you should be aware of before you attempt to move someone.
- Describe five ways to move a person.

After reading this chapter and completing the class activities, you should be able to:

- Demonstrate how to remove disposable latex-free gloves.

KEY TERMS

Abandonment: Ending the care of an injured or ill person without obtaining that person's consent or without ensuring that someone with equal or greater training will continue care.

Consent: Permission to receive emergency care granted by a competent adult either verbally or nonverbally.

Direct contact transmission: Mode of transmission of pathogens that occurs through directly touching infected blood or other potentially infectious materials (OPIM), or other agents such as chemicals, drugs or toxins.

Disease transmission: The passage of a disease from one person to another.

Implied consent: Legal concept that assumes a person would consent to receive emergency care if they were able or old enough to do so.

Indirect contact transmission: Mode of transmission of pathogens that occurs when a person touches objects that have the blood or other potentially infectious materials (OPIM) of an infected person, and that infected blood or OPIM enters the body through a correct entry site.

OPIM: Other potentially infectious materials such as body fluids (other than blood).

Personal protective equipment (PPE): The equipment and supplies that help prevent the responder from directly contacting infected materials; includes gloves, gowns, masks, shields and protective eyewear.

Standard precautions: Safety measures taken to prevent exposure to blood and OPIM when giving care to injured or ill persons; assumes that all body fluids, secretions and excretions (except sweat) are potentially infective.

Responding to Emergencies | **26** | Before Giving Care

Key Terms ▶

A list of key terms with their definitions also appears at the beginning of each chapter. You need to know these key terms and their meanings to understand the material in the chapters. These key terms are printed in ***boldface italics*** the first time they are explained in the chapter and also appear, defined, in the Glossary, located in the back of the textbook. Additional glossary terms appear in **boldface** within the chapter content.

Study Questions

1. Match each term with the correct definition.

   a. External bleeding   c. Pressure bandage   e. Arteries   g. Tourniquet

   b. Direct pressure   d. Internal bleeding   f. Veins

   ___ Using your gloved hand to apply pressure on the wound to control bleeding

   ___ Bleeding that can be seen coming from a wound

   ___ The escape of blood from an artery, vein or capillary inside the body

   ___ A tight band placed around an arm or leg to constrict blood vessels in order to stop blood flow to a wound

   ___ Blood vessels that carry blood from all parts of the body to the heart

   ___ Vessels that transport blood to the capillaries for distribution to the cells

   ___ A bandage applied snugly to maintain pressure on the wound to control bleeding

2. List two signs and symptoms of severe, life-threatening external bleeding.

3. Describe how to control severe, life-threatening external bleeding.

4. List five signs and symptoms of severe internal bleeding.

Use the following scenario to answer question 5.

The usual Saturday morning baseball game is in progress. A few spectators are standing around on the sidelines. As Milo takes a swing at a curve ball, he loses his grip on the bat, which flies several feet, hitting Chris hard on the thigh. Chris drops to the ground, clutching his leg. The skin where the leg was struck immediately becomes red and begins to swell.

5. What type of bleeding do you suspect Chris has?

For question 6, circle the letter of the correct answer.

6. A child has a deep cut on their arm. The child's face is moist and very pale. What would you do first?

   a. Have someone call 9-1-1 or the designated emergency number.

   b. Apply a hemostatic dressing to the wound.

   c. Place a cold pack on the affected arm.

   d. Apply pressure at the closest pressure point.

Answers are listed in the Appendix.

Responding to Emergencies | **149** | Bleeding

◀ Study Questions

At the end of each chapter is a series of study questions designed to test your retention and understanding of the chapter content and key terms. Completing these questions will help you determine how well you understand the material and also help you prepare for the final written exam. The answers to Study Questions are located in the Appendix of this textbook.

Ready to Respond?

READY TO RESPOND?

Think back to Mr. Getz in the opening scenario, and use what you have learned to respond to these questions:

1. Could atherosclerosis have led to Mr. Getz's collapse?
2. If Mr. Getz had experienced chest pain, how might stopping and resting have prevented his collapse?
3. Why is it important to know whether Mr. Getz may be suffering cardiac arrest?
4. If Mr. Getz is in cardiac arrest, why will CPR alone not sustain his life?

This feature includes application questions to challenge you to apply the information you have learned in the chapter and build a solution. The questions are based on the Learn and Respond scenario that appears at the beginning of the chapter. Answers to these questions can be found in the Appendix of this textbook.

What If...? ▶

This feature appears throughout each chapter and offers answers to some of the questions that participants may have as they learn about how to react in an emergency, especially regarding unexpected situations that may arise as you give care and information on how to deal with them.

What if... *I am giving chest compressions to a person in cardiac arrest and I hear a rib crack?*

In the adult population, particularly among older adults, rib and sternal (breastbone) fractures can be a complication of CPR. Making sure you use proper hand placement can minimize this risk. If you do hear a cracking sound and begin to feel crepitus (grinding) while compressing the chest, reassess your hand position and correct it as needed. Try to also remember that the potential benefits of CPR—namely, saving a life—outweigh the unpleasantness of a broken rib, which in most cases is not a life-threatening injury.

What if... *During CPR I lose count of the number of chest compressions I am performing and do more or less than the recommended 30 compressions?*

While 30 compressions is the recommended amount, performing 28 chest compressions in one cycle and 32 chest compressions in another cycle is not going to hurt the person's chances of survival. Rather, what is important is the chest compression rate and depth, which, for an adult, should be between 100 and 120 compressions per minute and at least 2 inches deep, while minimizing any interruptions.

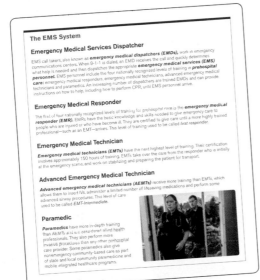

The EMS System

Emergency Medical Services Dispatcher

EMS call takers, also known as *emergency medical dispatchers (EMDs)*, work in emergency communications centers. When 9-1-1 is dialed, an EMD receives the call and quickly determines what help is needed and then dispatches the appropriate *emergency medical services (EMS) personnel.* EMS personnel include the four nationally recognized levels of training in *prehospital care:* emergency medical responders, emergency medical technicians, advanced emergency medical technicians and paramedics. An increasing number of dispatchers are trained EMDs and can provide instructions on how to help, including how to perform CPR, until EMS personnel arrive.

Emergency Medical Responder

The first of four nationally recognized levels of training for prehospital care is the *emergency medical responder (EMR)*. EMRs have the basic knowledge and skills needed to give emergency care to people who are injured or who have become ill. They are certified to give care until a more highly trained professional—such as an EMT—arrives. This level of training used to be called *first responder.*

Emergency Medical Technician

Emergency medical technicians (EMTs) have the next highest level of training. Their certification involves approximately 150 hours of training. EMTs take over the care from the responder who is initially at the emergency scene, and work on stabilizing and preparing the patient for transport.

Advanced Emergency Medical Technician

Advanced emergency medical technicians (AEMTs) receive more training than EMTs, which allows them to insert IVs, administer a limited number of lifesaving medications and perform some advanced airway procedures. This level of care used to be called *EMT-Intermediate.*

Paramedic

Paramedics have more in-depth training than AEMTs and are considered allied health professionals. They also perform more invasive procedures than any other prehospital care provider. Some paramedics also give nonemergency community-based care as part of state and local community paramedicine and mobile integrated healthcare programs.

◀ # Sidebars

Feature articles called sidebars enhance the information presented in the main body of the textbook. They present historical and current information and events that relate to the content of the chapter.

Smart Moves Prevention Boxes ▶

Applicable chapters include a boxed feature that outlines recommended preventive measures to avoid the injuries and/or illnesses discussed in the chapter.

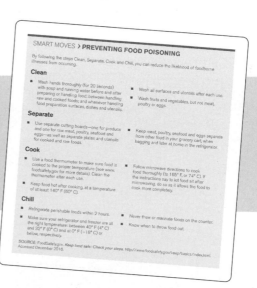

SMART MOVES > PREVENTING FOOD POISONING

By following the steps Clean, Separate, Cook and Chill, you can reduce the likelihood of foodborne illnesses from occurring.

Clean
- Wash hands thoroughly (for 20 seconds) with soap and running water before and after preparing or handling food; between handling raw and cooked foods; and whenever handling food preparation surfaces, dishes and utensils.
- Wash all surfaces and utensils after each use.
- Wash fruits and vegetables, but not meat, poultry or eggs.

Separate
- Use separate cutting boards—one for produce and one for raw meat, poultry, seafood and eggs—as well as separate plates and utensils for cooked and raw foods.
- Keep meat, poultry, seafood and eggs separate from other food in your grocery cart, when bagging and later at home in the refrigerator.

Cook
- Use a food thermometer to make sure food is cooked to the proper temperature (see www.foodsafety.gov for more details). Clean the thermometer after each use.
- Keep food hot after cooking, at a temperature of at least 140° F (60° C).
- Follow microwave directions to cook food thoroughly (to 165° F, or 74° C). If the instructions say to let food sit after microwaving, do so as it allows the food to cook more completely.

Chill
- Refrigerate perishable foods within 2 hours.
- Make sure your refrigerator and freezer are at the right temperature: between 40° F (4° C) and 32° F (0° C) and at 0° F (−18° C) or below, respectively.
- Never thaw or marinate foods on the counter.
- Know when to throw food out.

SOURCE: FoodSafety.gov. Keep food safe: Check your steps. http://www.foodsafety.gov/keep/basics/index.html. Accessed December 2016.

Tables

◀

Tables are included in many chapters. They summarize key concepts and information and may aid in studying.

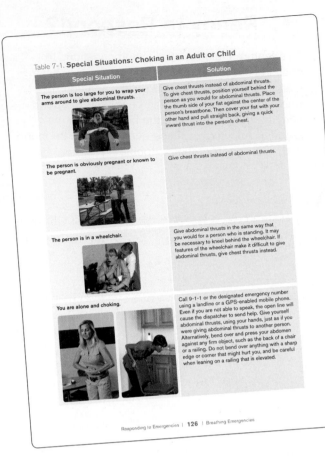

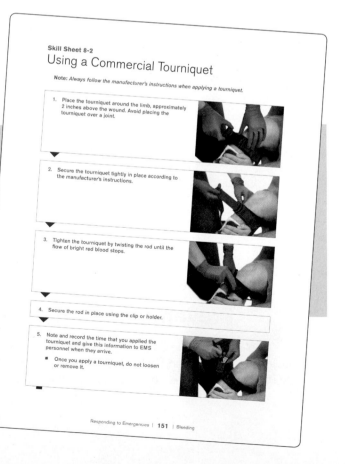

Skill Sheets ▶

At the end of certain chapters, Skill Sheets are available to give step-by-step directions for performing specific skills. Learning specific skills that you will need to give appropriate care for a person with an injury or sudden illness is an important part of this course. Photographs enhance each skill sheet.

Five Steps to Success: Study Tips While Using This Textbook

You should complete the following five steps for each chapter to gain the most from this textbook while studying from it:

1. Read the chapter Objectives before reading the chapter.

2. As you read the chapter, keep the Objectives in mind. When you finish, go back and review them.

3. Review figures and illustrations. Read captions and labels.

4. Answer the Ready to Respond? questions at the end of each chapter. Check your answers with those in the Appendix. If you cannot answer or do not understand the answers given, ask your instructor to help you with concepts or questions with which you are having difficulty.

5. Answer the Study Questions at the end of each chapter. Answer as many questions as you can without referring to the chapter. Then review the information covering any questions you were unable to answer, and try them again. Check your responses to the questions with the answers in the Appendix. If you have not answered a question appropriately, reread that part of the chapter to ensure that you understand why the answer is correct. This exercise will help you gauge how much information you are retaining and which areas you need to review. If, after rereading that part of the chapter, you still do not understand, ask your instructor to help you.

PART ONE

Introduction

1

IF NOT YOU ... WHO?

You and several friends are driving home after a softball game, when your lively game recap is suddenly interrupted by the sound of crashing metal. As you approach the intersection, you see a car that has swerved off the road and into a tree in an attempt to avoid another car that ran through the stop sign. You pull over a safe distance away from the crash and get out. As you approach the scene, you notice that the windshield is damaged. You can also see that the driver is motionless and bleeding from the forehead.

Learn and Respond ▶

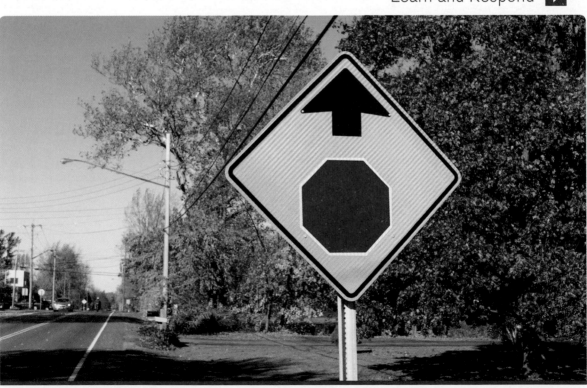

After reading this chapter, you should be able to:

- Describe two types of emergencies that require first aid.

- Describe your role in an emergency situation.

- Identify the most important action(s) you can take in an emergency.

- List six reasons that may prevent people from being willing to act in an emergency.

- Identify five ways bystanders can help at the scene of an emergency.

- Recognize the signs and symptoms of incident stress and when you may need help to cope.

KEY TERMS

Advanced emergency medical technician (AEMT): A person trained to give basic and limited advanced emergency medical care and transportation for critical and emergent patients who access the emergency medical services (EMS) system.

Emergency: A situation requiring immediate action.

Emergency medical dispatcher (EMD): A telecommunicator who has received special training to respond to a request for emergency medical services via 9-1-1 or a designated emergency number and to allocate appropriate resources to the scene of an emergency. Some EMDs are trained to provide prearrival medical instructions to a responder before emergency medical services (EMS) personnel arrive.

Emergency medical responder (EMR): A person trained in emergency care who may be called on to give such care as a routine part of their job until more advanced emergency medical services (EMS) personnel take over. EMRs often are the first trained professionals to respond to emergencies; also called "first responders."

Emergency medical services (EMS) personnel: Trained and equipped community-based personnel who give emergency care for injured or ill persons and who are often dispatched through 9-1-1 or a designated emergency number.

Emergency medical services (EMS) system: A network of professionals linked together to give the best care for people in all types of emergencies.

Emergency medical technician (EMT): A person who gives basic emergency medical care and transportation for critical and emergent patients who access the EMS system. EMTs are typically authorized to function after completing local and state certification requirements; formerly referred to as EMT-Basic.

First aid: The helping behaviors and initial care given for an acute injury or illness.

Good Samaritan laws: Laws that protect people against claims of negligence when they give emergency care in good faith without accepting anything in return.

Injury: Damage that occurs when the body is subjected to an external force, such as a blow, a fall, a collision, an electrical current or temperature extremes.

Lay responder: A layperson who is not trained to provide first aid, but who recognizes an emergency and decides to act.

(Continued)

┌─ KEY TERMS   continued

Life-threatening emergency: An injury or illness that impairs a person's ability to circulate oxygenated blood to all parts of the body and will likely cause death if not cared for immediately.

Non-life-threatening emergency: A situation that does not have an immediate impact on a person's ability to circulate oxygenated blood but still requires medical attention.

Paramedic: An allied health professional whose primary focus is to give advanced emergency medical care for critical and emergency patients who access the EMS system. Paramedics may also give nonemergency, community-based care based on state and local community paramedicine or mobile integrated healthcare programs.

Prehospital care: Emergency medical care given before a person arrives at a hospital or medical facility.

Sudden illness: A physical condition requiring immediate medical attention.

Trained lay responder: A layperson who is trained in basic emergency care (i.e., trained to give first aid), but who does not have special or advanced medical training, and is willing to act in an emergency.

Introduction

An **emergency** is a situation requiring immediate action. An emergency can happen at any place (on the road, in your home, where you work), to anyone (a friend, relative, stranger) and at any time. This text provides you with basic **first aid** information and skills so that you will be able to recognize and respond to any emergency appropriately by knowing how to give care to a person with an injury or sudden illness until more advanced care can be obtained. Your willingness to act and the care given may help save a life.

Types of Emergencies

There are two types of emergencies that require first aid: injury and sudden illness (usually referred to simply as illness). An **injury** is damage to the body from an external force, such as a broken bone from a fall. A **sudden illness** is a physical condition that requires immediate medical attention. Examples of sudden illness include a heart attack and a severe allergic reaction.

Emergencies can be further categorized as life-threatening and non-life-threatening. A **life-threatening emergency** is an injury or illness that impairs a person's ability to circulate oxygenated blood to all parts of the body and will likely cause death if not cared for immediately. A **non-life-threatening emergency** is a situation that does not have an immediate impact on a person's ability to circulate oxygenated blood but still requires medical attention. You will learn more about caring for life-threatening and non-life-threatening emergencies as you progress through this text.

Your Role in an Emergency

The **emergency medical services (EMS) system** is a network of professionals linked together to give the best care for people in all types of emergencies. Think of the EMS system as a chain made up of several links. Each link depends on the others for success. Without the involvement of **trained lay responders** such as you, the EMS system cannot function effectively. As a trained lay responder, your primary role in an emergency includes:

- Recognizing that an emergency exists.

- Being willing to act.

- Activating the EMS system by calling 9-1-1 or the designated emergency number.

- Giving care until EMS arrives and takes over or the situation resolves itself.

In the first few minutes of an emergency, a trained lay responder can provide help that can save a life or make the difference between a complete recovery and permanent disability. See The EMS System below for an overview of the roles played by professionals in responding to an emergency.

The EMS System

Emergency Medical Services Dispatcher

EMS call takers, also known as **emergency medical dispatchers (EMDs),** work in emergency communications centers. When 9-1-1 is dialed, an EMD receives the call and quickly determines what help is needed and then dispatches the appropriate **emergency medical services (EMS) personnel.** EMS personnel include the four nationally recognized levels of training in **prehospital care:** emergency medical responders, emergency medical technicians, advanced emergency medical technicians and paramedics. An increasing number of dispatchers are trained EMDs and can provide instructions on how to help, including how to perform CPR, until EMS personnel arrive.

Emergency Medical Responder

The first of four nationally recognized levels of training for prehospital care is the **emergency medical responder (EMR).** EMRs have the basic knowledge and skills needed to give emergency care to people who are injured or who have become ill. They are certified to give care until a more highly trained professional—such as an EMT—arrives. This level of training used to be called *first responder.*

Emergency Medical Technician

Emergency medical technicians (EMTs) have the next highest level of training. Their certification involves approximately 150 hours of training. EMTs take over the care from the responder who is initially at the emergency scene, and work on stabilizing and preparing the patient for transport.

Advanced Emergency Medical Technician

Advanced emergency medical technicians (AEMTs) receive more training than EMTs, which allows them to insert IVs, administer a limited number of lifesaving medications and perform some advanced airway procedures. This level of care used to be called *EMT-Intermediate.*

Paramedic

Paramedics have more in-depth training than AEMTs and are considered allied health professionals. They also perform more invasive procedures than any other prehospital care provider. Some paramedics also give nonemergency community-based care as part of state and local community paramedicine and mobile integrated healthcare programs.

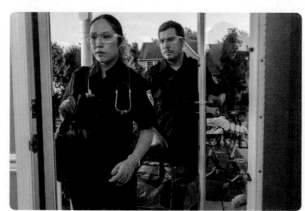

Preparing for an Emergency

By definition, emergencies are unexpected situations that require immediate action. But by expecting the unexpected and taking general steps to prepare, you can increase the likelihood of a positive outcome should an emergency situation arise.

By reading this textbook and participating in this American Red Cross Responding to Emergencies (RTE) course, you have taken an important first step in preparing for emergencies. You will learn the concepts and skills you need to recognize emergency situations and respond appropriately until advanced medical personnel arrive and take over. Once you have learned these concepts and skills, review and practice them regularly so that if you ever have to use them, you will be well prepared and have the confidence to respond.

Make sure you have ready access to items that will make it easier to respond to an emergency, should one occur. Keep a first aid kit in your home and vehicle (Box 1-1), and know the location of the first aid kit and automated external defibrillator (AED) in your workplace or community setting. Download the American Red Cross First Aid app to your mobile device so that you always have a first aid reference at your fingertips.

Box 1-1. **First Aid Kits**

You can purchase first aid kits and supplies from the Red Cross store (http://www.redcrossstore.org) or a local store. Whether you buy a first aid kit or assemble one yourself, make sure it has all of the items you may need. Check the kit regularly and replace any used or expired supplies. The Red Cross recommends that first aid kits include the following at a minimum:

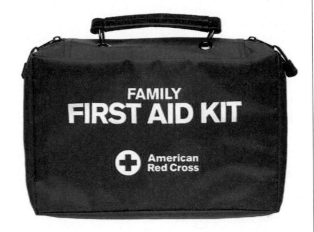

- 2 pairs of disposable latex-free gloves

- Latex-free adhesive bandages (3 of each of the following sizes):

    - 1 × 3 inches
    - ¾ × 3 inches
    - Large fingertip
    - Knuckle

- 8 sterile gauze pads (2 × 2 inches)

- 8 sterile gauze pads (4 × 4 inches)

- 1 roll of adhesive cloth tape (2½ yards × ⅜ inch)

- 4 roller bandages (2 inches or 3 inches × 4 yards)

- 4 roller bandages (4 inches × 4 yards)

- 1 elastic bandage (3 inches or 4 inches × 5 yards)

- 3 or 4 triangular bandages (40 inches × 40 inches × 56 inches)

- 1 36-inch malleable radiolucent splint

- 1 unit antibiotic ointment, cream or wound gel

- 4 sealable plastic bags (1 quart) or 2 chemical cold packs

- 5 antiseptic wipe packets

- 2 hydrocortisone ointment packets (approximately 1 gram each)

- 2 packets of chewable aspirin (81 mg each)

- 1 space blanket

- 1 CPR breathing barrier (with one-way valve)

- 1 pair of utility shears or scissors

- Oral thermometer (non-mercury/non-glass)

- Tweezers

- First aid manual

For a list of the recommended contents for a workplace first aid kit, see ANSI/ISEA Z308. 1-2015—*American National Standard for Minimum Requirements for Workplace First Aid Kits and Supplies.*

Keep a current list of emergency telephone numbers in your mobile phone, by the telephones in your home and workplace, and in your first aid kit. Most people in the United States call 9-1-1 for help in emergencies. But in some areas of the United States and in many workplaces, you many need to dial a designated emergency number instead. If you live or work in an area where 9-1-1 is *not* the number you should call in an emergency, make sure you know what the designated emergency number is.

Also include the numbers for the police department, fire department and the national Poison Help line (1-800-222-1222) on your list. Teach everyone in your home how and when to use these numbers.

Take steps to make it easier for EMS personnel and others to help you should an emergency occur:

- Make sure your house or apartment number is large, easy to read and well lit at night. Numerals are easier to read than spelled-out numbers.

- Keep relevant medical information, such as a list of the medications that each family member takes, in an accessible place (for example, on the refrigerator door and in your wallet or mobile phone).

- If you have a chronic medical condition such as diabetes, epilepsy or allergies, consider wearing a medical identification tag to alert responders to the presence of the condition in case you are not able to (Figure 1-1, A). You can also create a digital medical identification tag in your mobile phone that can be accessed without unlocking the phone (Figure 1-1, B). In addition to information about chronic medical conditions, blood type and so on, you can enter contact information for the person you would want contacted on your behalf in case of an emergency.

In a life-threatening emergency, every second counts. By preparing for emergencies, you can help ensure that care begins as soon as possible—for yourself, a family member, a co-worker or a member of your community.

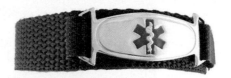

A

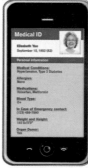

B

Figure 1-1, A–B. A medical identification tag, **A,** or an app on your phone, **B,** can give responders important information about you in case you are not able to. *Photos: N-StyleID.com*

Recognizing an Emergency

The ability to recognize that an emergency has occurred is the first step toward taking appropriate action. You may become aware of an emergency from certain indicators, including:

- Unusual sounds.

- Unusual sights.

- Unusual odors.

- Unusual appearance or behaviors.

Box 1-2 provides examples for each of these indicators. See also Figure 1-2.

Your own personal safety is a top priority. Always put your own safety first if you smell an unusual or very strong odor because many fumes are poisonous. An unusual odor on a person's breath may also be a clue to an emergency situation. A person experiencing a diabetic emergency, for example, may have a sweet breath odor that can be mistaken for the smell of alcohol. You will learn about diabetic emergencies in Chapter 15.

It may also be difficult to tell if someone's appearance or behavior is unusual, particularly if it is a stranger. If you see someone collapse to the floor, they obviously require your immediate attention. You will not know if your help is needed until you check the scene and approach the person. The person may merely have slipped and may not need your immediate help. On the other hand, the person may be unresponsive and need immediate medical assistance.

Box 1-2. **Signs of an Emergency**

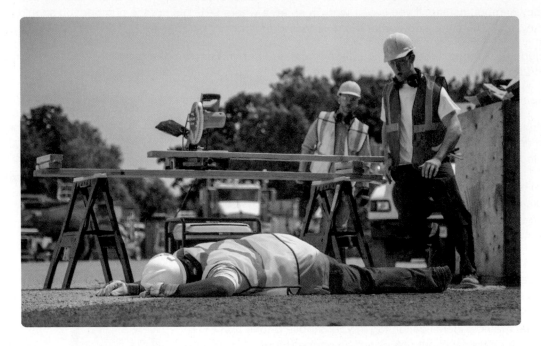

Unusual Sounds

- Screaming, moaning, yelling or calls for help
- Sudden, loud noises such as breaking glass, crashing metal or screeching tires
- A change in the sound(s) made by machinery or equipment
- The sound of an explosion or falling ladder
- Unusual silence

Unusual Sights

- A stopped vehicle on the roadside or a car that has run off the road
- Downed electrical wires
- Sparks, smoke or fire
- A person who collapses or is lying motionless
- Signs or symptoms of injury or illness, such as profuse sweating for no apparent reason or an uncharacteristic skin color
- Spilled medication or an empty medication container
- An overturned pot in the kitchen

Unusual Odors

- A foul or unusually strong chemical odor
- The smell of smoke
- The smell of gas
- An unrecognizable odor
- An inappropriate odor (e.g., a sickly sweet odor on a person's breath)

Unusual Appearance or Behaviors

- Unresponsiveness
- Confusion, drowsiness or unusual behavior
- Personality or mood changes (e.g., agitation in a person who is normally calm or irritability in a person who is normally pleasant)
- Trouble breathing
- Sudden collapse, slip or fall
- Clutching the chest or throat
- A person doubled over in pain
- Slurred, confused or hesitant speech
- Sweating for no apparent reason
- Uncharacteristic skin color
- Inability to move a body part

Deciding to Take Action

Once you recognize an emergency situation, you must decide to take action. In an emergency, deciding to act is not always as simple as it sounds. Some people are slow to act in an emergency because they panic, are not exactly sure what to do or think someone else will take action. But in an emergency situation, your decision to take action and be willing to act could make the difference between life and death for the person who needs help.

Your decision to act in an emergency should be guided by your own values and by your knowledge of the risks that may be present. However, even if you decide not to give care, you should at least call 9-1-1 or the designated emergency number to get emergency medical help to the scene.

Willingness to Act

Sometimes people recognize an emergency but are reluctant to act. People have various reasons for hesitating or not acting. Common reasons people give for not acting include:

- Being uncertain that an emergency actually exists.

- Being afraid of giving the wrong care or inadvertently causing the person more harm.

- Assuming that the situation is already under control.

- Squeamishness related to unpleasant sights, sounds or smells.

- Fear of catching a disease.

- Fear of being sued.

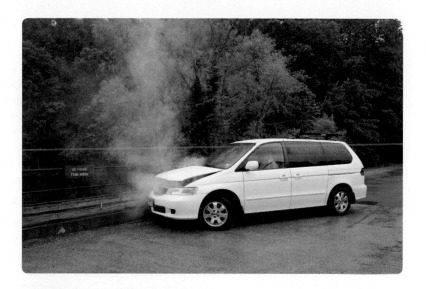

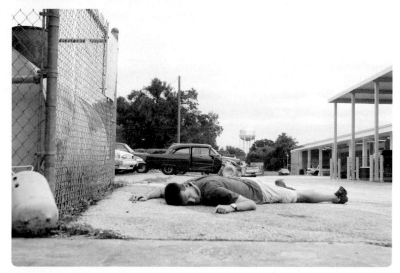

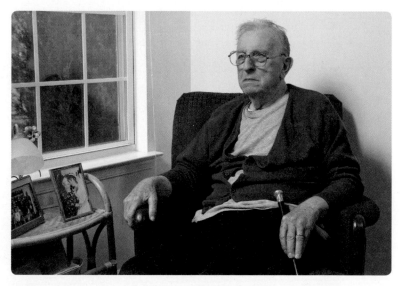

Figure 1-2. Unusual sounds, sights or behaviors are some of the indicators of an emergency.

Many different fears and concerns can cause a person to hesitate to respond in an emergency. Understanding these fears and concerns can help you to overcome them:

- **Being uncertain that an emergency actually exists.** Sometimes people hesitate to take action because they are not sure that the situation is a real emergency and do not want to waste the time of the EMS personnel. If you are not sure what to do, err on the side of caution and call 9-1-1 or the designated emergency number.

- **Being afraid of giving the wrong care or inadvertently causing the person more harm.** Getting trained in first aid can give you the confidence, knowledge and skills you need to respond appropriately to an emergency. If you are not sure what to do, call 9-1-1 or the designated emergency number and follow the EMS dispatcher's instructions. The worst thing to do is nothing.

- **Assuming that the situation is already under control.** Although there may be a crowd of people around the injured or ill person, it is possible that no one has taken action. If no one is giving care or directing the actions of bystanders, you can take the lead (Figure 1-3). If someone else is already giving care, confirm that someone has called 9-1-1 or the designated emergency number and ask how you can be of help.

- **Squeamishness related to unpleasant sights, sounds or smells.** Many people feel faint or nauseated when confronted with upsetting sights, sounds or smells, such as blood, vomit or a traumatic injury. You may have to turn away for a moment and take a few deep breaths to regain your composure before you can give care. If you still are unable to give care, you can volunteer to help in other ways, such as by calling 9-1-1 or the designated emergency number and bringing necessary equipment and supplies to the scene.

- **Fear of catching a disease.** In today's world, the fear of contracting a communicable disease while giving care to another person is a real one. However, although it is possible for diseases to be transmitted in a first aid situation, it is extremely unlikely that you will catch a disease this way. Taking additional precautions, such as putting on disposable latex-free gloves and using a CPR breathing barrier, can reduce your risk even further.

- **Fear of being sued.** Sometimes people hesitate to get involved because they are worried about liability. In fact, lawsuits against *lay responders* (nonprofessionals who give care in an emergency situation) are highly unusual and rarely successful. The majority of states and the District of Columbia have *Good Samaritan laws* that protect people against claims of negligence when they give emergency care in good faith without accepting anything in return. For more information on Good Samaritan laws, see Chapter 3.

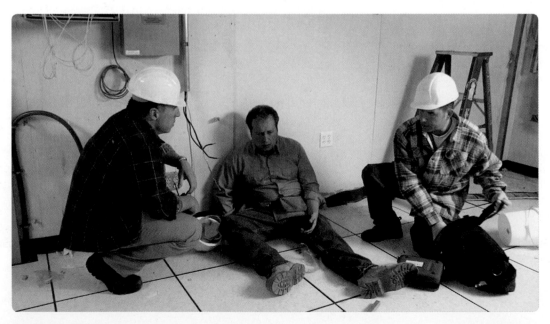

Figure 1-3. A bystander can help you respond to an emergency in many ways.

What if... *I really don't know what is wrong with the person I am trying to help, or how serious their injury is?*

Lay responders decide not to act for many reasons; fear of not knowing what to do or of doing something wrong is normally at the top of the list. Rest assured, however, that regardless of your knowledge and skill level, you can always help by taking one simple but important step in an emergency: calling 9-1-1 or the designated emergency number. After that, if you are uncomfortable with actually performing any emergency care, providing comfort and reassurance and controlling the scene would be the next best things you can do.

What if... *I mistakenly call 9-1-1 or the designated emergency number from a landline phone?*

In either case if you were to dial 9-1-1 accidentally—do not hang up! Instead, explain to the call taker what happened. In the case of a call coming in on an E9-1-1 line, if you were to hang up before speaking with the call taker, it would trigger an automatic call back. If the dispatcher was unable to reach anyone, appropriate personnel would be sent to investigate the situation, potentially tying up valuable resources.

What if... *I only have a mobile phone at home, and not a landline? Will I still have access to 9-1-1?*

Yes. Throughout the United States, mobile phones can access the 9-1-1 system as long there is a wireless signal. Most wireless public safety answering points (PSAPs) have the ability to locate the phone's location, but this can take some time so it is critical to tell the call taker your exact location to speed up the response.

Finally, if you do need to call 9-1-1, remember not to hang up until you are sure the dispatcher has all of the information necessary to send help to exactly where it is needed.

Your willingness to act in an emergency should be guided by your own values and by your knowledge of the risks that may be present. However, even if you decide not to give care, you should at least call 9-1-1 or the designated emergency number to get emergency medical help to the scene if it is warranted.

Activating the EMS System

Calling 9-1-1 or the designated emergency number is the most important action you and other trained lay responders can take in an emergency. Early arrival of EMS personnel increases the person's chances of surviving a life-threatening emergency. Remember, some facilities, such as hotels, office and university buildings and some stores, require you to dial a 9 or some other number to get an outside line before you dial 9-1-1 (e.g., 9-9-1-1). There are also a few areas that still are without access to a 9-1-1 system and use either a 7- or 10-digit emergency number instead. Becoming familiar with your local system is important so you are ready when an emergency occurs.

When you dial 9-1-1 or the designated emergency number, your call will normally be answered by a 9-1-1 call taker. It is important to stay calm and listen to the call taker's questions. The most important information you can share with the call taker is the location of the emergency so that public safety resources can be dispatched while other information is gathered and any prearrival instructions can be given. Based on the nature of the emergency, you may be transferred by the call taker to an EMD or a dispatcher, if appropriate. The EMD will ask you a series of questions in order to ensure that the most appropriate response is sent to the location of the emergency.

You should not hang up until directed by the EMD. Once EMS personnel are on the way, the EMD may stay on the line and give you prearrival instructions to assist you with lifesaving techniques until EMS personnel take over (Figure 1-4).

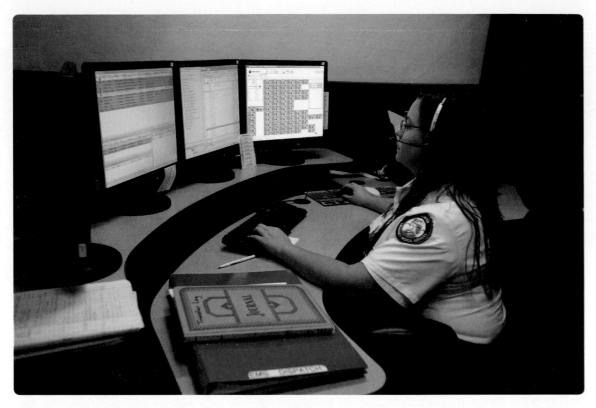

Figure 1-4. Many EMDs give prearrival instructions for what to do before EMS personnel arrive.

Giving Care Until Help Arrives

There are many actions you, other trained lay responders or bystanders can take before EMS personnel arrive. Always follow the prearrival instructions provided by the EMD. These instructions may range from taking actions that make the scene safer and more accessible to EMS personnel (e.g., confining household pets, turning on extra lights, gathering the person's medications) to giving care. You will learn to give more advanced care for an injured or ill person as you progress through this course.

In general, you should give appropriate care to an injured or ill person until one or more of the following occurs:

- Another trained responder or EMS personnel take over.

- You are alone and you need to call 9-1-1 or the designated emergency number after giving initial care in a Care First situation (see Box 2-3 in Chapter 2).

- You are too exhausted to continue.

- The scene becomes unsafe.

- The person you are helping is awake and alert and asks you to stop giving care.

Incident Stress

After responding to an emergency involving a serious injury, illness or death, it is not unusual to experience acute stress. Sometimes, people who have given first aid or performed CPR in these situations feel that they are unable to cope with the stress. This feeling is known as incident stress. If not appropriately managed, this acute stress may lead to a serious condition called post-traumatic stress disorder.

Signs and Symptoms of Incident Stress Reactions

Some effects may appear right away, whereas others may take longer to develop. Signs and symptoms of incident stress include:

- Anxiousness and inability to sleep.
- Nightmares.
- Restlessness and other problems.
- Confusion.
- Lower attention span.
- Poor concentration.
- Denial.
- Guilt.

- Depression.
- Anger.
- Nausea.
- Change in interactions with others.
- Increased or decreased eating.
- Uncharacteristic, excessive humor or silence.
- Unusual behavior.
- Difficulty performing one's job.

Coping with Incident Stress

Incident stress may require professional help to prevent post-traumatic stress from developing. Other things that you may do to help reduce stress include using relaxation techniques, eating a balanced diet, avoiding alcohol and drugs, getting enough rest, and participating in some type of physical exercise or activity.

If you recognize these signs or symptoms in yourself or another responder, it is important to seek help from a trained mental healthcare professional.

Summary

An emergency can happen at any place, to anyone and at any time. The EMS system is a network of community resources and medical personnel that give emergency care to injured or ill persons. However, the EMS system cannot function properly without the actions of a trained lay responder like you. By learning to recognize an emergency and, more importantly, being willing to act (calling 9-1-1 or the designated emergency number and giving care), you can help save the life of a person with an injury or sudden illness. Once you have taken care of the injured or ill person, remember to also consider your own feelings about the emergency situation and take signs and symptoms of incident stress seriously if any are present.

In the following chapters, you will learn how to manage different kinds of emergencies. You will learn emergency action steps that you can apply to any emergency situation, and how to give care in both life-threatening and non-life-threatening situations.

READY TO RESPOND? ❯

Think back to the car crash in the opening scenario, and use what you have learned to respond to these questions:

1. What immediate steps could you and your friends who were first on the scene at the car crash take?

2. As you approach the car and the injured person, you begin to feel faint and nauseated, and are not sure you can proceed any further. How can you still help?

Study Questions

1. **In each of the following three scenarios, circle the indicators of a potential emergency.**

    a. I was fixing sandwiches and talking with my next-door neighbor, Mrs. Roberts, who had come by to borrow a book. My 3-year-old, Jenny, was in her room playing with some puzzles. As Mrs. Roberts got up to leave, I heard a loud thump and a shriek from upstairs.

    b. I was on the bus headed for work. A man from the back of the bus came down the aisle, and I noticed that he was moving unsteadily. It was cold in the bus, but I noticed he was sweating and looked very pale. "I don't know where I am," I heard him mumble to himself.

    c. On my way into the grocery store from the parking lot, I heard the loud screech of tires and the crash of metal. I saw that a car had struck a telephone pole, causing the telephone pole to lean at an odd angle. Wires were hanging down from the pole onto the street. It was very frightening.

2. **List the six common fears or concerns that prevent people from taking action at the scene of an emergency.**

3. **How can a trained lay responder overcome any one of these fears or concerns listed in question 2?**

4. **Match each item with the correct phrase.**

    a. First aid

    b. Lay responder

    c. Emergency

    d. Sudden illness

    e. EMS system

    f. Common fears and concerns

    _____ A situation requiring immediate action

    _____ A network of community resources and medical personnel that gives emergency care to a person with an injury or sudden illness

    _____ Immediate care given to a person with an injury or sudden illness until more advanced care can be obtained

    _____ A physical condition, such as a heart attack, requiring immediate medical attention

    _____ A layperson (someone who does not have special or advanced medical training or skill) who recognizes an emergency and is willing to act

    _____ Reasons for not acting or for hesitating to act in an emergency situation

5. **Identify five ways bystanders can help at the scene of an emergency.**

Answers are listed in the Appendix.

2 RESPONDING TO AN EMERGENCY

As you arrive at your friend's house one Saturday morning, you are surprised that your friend is not in his usual spot—in the driveway tinkering with the antique car he is currently restoring. It's a little chilly today, though, and you hear music coming from the garage, so you figure your friend is in the garage. When you open the garage door to say hello, you are not prepared to find your friend lying on the floor apparently unresponsive. You need to do something, but what?

Learn and Respond ❯

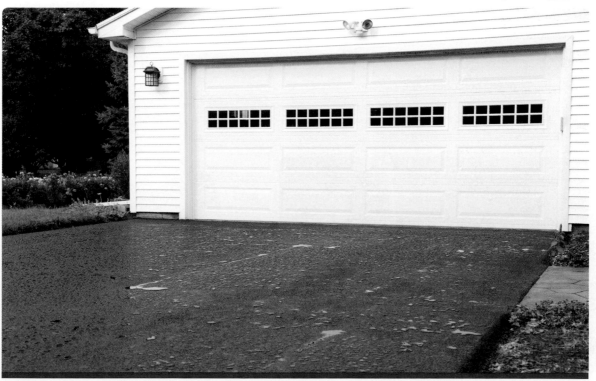

Introduction

An emergency scene can be overwhelming. It poses questions that demand immediate answers. What should I do first? Where can I get help? What can I do to help the injured or ill person? By learning how to check an emergency scene and prioritize your actions, you will be able to respond effectively in any emergency situation.

Taking Action: The Emergency Action Steps

In any emergency situation, there are three simple steps to take to guide your actions. If you ever feel nervous or confused, remember these three *emergency action steps* to get you back on track:

1. **CHECK** the scene and the person.

2. **CALL** 9-1-1 or the designated emergency number.

3. **CARE** for the person.

Check

First, check the scene. Then check the person.

Check the Scene

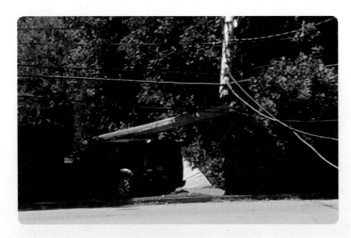 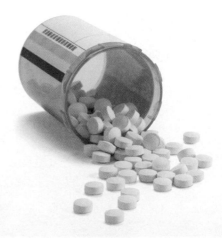

Photo: Jonathan L. Epstein, MEMS

Before rushing to help an injured or ill person, conduct a **scene size-up** and form an initial impression. Try to answer these questions:

- Is the scene safe to enter?
- What happened?
- How many people are involved?

- What is your initial impression about the nature of the person's injury or illness?
- Is anyone else available to help?

- **Is the scene safe to enter?** Check for hazards that could jeopardize your safety or the safety of bystanders, such as fire, downed electrical wires, spilled chemicals, an unstable building or traffic. Do not enter bodies of water unless you are specifically trained to perform in-water rescues (Box 2-1). Avoid entering confined areas with poor ventilation and places where natural gas, propane or other substances could explode. Do not enter the scene if there is evidence of criminal activity or the person is hostile or threatening suicide. If these or other dangers threaten, stay at a safe distance and call 9-1-1 or the designated emergency number immediately. Once professional responders make the scene safe, you can offer your assistance as appropriate.

Box 2-1. **Reach or Throw, Don't Go!**

Never go into water or onto ice in an attempt to rescue a person who is in trouble. Instead, get help from a trained responder, such as a lifeguard, to get the person out of the water as quickly and safely as possible.

Reaching and throwing assists are the safest assists for responders who are not professionally trained lifeguards to use to help a person who is in trouble in the water. When doing a reaching or throwing assist:

- Talk to the person and let the person know help is coming.

- Tell the person what they can do to help with the rescue, such as grasping a line or other floating device. Use gestures to communicate with the person if it is too noisy or if the person is too far away to hear.

- Encourage the person to move toward safety by kicking their legs or stroking with their arms. Some people are able to reach safety by themselves with calm encouragement from a person on the deck or shore.

Reaching assist. To do a reaching assist, use any available object that will extend your reach and give the person something to grab onto (such as a pole, an oar or paddle, a branch or a towel). Extend the object to the person, tell them to hold on and pull the person to safety. If no equipment is available and you are close enough, you may be able to perform a reaching assist by extending your arm to the person. You can also perform a reaching assist

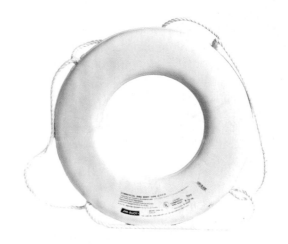

from a position within the water by extending an arm or a leg to the person, if you are already in the water and you have something secure to hold onto.

Throwing assist. A throwing assist involves throwing a floating object to the person so that they can grasp it and be pulled to safety. A floating object with a line attached (such as a ring buoy) is ideal for a throwing assist; however, a line or an object that floats (such as a life jacket or cooler) can be used instead.

Wading assist. A wading assist involves wading into the water and using a reaching assist to help pull the person to safety. Only use a wading assist in water that is less than chest deep. If a current or soft bottom makes wading dangerous, do not enter the water. For your own safety, wear a life jacket if one is available and take something to extend to the person, such as a ring buoy, branch, pole or paddle.

- **What happened?** Take note of anything that might tell you the cause of the emergency. If the person is unresponsive and there are no witnesses, your check of the scene may offer the only clues as to what happened. Use your senses to detect anything out of the ordinary, such as broken glass, a spilled bottle of medication, or an unusual smell or sound. Keep in mind that the injured or ill person may not be exactly where they were when the injury or illness occurred—someone may have moved the person, or the person may have moved in an attempt to get help.

- **How many people are involved?** Look carefully for more than one injured or ill person. A person who is moving or making noise or who has very visible injuries will likely attract your attention right away, but there may be a person who is silent and not moving or a person obscured by debris or wreckage that you do not notice at first. It is also easy to overlook a small child or an infant. In an emergency with more than one injured or ill person, you may need to prioritize care (in other words, decide who needs help first).

- **What is your initial impression about the nature of the person's injury or illness?** Before you reach the person, try to form an initial impression about the person's condition and what is wrong. For example, does the person seem alert, or confused or sleepy? Look at the person's skin—does it appear to be its normal color, or does it seem pale, ashen (gray) or flushed? Is the person moving, or motionless? Does the person have any immediately identifiable injuries? Look for signs of a life-threatening injury or illness, such as unresponsiveness, trouble breathing or severe bleeding. If you see severe, life-threatening bleeding, use the resources available to you to control the bleeding as soon as possible (see Chapter 8).

- **Is anyone else available to help?** Take note of bystanders who can be of assistance. A bystander who was there when the emergency occurred or who knows the injured or ill person may be able to provide valuable information about the situation or the person. Bystanders can also assist in other ways, such as by calling 9-1-1 or the designated emergency number, waiting for EMS personnel and leading them to the site of the emergency, getting needed items (such as an AED and first aid kit), controlling crowds, and reassuring the injured or ill person.

What if... I am trying to help out an injured neighbor, but the family dog starts acting aggressively towards me when I enter the house? Should I try to enter anyway?

An aggressive animal is complex and unpredictable, and the potential consequences of being attacked by such an animal can be serious. You should not risk becoming injured yourself, complicating the emergency further. Instead of continuing into the house, immediately call 9-1-1 or the designated emergency number from a safe place, and explain that you need to report an emergency and that there is an aggressive animal blocking your access to the injured person. The dispatcher will make sure that the appropriate resources are dispatched to the scene to handle the full situation safely and appropriately. The same would be true if you encountered downed power lines, falling rocks, fire, smoke or the like.

What if... I am helping on the scene of a car crash in which a downed power line has fallen on someone's car and is touching the ground? Should I help the person exit the car?

No! The person should stay in the car. When a person is in the vehicle, they are not a part of the electricity's path to the ground; therefore, the car is the safest place to be under the circumstances. Have the person wait in the car until public safety professionals or qualified electrical workers turn the power off. At the same time, you should stay in a safe location while waiting for help to arrive. Electricity can spread out through the ground in a circle from any downed line, making more than just the vehicle electrically charged.

Check the Person

When you reach the person, you can conduct a more thorough check to determine what is wrong and what care is needed.

If the person is awake and alert, obtain consent (you will learn about consent in Chapter 3) and then begin to gather additional information about the nature of the person's injury or illness. Chapter 5 provides more detail about how to check a person who is responsive.

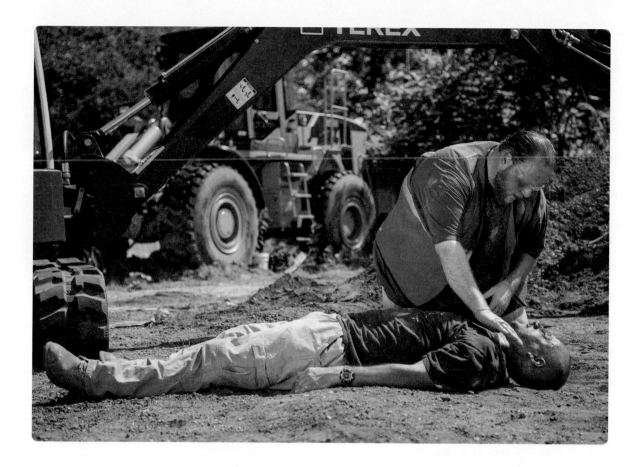

If the person appears to be unresponsive, shout, using the person's name if you know it. If there is no response, tap the person's shoulder (if the person is an adult or child) or the bottom of the person's foot (if the person is an infant) and shout again while checking for normal breathing. Check for responsiveness and breathing for no more than 5 to 10 seconds. If the person does not respond to you in any way (such as by moving, opening their eyes or moaning) and the person is not breathing or is only gasping, the person is unresponsive. If the person responds and is breathing normally, the person is responsive but may not be fully awake. Give care according to the conditions that you find and your level of knowledge and training.

Unresponsiveness, trouble breathing and severe bleeding are all signs of a life-threatening emergency. If your initial check of the person reveals these or any other life-threatening conditions (see Box 2-2), make sure that someone calls 9-1-1 or the designated emergency number right away. Also have someone bring an AED and a first aid kit, if these items are available.

Call

If you decide it is necessary to summon EMS personnel (see Box 2-2), make the call quickly and return to the person. If possible, ask someone else to make the call so that you can begin giving care. The person making the call should be prepared to give the dispatcher the following information:

- The location of the emergency (the address, or nearby intersections or landmarks if the address is not known)

- The nature of the emergency (e.g., whether police, fire or medical assistance is needed)

- The telephone number of the phone being used

- A description of what happened

- The number of injured or ill people

- What help, if any, has been given so far, and by whom

Box 2-2. When to Activate the EMS System

Call 9-1-1 or the designated emergency number for any of the following emergency situations and conditions.

Emergency Situations

- An injured or ill person who needs medical attention and cannot be moved

- Fire or explosion

- Downed electrical wires

- Swiftly moving or rapidly rising flood waters

- Drowning

- Presence of poisonous gas

- Serious motor-vehicle collision

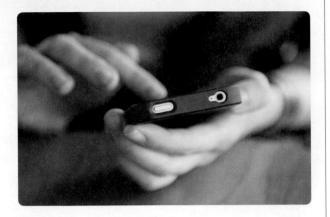

Emergency Conditions

- Unresponsiveness or an altered level of consciousness (LOC), such as drowsiness or confusion

- Breathing problems (trouble breathing or no breathing)

- Chest pain, discomfort or pressure lasting more than a few minutes that goes away and comes back or that radiates to the shoulder, arm, neck, jaw, stomach or back

- Persistent abdominal pain or pressure

- Severe external bleeding (bleeding that spurts or gushes steadily from a wound)

- Vomiting blood or passing blood

- Severe (critical) burns

- Suspected poisoning that appears to be life threatening

- Seizures

- Signs or symptoms of a stroke (e.g., drooping of the face on one side; sudden weakness on one side of the body; sudden slurred speech or difficulty speaking; or a sudden, severe headache)

- Suspected or obvious injuries to the head, neck or spine

- Suspected or obvious broken bone

PHOTO: Hammonds/Shutterstock.com

The caller should stay on the phone until the dispatcher tells the caller it is all right to hang up. The dispatcher may need more information. Many dispatchers are also trained to give first aid and CPR instructions over the phone, which can be helpful if you are unsure of what to do or need to be reminded of the proper care steps.

If you are alone and there is no one to send to call 9-1-1 or the designated emergency number, you may need to decide whether to call first or give care first (Box 2-3). Call First situations are likely to be cardiac arrest. In cardiac arrest, the priority is getting help on the scene as soon as possible because early access to EMS personnel and an AED increases the person's chances for survival. Care First situations include breathing emergencies and severe, life-threatening bleeding. In these situations, there are immediate actions that you can take at the scene that may prevent the person's condition from worsening. After you take these actions, call 9-1-1 or the designated emergency number to get advanced medical help on the way.

Box 2-3. **Call First or Care First?**

Most of the time, you will call first and then give care. But if you are alone, you must decide whether to call first or care first.

If you are ALONE:

CALL First (call 9-1-1 or the designated emergency number before giving care) for:

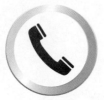

- Any person about 12 years or older who is unresponsive.

- A child or an infant whom you witnessed suddenly collapse.

- An unresponsive child or infant known to have heart problems.

CARE First (give immediate care, then call 9-1-1 or the designated emergency number) for:

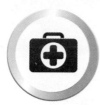

- An unresponsive infant or child younger than about 12 years whom you did not see collapse.

- A person who is choking.

- A person who is experiencing a severe allergic reaction (anaphylaxis) and has an epinephrine auto-injector.

- A person who has severe, life-threatening bleeding.

As a trained lay responder, your top priority is to ensure that the person receives more advanced care as soon as possible. The EMS system works more effectively if you can give information about the person's condition when the call is placed. This information helps to ensure that the person receives proper medical care as quickly as possible. Make the call quickly and return to caring for the person. If possible, ask a bystander to make the call.

Care

The final emergency action step is to give care according to the conditions that you find and your level of knowledge and training. Always care for life-threatening conditions before those that are not life threatening. For example, a breathing emergency would take priority over an injured (e.g., deformed) leg. Follow these general guidelines:

- Do no further harm.

- Monitor the person's breathing and level of consciousness.

- Help the person rest in the most comfortable position.

- Keep the person from getting chilled or overheated.

- Reassure the person by telling them that you will help and that EMS personnel have been called (if appropriate).

- Give care consistent with your knowledge and training as needed, and continue to watch for changes in the person's condition.

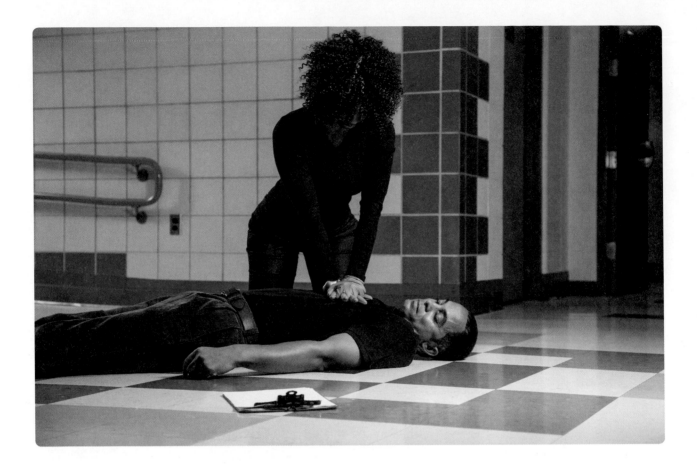

Generally speaking, you should avoid moving an injured or ill person to give care. Unnecessary movement can cause additional injury and pain and may complicate the person's recovery. However, under the following three conditions, it would be appropriate to move an injured or ill person:

- You must move the person to protect them from immediate danger (such as fire, flood or poisonous gas). However, you should attempt this only if you can reach the person and remove them from the area without endangering yourself.

- You must move the person to reach another person who may have a more serious injury or illness.

- You must move the person to give proper care. For example, it may be necessary to move a person who needs CPR onto a hard, flat surface.

If you must move the person, use one of the techniques described in Emergency Moves in Chapter 3.

Transporting the Person Yourself

If the person does not have a life-threatening injury or illness, you may decide to take the injured or ill person to a medical facility yourself instead of calling for EMS personnel. Never transport a person yourself if the person has or may develop a life-threatening condition, if you are unsure of the nature of the injury or illness, or if the trip may aggravate the injury or cause additional injury.

If you decide it is safe to transport the person yourself, be sure you know the quickest route to the nearest medical facility capable of handling emergency care. Ask someone to come with you to help keep the person comfortable and monitor the person for changes in condition so that you can focus on driving. Remember to obey traffic laws. No one will benefit if you are involved in a motor-vehicle collision or get a speeding ticket on your way to the medical facility.

Discourage an injured or ill person from driving themself to the hospital. An injury may restrict movement, or the person may become faint. The sudden onset of pain may be distracting. Any of these conditions can make driving dangerous for the person, passengers, other drivers and pedestrians.

Adult, Child or Infant?

While you would not normally think of a 14-year-old boy as an adult, or you might consider a 1-year-old still more of a baby than a child, the definitions when it comes to giving emergency care are different.

For purposes of first aid, follow these guidelines:

- An adult is defined as someone about age 12 (adolescent) or older.

- A child is someone between the ages of 1 and 12.

- An infant is someone younger than 1 year.

When using an AED:

- A child is considered to be someone between the ages of 1 and 8 years or weighing less than 55 pounds.

Summary

Emergency situations are often confusing and frightening. To take appropriate actions in any emergency, follow the three basic emergency action steps: **CHECK—CALL—CARE. CHECK** the scene by performing a scene size-up and then check the person, **CALL** 9-1-1 or the designated emergency number to activate the EMS system and **CARE** for the person until EMS personnel arrive.

READY TO RESPOND? ❯

Think back to the scene in the garage in the opening scenario, and use what you have learned to respond to these questions:

1. What dangers could exist in the garage?

2. What specific factors in the garage could influence your decision to move or not move your friend?

3. After checking the scene in the garage and moving your friend to safety if needed, what would you do next? Why?

Study Questions

1. List the emergency action steps.

Answer questions 2–5 based on the scenario below.

You are driving along the interstate. It is getting dark. Rain has been falling steadily and is now beginning to freeze. Suddenly a tractor-trailer that you can see in the distance ahead of you begins to sway and slide, then jackknifes and crashes onto its left side. Drivers put on their brakes and swerve, and by some miracle, everyone close by manages to avoid crashing into the fallen truck or each other. You pull onto the median and stop a safe distance behind the truck.

2. List the possible dangers to be aware of at the scene of this emergency.

3. Describe the actions you should take if you determine that the scene is unsafe.

4. You check the driver and discover that the driver is unresponsive. You tell a bystander to call 9-1-1. List the information that the bystander should have when calling 9-1-1.

5. Describe the actions you would take if no one else was available to help.

Answers are listed in the Appendix.

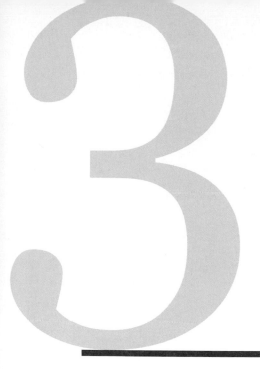

3 BEFORE GIVING CARE

You are about to head out for a jog from the parking lot of a local recreation area when you see a group of kids come running off the trail. One boy suddenly pitches forward after tripping on his shoelace and lands right on his hands and face on the pavement. You'd be surprised if he's not scraped up pretty good, so you quickly grab your first aid kit from the car and hurry over to see how you can help. A moment later, his grandfather emerges from the trail and runs to his side.

Learn and Respond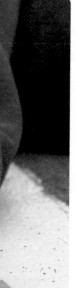

After reading this chapter, you should be able to:

- List four conditions that must be present for disease transmission to occur.

- Identify two ways in which a pathogen can enter the body.

- Describe how to minimize the risk of disease transmission when giving care in a situation that involves visible blood.

- Describe the difference between consent and implied consent.

- Describe the purpose of Good Samaritan laws.

- List three situations in which moving a person is necessary.

- List seven limitations you should be aware of before you attempt to move someone.

- Describe five ways to move a person.

After reading this chapter and completing the class activities, you should be able to:

- Demonstrate how to remove disposable latex-free gloves.

KEY TERMS

Abandonment: Ending the care of an injured or ill person without obtaining that person's consent or without ensuring that someone with equal or greater training will continue care.

Consent: Permission to receive emergency care granted by a competent adult either verbally or nonverbally.

Direct contact transmission: Mode of transmission of pathogens that occurs through directly touching infected blood or other potentially infectious materials (OPIM), or other agents such as chemicals, drugs or toxins.

Disease transmission: The passage of a disease from one person to another.

Implied consent: Legal concept that assumes a person would consent to receive emergency care if they were able or old enough to do so.

Indirect contact transmission: Mode of transmission of pathogens that occurs when a person touches objects that have the blood or other potentially infectious materials (OPIM) of an infected person, and that infected blood or OPIM enters the body through a correct entry site.

OPIM: Other potentially infectious materials such as body fluids (other than blood).

Personal protective equipment (PPE): The equipment and supplies that help prevent the responder from directly contacting infected materials; includes gloves, gowns, masks, shields and protective eyewear.

Standard precautions: Safety measures taken to prevent exposure to blood and OPIM when giving care to injured or ill persons; assumes that all body fluids, secretions and excretions (except sweat) are potentially infective.

Introduction

As a trained lay responder, you have made an important decision to help an injured or ill person. However, in any emergency situation your top priority is to ensure your own safety. In this chapter, you will learn how to protect yourself from disease transmission, as well as how to properly move a person in a way that is safe for both the person and you. In addition, this chapter provides you with some basic legal information you need to know before giving care.

Preventing Disease Transmission

Bloodborne pathogens, such as bacteria and viruses, are present in blood and ***other potentially infectious materials (OPIM)*** and can cause disease. They are acquired from other people, animals, insects or things that have been in contact with the pathogen. Because some infectious diseases such as hepatitis and human immunodeficiency virus (HIV) are very serious, you must learn how to protect yourself and others from ***disease transmission,*** or the passage of disease from one person to another, while helping a person who has been injured or is ill.

How Diseases Spread

The disease process begins when a **pathogen** (e.g., a **bacteria** or **virus**) enters the body. When pathogens enter the body, they can sometimes overpower the body's natural defense systems and cause illness. This type of illness is called an **infection.** Most infectious diseases are caused by bacteria and viruses.

Bacteria are everywhere. They do not depend on other organisms for life and can live outside the human body. Most bacteria do not infect humans. Those that do may cause serious illness. Bacterial meningitis and **tetanus** are examples of diseases caused by bacteria. The body's ability to fight infection depends on its immune system. In a person with a healthy immune system, a bacterial infection is often avoided. However, another person may have difficulty fighting infection caused by bacteria. When an infection is present, physicians may prescribe antibiotics that either kill the bacteria or weaken them enough for the body to get rid of them. Commonly prescribed antibiotics include penicillin, erythromycin and tetracycline.

Unlike bacteria, viruses such as the flu, Ebola and Zika depend on other organisms to live and reproduce. Viruses can cause many diseases, including the common cold (caused by the rhinovirus), hepatitis and HIV. Once in the body, viruses may be difficult to eliminate because very few medications are effective against viral infections. Although there are some medications that kill or weaken viruses, the body's own immune system is the main defense against them.

How Bloodborne Pathogens Spread

For any disease to be spread, including bloodborne disease, all four of the following conditions must be met:

- A pathogen is present.

- There is sufficient quantity of the pathogen present to cause disease.

- The pathogen passes through the correct entry site (i.e., eyes, mouth and other mucous membranes or skin pierced or broken by cuts, abrasions, bites and sharp objects).

- A person is susceptible to the pathogen.

To understand how infections occur, think of these four conditions as pieces of a puzzle. All of the pieces have to be in place for the picture to be complete. If any one of these conditions is missing, an infection cannot occur (Figure 3-1).

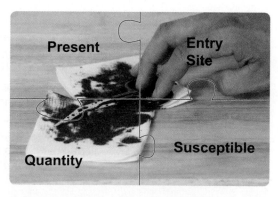

Figure 3-1. If any one of these conditions is missing, infection will not occur.

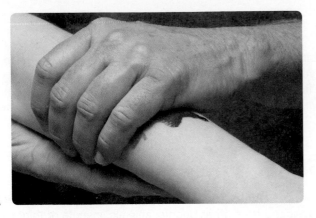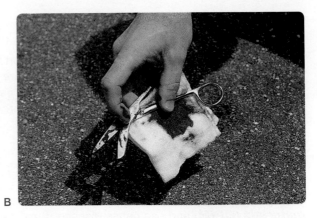

A   B

Figure 3-2. A, Example of direct contact transmission. **B,** Example of indirect contact transmission.

Bloodborne pathogens such as hepatitis B virus (HBV), hepatitis C virus (HCV) and HIV can spread from person to person through ***direct contact transmission*** and ***indirect contact transmission*** with infected blood or OPIM. HBV, HCV and HIV are not spread by food or water or by casual contact such as hugging or shaking hands.

Direct contact transmission occurs when the infected blood or OPIM from one person enters another person's body at a correct entry site. For example, direct transmission can occur through infected blood splashing in the eye or by directly touching body fluids from an infected person (Figure 3-2, A).

Indirect contact transmission can occur when a person touches an object that contains the blood or OPIM of an infected person, and that infected blood or OPIM enters the body through a correct entry site. These objects include soiled dressings, equipment and work surfaces that are contaminated with an infected person's blood or OPIM. For example, indirect contact transmission can occur when a person picks up blood-soaked bandages with a bare hand and the pathogens enter through a break in the skin on the hand (Figure 3-2, B).

Standard Precautions When Giving Care

Standard precautions are safety measures taken to prevent exposure to blood and OPIM when giving care to injured or ill persons. This approach to infection control means that you should consider all body fluids and substances as infectious. These precautions and practices include personal hygiene, using ***personal protective equipment (PPE),*** using proper equipment for cleaning and disinfecting contaminated surfaces and properly disposing of contaminated materials (e.g., use of biohazard bags).

Personal Hygiene

Good personal hygiene habits, such as frequent hand washing, are the best way to prevent disease transmission (Figure 3-3). You should always wash your hands thoroughly with soap and warm running water when you have finished giving care, even if you wore disposable latex-free gloves. If time permits, wash your hands before giving care in non-emergent situations. Wash for a minimum of 20 seconds and make sure to cover all surfaces of both hands: your wrists, the palms and backs of your hands, in between your fingers and underneath your fingernails.

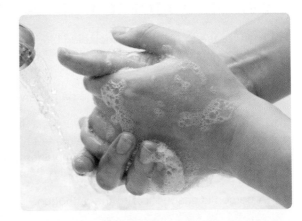

Figure 3-3. Thorough hand washing after giving care helps to protect you against disease. *Photo: Gang Lui/ Shutterstock.com*

To wash your hands correctly, you should:

- Wet your hands with warm water.
- Apply soap to your hands.
- Rub your hands vigorously for at least 20 seconds, covering all surfaces of the hands and fingers.
  - Use warm running water.
  - Scrub nails by rubbing them against the palms of your hands.
- Rinse your hands with water.
- Dry your hands thoroughly with a clean paper towel.
- Turn off the faucet using the paper towel.

If soap and water are not available, you may use an alcohol-based hand sanitizer to decontaminate your hands. When using an alcohol-based hand sanitizer, use the amount of product recommended by the manufacturer. Rub it thoroughly over all surfaces of your hands, including your nails and in between your fingers, until the product dries. Wash your hands with soap and water as soon as you have access to hand-washing facilities.

Safety First! Alcohol-based hand sanitizers may not be as effective if your hands are visibly soiled with dirt or body fluids. In addition, although using an alcohol-based hand sanitizer properly will reduce the number of pathogens on your hands, it may not eliminate all pathogens. For these reasons, always wash your hands with soap and water as soon as you can, even if you used an alcohol-based hand sanitizer! Also, always keep alcohol-based hand sanitizers out of the reach of children.

Personal Protective Equipment

Personal protective equipment (PPE) is equipment used to prevent pathogens from contaminating your skin, mucous membranes or clothing. Articles of PPE that are commonly used when giving first aid care include disposable latex-free gloves and CPR breathing barriers. Face masks and protective eyewear are other types of PPE that may be used in a first aid situation.

Safety First! Be prepared by having a first aid kit handy and adequately stocked with PPE. You can also carry a keychain kit containing a pair of disposable latex-free gloves and a breathing barrier so that you always have this equipment readily available.

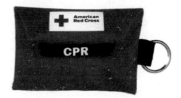

Disposable Latex-Free Gloves

Disposable latex-free gloves are meant to be worn once and then discarded. Never clean or reuse these gloves. Disposable latex-free gloves should fit properly and be free of rips or tears. Wear disposable latex-free gloves:

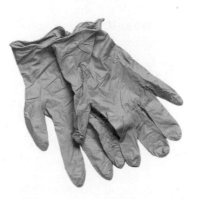

- When giving care, especially whenever there is a possibility that you will come in contact with a person's blood or OPIM.
- When there is a break in the skin on your own hands (cover any cuts, scrapes or sores before putting on the gloves).
- When you must handle items or surfaces soiled with blood or OPIM.

When you are wearing gloves, try to limit how much you touch other surfaces with your gloved hands. Pathogens from your soiled gloves can transfer to other items or surfaces that you touch, putting the next person who handles the item or touches the surface at risk for infection. If possible, remove soiled gloves and replace them with a clean pair before touching other surfaces or equipment in your first aid kit. When you are finished giving care, remove your gloves using proper technique to avoid contaminating your own skin, dispose of the gloves properly and wash your hands. When multiple people are in need of care, remove your gloves, wash your hands and replace your gloves with a clean pair before assisting the next person.

Safety First! Because many people are allergic to latex, the American Red Cross recommends the use of disposable latex-free gloves. Nitrile gloves are preferred over other types of disposable latex-free gloves, such as those made of vinyl.

CPR Breathing Barriers

CPR breathing barriers are used to protect you from contact with blood and OPIM, such as saliva, as you give rescue breaths. Breathing barriers also protect you from breathing the air that the person exhales. The most basic and portable type of breathing barrier is a face shield, a flat piece of thin plastic that you place over the person's face, with the opening over the person's mouth. The opening contains a filter or a valve that protects you from coming into contact with the person's body fluids and exhaled air. A pocket mask is a transparent, flexible device that creates a tight seal over the person's nose and mouth to allow you to give rescue breaths without making mouth-to-mouth contact or inhaling exhaled air. Breathing barriers sized specifically for children and infants are available. Always use equipment that is sized appropriately for the injured or ill person.

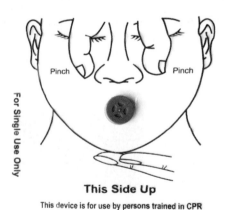

For Single Use Only

Pinch   Pinch

This Side Up

This device is for use by persons trained in CPR

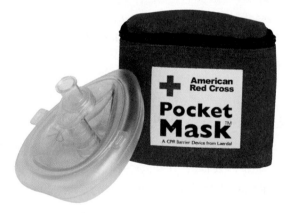

American Red Cross

Pocket Mask™

A CPR Barrier Device from Laerdal

What if... *I need to help someone who is bleeding severely, but there are no disposable latex-free gloves available to protect me against bloodborne pathogens?*

Protecting yourself and others from disease transmission, especially in the presence of visible blood, requires the use of standard precautions. However, if PPE, such as disposable latex-free gloves, is not readily available, a person who is awake and alert may be able to apply direct pressure to their own wound. If that is not an option, consider the use of items such as a plastic sandwich bag, plastic wrap or a plastic shopping bag. While not "ideal," any of these can help to minimize exposure to blood and OPIM.

Additional Precautions

When giving care, you should also take the following precautions to protect yourself and the person you are helping:

- Do not eat, drink or touch your mouth, nose or eyes when giving care or before you wash your hands after care is given.

- Avoid handling any of your personal items, such as pens or combs, while giving care or before you wash your hands.

- Ensure that you clean and disinfect anything you may have touched inadvertently with contaminated gloves such as door knobs, phones or other equipment.

- Do not touch objects that may be soiled with blood or OPIM.

Cleaning Up After Giving Care or a Blood Spill

Thoroughly clean and disinfect all surfaces that may have come into contact with the injured or ill person as well as any materials that may have become contaminated while giving care.

If a blood spill occurs:

- Clean up the spill immediately or as soon as possible after the spill occurs.

- Use disposable latex-free gloves and other PPE when cleaning up spills.

- Wipe up the spill with paper towels or other absorbent materials (Figure 3-4).

  ○ If the spill is mixed with sharp objects, such as broken glass or needles, do not pick these up with your hands. Use tongs, a broom and dustpan or two pieces of cardboard to scoop up the sharp objects.

- After the area has been wiped up, flood the area with an appropriate disinfectant, such as a fresh solution of approximately 1½ cups of liquid chlorine bleach to 1 gallon of fresh water (1 part bleach per 9 parts water). Let stand for at least 10 minutes.

- Dispose of the contaminated material used to clean up the spill in a labeled biohazard container.

- Contact your worksite safety representative or your local health department regarding the proper disposal of potentially infectious materials.

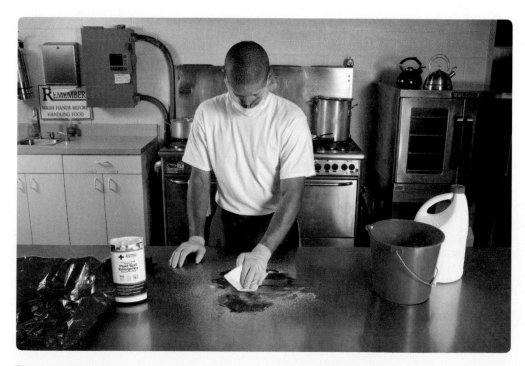

Figure 3-4. When cleaning up a blood spill, follow all standard precautions.

If You Are Exposed

If you are exposed to blood or OPIM (e.g., a person's blood gets into a cut on your hand, bloody saliva splashes into your mouth or eyes), take the following steps immediately:

- Clean the contaminated area thoroughly with soap and water.

- Flush splashes of blood or OPIM in the mouth or nose with water.

- If the eyes are involved, irrigate with clean water, saline or sterile irrigants for 20 minutes.

Be sure to notify a police officer or other professional on the scene, such as a firefighter or emergency medical services (EMS) personnel, or your healthcare provider, that you have been exposed. Seek immediate medical attention.

Legal Considerations

Obtaining Consent to Help

Before giving first aid care, you must obtain **consent** (permission) from the injured or ill person (or the person's parent or guardian if the person is a minor) (Figure 3-5). To obtain consent:

- State your name.

- State the type and level of training that you have (such as training in first aid or CPR).

- Explain what you think is wrong.

- Explain what you plan to do.

- Ask if you may help.

With this information, an injured or ill person can grant consent for care. Someone who is unresponsive, confused or mentally impaired may not be able to grant consent. In these cases, the law assumes the person would give consent if they were able to do so. This is called **implied consent.** Implied consent also applies when a minor needs emergency medical assistance and the minor's parent or guardian is not present.

An injured or ill person may refuse care, even if they desperately need it. A parent or guardian also may refuse care for a minor in their care. You must honor the person's wishes. Explain to the person why you believe care is necessary, but do not touch or give care to the person if care was refused. If you believe the person's

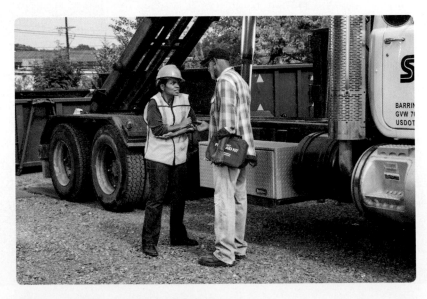

Figure 3-5. Obtain consent before giving care.

condition is life threatening, call EMS personnel to evaluate the situation. If the person gives consent initially but then withdraws it, stop giving care and call for EMS personnel if you have not already done so.

If you do not speak the same language as the injured or ill person, obtaining consent may be challenging. Find out if someone else at the scene can serve as a translator. If a translator is not available, do your best to communicate with the person by using gestures and facial expressions. When you call 9-1-1 or the designated emergency number, explain that you are having difficulty communicating with the person, and tell the dispatcher which language you believe the person speaks. The dispatcher may have someone available who can help with communication.

> **What if...** *A person in obvious need of help refuses care—but then becomes unresponsive?*
>
> *An injured person who is competent has the legal right to refuse first aid care from a trained lay responder, public safety personnel or a healthcare provider. As taught in this chapter, you should at least call 9-1-1 or the designated emergency number, even if the person will not let you give care yourself. If while waiting for additional help to arrive that person becomes unresponsive and is critically injured, the rules of implied consent should be followed. Implied consent assumes that the person would want care for a life-threatening condition if they could give consent.*

Abandonment

Just as you must obtain the injured or ill person's consent before beginning care, you must also continue to give care once you have begun. Once you have started emergency care, you are legally obligated to continue that care until a person with equal or higher training relieves you, you are physically unable to continue or the person refuses care. Usually, your obligation for care ends when more advanced medical professionals take over. If you stop your care before that point without a valid reason, such as leaving momentarily to get the proper equipment, you could be legally responsible for the ***abandonment*** of a person in need (Box 3-1).

Box 3-1. **Good Samaritan Laws**

Good Samaritan laws, which protect the responder from financial liability, were developed to encourage people to help others in emergency situations. They assume a responder will do their best to save a life or prevent further injury. Good Samaritan laws require the responder to use common sense and a reasonable level of skill, and to give only the type of emergency care for which the responder is trained. Good Samaritan laws usually protect responders who act the way a "reasonable and prudent person" would act if that person were in the same situation. For example, a reasonable and prudent person would:

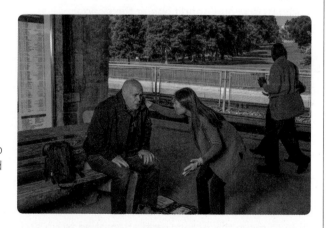

- Move a person only if the person's life were in danger.

- Ask a responsive person (or the parent or guardian of a minor) for permission to help (consent) before giving care.

- Check the person for life-threatening conditions before giving further care.

- Call 9-1-1 or the designated emergency number.

- Continue to give care until more highly trained personnel take over.

If a lay responder's actions were grossly negligent or reckless, or if the responder abandoned the person after starting care, Good Samaritan laws may not protect the responder. For more information about your state's Good Samaritan law(s), conduct an Internet search or contact a legal professional.

What if... *I help someone who ends up needing surgery to repair the injury? Can I be sued for giving care?*

Lay responders in most, if not all, states may be protected by their respective state's Good Samaritan law(s). If you use common sense and a reasonable level of skill to give only the type of emergency care for which you are trained, Good Samaritan laws will most likely protect you. Please refer to your state's Good Samaritan law(s) for further details.

Reaching and Moving a Person

Usually, when you give first aid, you will not face hazards that require moving the person immediately. In most cases, you can follow the emergency action steps by checking the scene and the person, calling 9-1-1 or the designated emergency number and caring for the person where you find them. In fact, one of the most dangerous threats to a seriously injured or ill person is unnecessary movement. Movement can lead to further injury and pain, and can complicate recovery. For example, if the person has a fracture of the leg, movement could result in the end of the bone tearing the skin. Soft tissue damage, damage to nerves, blood loss and infection all could result unnecessarily.

However, there are some situations in which moving the person would be appropriate. You should move a person only when you can do so safely and only in one of the following three situations:

- When you must move the person to protect them from immediate danger (such as fire, flood or poisonous gas). However, you should attempt this only if you can reach the person and remove them from the area without endangering yourself.

- When you must move the person to reach another person who may have a more serious injury or illness.

- When you must move the person to give proper care. For example, it may be necessary to move a person who needs CPR onto a hard, flat surface.

Before you act, consider the following limitations to moving one or more persons quickly and safely:

- Any dangerous conditions at the scene

- The size of the person

- The distance the person must be moved

- Your physical ability

- Whether others (bystanders) can help you

- The person's condition

- Any aids or equipment to facilitate moving the person at the scene

Considering these limitations will help you decide how to proceed. For example, if you are injured, you may be unable to move the person, and attempting to do so will only risk making the situation worse. If you become part of the problem, EMS personnel will have one more person to rescue.

To protect yourself and the person, follow these guidelines when moving a person:

- Use your legs, not your back, when you bend.

- Bend at the knees and hips, and avoid twisting your body.

- Maintain a firm grip on the person.

- Walk forward when possible, taking small steps and looking where you are going to maintain a firm footing.

- Avoid twisting or bending anyone with a possible head, neck or spinal injury.

- Do not move a person who is too large to move comfortably.

- Use good posture.

Gaining Access

Sometimes you cannot give care because the person is inaccessible. One example is a situation in which someone is able to call for help but is unable to unlock the door of the home or office. A person may also be inaccessible in a motor vehicle collision. Vehicle doors are sometimes locked or crushed, windows may be rolled up or the vehicle may be unstable. Fire, water or other obstacles may prevent you from safely reaching the person.

During the scene size-up, begin to think of how to safely gain access to the person. If you cannot reach the person, you may not be able to give care. But remember, when attempting to reach a person, your safety is the most important consideration. Protect yourself and the person by doing only what you are trained to do and by using equipment appropriate for the situation. In traffic-related incidents, items such as reflective markers or flares and flashlights may help keep you and the scene visible to oncoming traffic.

Emergency Moves

Generally speaking, you should avoid moving an injured or ill person to give care. Unnecessary movement can cause additional injury and pain and may complicate the person's recovery.

If you must move a person in an emergency situation, the goal is to do so without injuring yourself or causing additional injury to the person. The following common emergency moves can be done by one or two people and with minimal or no equipment. The situation will dictate which move you should use (Table 3-1).

Table 3-1. **Emergency Moves**

Move	When to Use It	How to Do It
Walking Assist 	To move a person who can walk but needs help*	1. Place the person's arm around your shoulder or waist (depending on how tall the person is), and hold it in place with one hand. 2. Support the person with your other hand around the person's waist. (Another responder can also support the person in the same way on the other side.)

(*Continued*)

Table 3-1. continued

Move	When to Use It	How to Do It
Two-Person Seat Carry	To move a responsive person who is not seriously injured*	1. Put one arm under the person's thighs and the other across their back, under the arms. Have a second responder do the same. 2. Interlock your arms with the other responder's arms under the person's legs and across the person's back. 3. Lift the person in the "seat" formed by your interlocked arms.
Clothes Drag	To move a responsive or an unresponsive person who may have a head, neck or spinal injury	1. Grasp the person's shirt behind the neck, gathering enough material so that you have a firm grip. 2. Cradle the person's head with the shirt and your hands, and pull the person to safety.
Blanket Drag	To move a responsive or an unresponsive person	1. Fold the blanket in half lengthwise, and place it so that the fold is alongside the person's body. 2. Take the top layer of the folded blanket, and roll it toward the person's body. 3. Position yourself so that the person is between you and the blanket. 4. Put one hand on the person's shoulder and the other on their hip and roll the person onto their side, toward you, and then pull the blanket toward you so that it is against the person's body. 5. Roll the person onto their back, onto the blanket. 6. Pull the side of the blanket that was rolled up toward yourself, so that the person is in the middle of the blanket. 7. Gather the blanket at the person's head and pull the person to safety.

(Continued)

Table 3-1. continued

Move	When to Use It	How to Do It
Ankle Drag	To move a person who is too large to move another way	1. Cross the person's arms over their chest. 2. Firmly grasp the person's ankles. 3. Move backward, pulling the person in a straight line and being careful not to bump the person's head.

*Do not use this emergency move if you suspect that the person has a head, neck or spinal injury.

Summary

In any emergency situation, your top priority is to ensure your own safety. Protect yourself from disease transmission by wearing PPE, such as disposable latex-free gloves and breathing barriers, and following good personal hygiene practices, such as hand washing. Always check the scene for safety during the scene size-up before you approach a person, and be sure to obtain consent from an adult person who is awake and alert. If a person does not give consent, do not give care, but do call 9-1-1 or the designated emergency number. Never move a person unless the scene is or becomes unsafe. If you must move a person, be sure to do so in a manner that is safe for you and will not cause the person any further harm. By thinking before you give care, you will not only be ensuring the safety of the person but also your own.

> **READY TO RESPOND?** ❯
>
> Think back to the boy in the opening scenario, and use what you have learned to respond to these questions:
>
> 1. What steps should you take before beginning to give care?
>
> 2. What steps will help to prevent disease transmission after giving care?

Study Questions

For questions 1–5, circle the letter of the correct answer.

1. **Disease transmission from a person to a responder requires four conditions to be present. Which of the following is NOT one of these four?**

   a. The person may or may not be infected with a disease.

   b. The responder must be susceptible to the pathogen.

   c. There must be enough of the pathogen present to cause infection.

   d. The pathogen passes through a correct entry site.

(Continued)

2. You are giving first aid to a child who has fallen off a bike. An untrained bystander who is not wearing gloves picks up the gauze with blood on it. The bystander's action is an example of exposure through—

   a. Direct contact.   b. Bacterial contact.   c. Viral contact.   d. Indirect contact.

3. Safety measures you can use to prevent disease transmission include—

   a. Calling 9-1-1 or the designated emergency number.
   b. Using PPE such as disposable latex-free gloves.
   c. Correctly removing disposable latex-free gloves worn while giving care, and then wiping up a blood spill with a paper towel.
   d. Monitoring the person until EMS personnel arrive.

4. To obtain a person's consent to give care, you must tell the person—

   a. Your level of training.
   b. Your age.
   c. A diagnosis of the problem.
   d. Your job.

5. Which would you use to move a person with a suspected head, neck or spinal injury?

   a. Pack-strap carry   b. Walking assist   c. Clothes drag   d. Two-person seat carry

6. List three situations in which it may be necessary to move a person.

7. List four of the limitations you should consider before attempting to move a person in an emergency.

8. List at least five of the seven guidelines to follow when moving a person in an emergency.

9. Name five common types of emergency moves.

Answers are listed in the Appendix.

Skill Sheet 3-1

Removing Disposable Latex-Free Gloves

1. Pinch the palm side of one glove on the outside near your wrist.

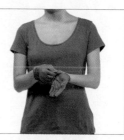

2. Pull the glove toward your fingertips, turning it inside out as you pull it off your hand.

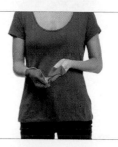

3. Hold the glove in the palm of your other (still-gloved) hand.

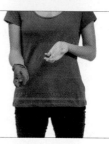

4. Carefully slip two fingers under the wrist of the other glove. Avoid touching the outside of the glove.

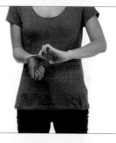

5. Pull the glove towards your fingertips, turning it inside out as you pull it off your hand. The other glove is now contained inside.

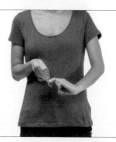

6. Dispose of the gloves properly and wash your hands.

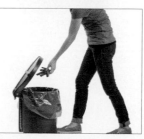

PART TWO

Assessment

4

THE HUMAN BODY

You are helping your brother Jim with some home renovations when he bangs his head hard on a low beam and falls to the ground. He is unresponsive and bleeding from the spot where he struck his head. When you call 9-1-1 from your mobile phone, the call taker tells you an ambulance is on the way and instructs you to take steps to control the bleeding and monitor Jim's breathing. "Why watch his breathing?" you wonder, since he injured his head, not his chest.

Learn and Respond >

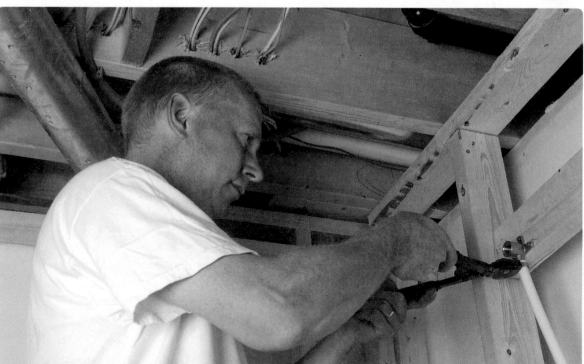

After reading this chapter, you should be able to:

- Identify various anatomical terms commonly used to refer to the body.

- Describe various body positions.

- Describe the major body cavities.

- Identify the eight body systems and the major structures in each system.

- Give examples of how body systems work together.

KEY TERMS

Anatomy: The study of structures, including gross anatomy (structures that can be seen with the naked eye) and microscopic anatomy (structures seen under the microscope).

Body system: A group of organs and other structures that work together to carry out specific functions.

Cells: The basic units that combine to form all living tissue.

Circulatory system: A group of organs and other structures that carry blood and other nutrients throughout the body and remove waste.

Digestive system: A group of organs and other structures that digest food and eliminate waste.

Endocrine system: A group of organs and other structures that regulate and coordinate the activities of other systems by producing chemicals (hormones) that influence tissue activity.

Genitourinary system: A group of organs and other structures that eliminate waste and enable reproduction.

Integumentary system: A group of organs and other structures that protect the body, retain fluids and help to prevent infection.

Musculoskeletal system: A group of tissues and other structures that support the body, protect internal organs, allow movement, store minerals, manufacture blood cells and create heat.

Nervous system: A group of organs and other structures that regulate all body functions.

Organ: A structure of similar tissues acting together to perform specific body functions.

Physiology: How living organisms function (e.g., movement and reproduction).

Respiratory system: A group of organs and other structures that bring air into the body and remove waste through a process called breathing, or respiration.

Tissue: A collection of similar cells acting together to perform specific body functions.

Vital organs: Those organs whose functions are essential to life, including the brain, heart and lungs.

Introduction

As a trained lay responder, you do not need to be an expert in human body structure and function to give effective care. Neither should you need a medical dictionary to effectively describe an injury. However, knowing some basic anatomical terms, and understanding what the body's structures are and how they work, will help you more easily recognize and understand injuries and illnesses, and more accurately communicate with emergency medical services (EMS) personnel about a person's condition.

As you will learn in this chapter, body systems do not function independently. Each system depends on other systems to function properly. When your body is healthy, your body systems work well together. But an injury or illness in one body part or system will often cause problems in others. Knowing the location and function of the major organs and structures within each body system will help you to more accurately assess a person's condition and give the best care.

To remember the location of body structures, it helps to visualize the structures that lie beneath the skin. The structures you can see or feel are reference points for locating the internal structures you cannot see or feel. Using reference points will help you describe the location of injuries and other conditions you may find. This chapter provides you with an overview of important reference points and terminology, while also focusing on body structure *(anatomy)* and function *(physiology)* of the eight body systems.

Anatomical Terms

While it is not a must to use correct anatomical terms when providing EMS personnel with information about a person you are helping, you may hear some of the following words being used. As mentioned in the introduction, knowing what they mean and how to use them properly can help you provide more accurate information to an EMS dispatcher, or when handing over care of a person to EMS personnel.

Directions and Locations

When discussing where a person is experiencing signs and symptoms of an injury or illness, the following anatomical terms are helpful to know (Figure 4-1, A–B):

- **Anterior/posterior:** Any part toward the front of the body is anterior; any part toward the back is posterior.

- **Superior/inferior:** Superior describes any part toward the person's head; inferior describes any part toward the person's feet.

- **Frontal or coronal plane:** That which divides the body vertically into two planes, anterior (the person's front) and posterior (the person's back).

- **Sagittal or lateral plane:** That which divides the body vertically into right and left planes.

- **Transverse or axial plane:** That which divides the body horizontally, into the superior (above the waist) and inferior (below the waist) planes.

- **Medial/lateral:** The terms medial and lateral refer to the midline, an imaginary line running down the middle of the body from the head to the ground, and creating right and left halves. Any part toward the midline is medial; any part away from the midline is lateral.

- **Proximal/distal:** Proximal refers to any part close to the trunk (chest, abdomen and pelvis); distal refers to any part away from the trunk and nearer to the extremities (arms and legs).

- **Superficial/deep:** Superficial refers to any part near the surface of the body; deep refers to any part far from the surface.

- **Internal/external:** Internal refers to the inside and external to the outside of the body.

- **Right/left:** Right and left always refer to the person's right and left, not the responder's right and left.

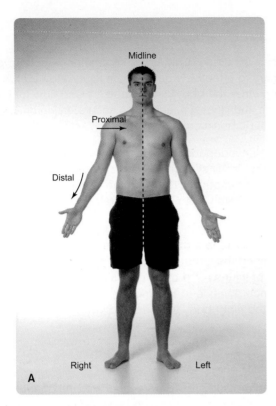

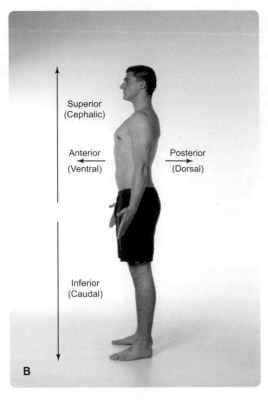

Figure 4-1, A–B. A, Any part of the body toward the midline is medial; any part away from the midline is lateral. Any part close to the trunk is proximal; any part away from the trunk is distal. **B,** Anterior refers to the front part of the body; posterior refers to the back of the body. Superior refers to anything toward the head; inferior refers to anything toward the feet. *Photos: courtesy of the Canadian Red Cross*

Movements

Flexion is the term used to describe flexing or a bending movement, such as bending at the knee or making a fist. Extension is the opposite of flexion—that is, a straightening movement (Figure 4-2). The prefix "hyper" used with either term describes movement beyond the normal position.

Positions

As a trained lay responder, you will often have to describe a person's position to the EMS call taker or other personnel at the public safety answering point (PSAP). Using correct terms will help you communicate the extent of a person's injury quickly and accurately. Terms used to describe body positions include:

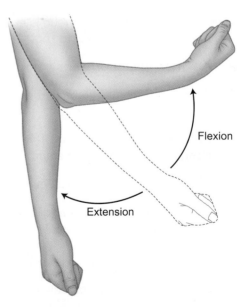

Figure 4-2. Flexion and extension.

- **Anatomical position.** This position, where the person stands with body erect and arms down at the sides, palms facing forward, is the basis for all medical terms that refer to the body.

- **Supine position.** The person is lying face-up on their back (Figure 4-3, A).

- **Prone position.** The person is lying face-down on their stomach (Figure 4-3, B).

- **Right and left lateral recumbent position.** The person is lying on their left or right side (Figure 4-3, C).

- **Fowler's position.** The person is lying on their back, with the upper body elevated at a 45° to 60° angle (Figure 4-3, D).

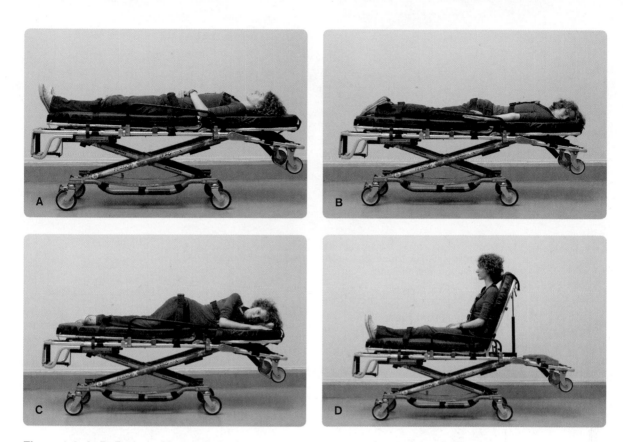

Figure 4-3, A–D. Body positions include: **A,** supine position; **B,** prone position; **C,** right and left lateral recumbent position; and **D,** Fowler's position.

Body Cavities

The organs of the body are located within hollow spaces in the body referred to as body cavities (Figure 4-4). The five major body cavities include the:

- **Cranial cavity.** Located in the head and protected by the skull. It contains the brain.

- **Spinal cavity.** Extends from the bottom of the skull to the lower back, is protected by the vertebral (spinal) column and contains the spinal cord.

- **Thoracic cavity (chest cavity).** Located in the trunk between the diaphragm and the neck, and contains the lungs and heart. The rib cage, sternum and the upper portion of the spine protect it. The diaphragm separates this cavity from the abdominal cavity (Figure 4-5).

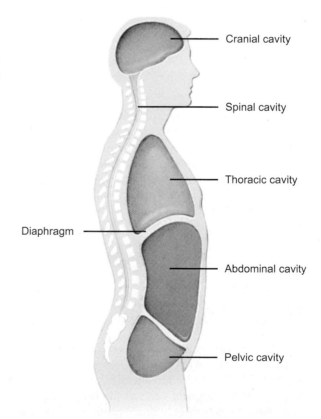

Figure 4-4. The five major body cavities.

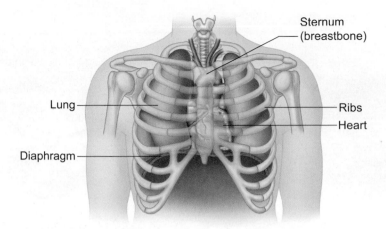

Figure 4-5. The thoracic cavity is located in the trunk between the diaphragm and the neck.

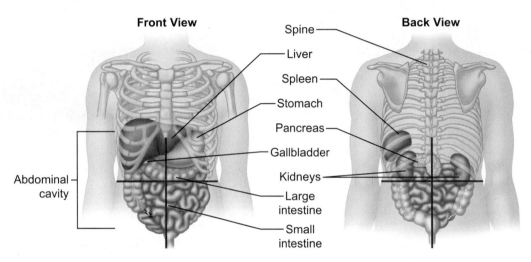

Figure 4-6. The abdominal cavity contains the organs of digestion and excretion.

- **Abdominal cavity.** Located in the trunk below the chest cavity, between the diaphragm and the pelvis. It is described using four quadrants created by imagining a line from the breastbone down to the lowest point in the pelvis and another one horizontally through the navel. This creates the right and left, upper and lower quadrants. The abdominal cavity contains the organs of digestion and excretion, including the liver, gallbladder, spleen, pancreas, kidneys, stomach and intestines (Figure 4-6).

- **Pelvic cavity.** Located in the pelvis, and is the lowest part of the trunk. Contains the bladder, rectum and internal female reproductive organs. The pelvic bones and the lower portion of the spine protect it.

Further description of the major organs and their functions are in the next section of this chapter and in later chapters.

Body Systems

The human body is a miraculous machine. It performs many complex functions, each of which helps us live. The human body is made up of billions of different types of **cells** that contribute in special ways to keep the body functioning normally. Similar cells form together into **tissues,** and these in turn form together into **organs. Vital organs** such as the brain, heart and lungs are organs whose function are essential for life. Each **body system** contains a group of organs and other structures that are specially adapted to perform specific body functions needed for life (Table 4-1).

Table 4-1. **Body Systems**

System	Major Structures	Primary Function	How the System Works with Other Body Systems
Musculoskeletal System	Bones, ligaments, muscles and tendons	Provides body's framework; protects internal organs and other underlying structures; allows movement; produces heat; manufactures blood components	Provides protection to organs and structures of other body systems; muscle action is controlled by the nervous system
Respiratory System	Airway and lungs	Supplies the body with oxygen, and removes carbon dioxide and other impurities through the breathing process	Works with the circulatory system to provide oxygen to cells; is under the control of the nervous system
Circulatory System	Heart, blood and blood vessels	Transports nutrients and oxygen to body cells and removes waste products	Works with the respiratory system to provide oxygen to cells; works in conjunction with the urinary and digestive systems to remove waste products; helps give skin color; is under control of the nervous system
Nervous System	Brain, spinal cord and nerves	One of two primary regulatory systems in the body; transmits messages to and from the brain	Regulates all body systems through a network of nerve cells and nerves
Integumentary System	Skin, hair and nails	An important part of the body's communication network; helps prevent infection and dehydration; assists with temperature regulation; aids in production of certain vitamins	Helps to protect the body from disease-producing organisms; together with the circulatory system, helps to regulate body temperature under control of the nervous system; communicates sensation to the brain by way of the nerves
Endocrine System	Glands	Secretes hormones and other substances into the blood and onto skin	Together with the nervous system, coordinates the activities of other systems
Digestive System	Mouth, esophagus, stomach and intestines	Breaks down food into a usable form to supply the rest of the body with energy	Works with the circulatory system to transport nutrients to the body and remove waste products
Genitourinary System	Uterus, genitalia, kidneys and bladder	Performs the processes of reproduction; removes wastes from the circulatory system and regulates water balance	Assists in regulating blood pressure and fluid balance

For example, the ***circulatory system*** consists of the heart, blood and blood vessels. This system keeps all parts of the body supplied with oxygen-rich blood. For the body to work properly, all of the following systems must work well together:

- Musculoskeletal
- Respiratory
- Circulatory
- Nervous

- Integumentary
- Endocrine
- Digestive
- Genitourinary

The Musculoskeletal System

The ***musculoskeletal system*** is a combination of two body systems, the muscular and skeletal systems, and consists of the bones, muscles, ligaments and tendons. This system performs the following functions:

- Supports the body
- Protects internal organs
- Allows movement

- Stores minerals
- Produces blood cells
- Produces heat

The adult body has 206 bones. Bone is hard, dense tissue that forms the skeleton. The skeleton forms the framework that supports the body. Where two or more bones join, they form a joint. Fibrous bands called ligaments usually hold bones together at joints. Bones vary in size and shape, allowing them to perform specific functions. Tendons connect muscles to bone.

The Muscular System

The muscular system allows the body to move. Muscles are soft tissues. The body has more than 600 muscles, most of which are attached to bones by strong tissues called tendons (Figure 4-7). Muscle tissue has the ability to contract (become shorter and thicker) when stimulated by an electrical or nerve impulse. Muscle cells, called fibers, are usually long and threadlike and are packed closely together in bundles, which are bound together by connective tissue.

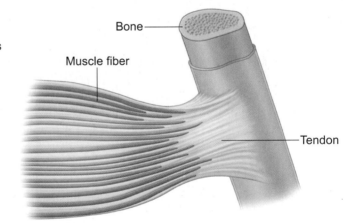

Figure 4-7. Most of the body's muscles are attached to bones by tendons. Muscle cells, called fibers, are long and threadlike.

There are three basic types of muscles, including:

- **Skeletal.** Skeletal, or voluntary, muscles are under the control of the brain and nervous system. These muscles help give the body its shape and make it possible to move when we walk, smile, talk or move our eyes.

- **Smooth.** Smooth muscles, also called involuntary muscles, are made of longer fibers and are found in the walls of tube-like organs, ducts and blood vessels. They also form much of the intestinal wall.

- **Cardiac.** Cardiac muscles are only found in the walls of the heart and share some of the properties of the other two muscle types: they are smooth (like the involuntary muscles) and striated (string-like, like the voluntary muscles). They are a special type of involuntary muscle that controls the heart. Cardiac muscles have the unique property of being able to generate their own impulse independent of the nervous system.

The Skeletal System

The skeleton is made up of six sections: the skull, spinal column, thorax, pelvis, and upper and lower extremities (Figure 4-8).

- **The skull:** The skull is made up of two main parts: the cranium and the face. The cranium is made up of broad, flat bones that form the top, back and sides, as well as the front, which house the brain. Thirteen smaller bones make up the face, as well as the hinged lower jaw, or mandible, which moves freely.

- **The spinal column:** The spinal column, or spine, houses and protects the spinal cord. It is the principal support system of the body. The spinal column is made up of 33 small bones called vertebrae, 24 of which are movable. They are divided into five sections of the spine: 7 cervical (neck), 12 thoracic (upper back), 5 lumbar (lower back), and 9 sacral (lower spine with fused vertebrae) and coccyx (tailbone) (Figure 4-9).

- **The thorax:** The thorax, also known as the chest, is made up of 12 pairs of ribs, the sternum (breastbone) and the thoracic spine. Ten pairs of ribs are attached to the sternum with cartilage while the bottom two pairs are connected only to the vertebrae in the back. Together, these structures protect the heart and lungs, and portions of other organs such as the spleen and liver.

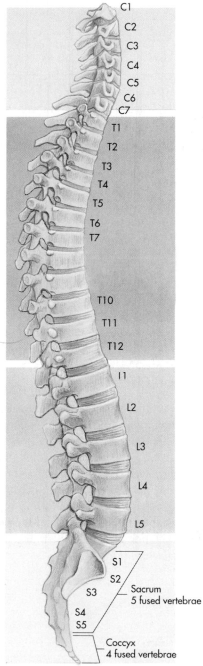

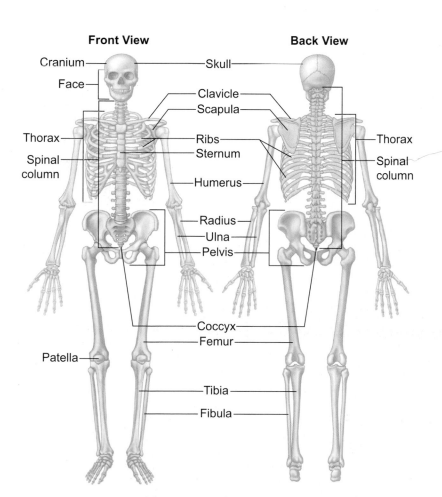

Front View   **Back View**

Cranium — Skull
Face
Clavicle
Scapula
Thorax — Ribs — Thorax
Spinal column — Sternum — Spinal column
Humerus
Radius
Ulna
Pelvis
Coccyx
Femur
Patella
Tibia
Fibula

Figure 4-8. The six parts of the skeleton are the skull, the spinal column, the thorax, the pelvis, and the upper and lower extremities.

Figure 4-9. The spinal column is divided into five sections: cervical, thoracic, lumbar, sacral and coccyx.

- **The pelvis:** The pelvis, also known as the hip bones, is made up of several bones, including the ilium, pubis and ischium. The pelvis supports the intestines, and contains the bladder and internal reproductive organs.

- **Upper extremities:** The upper extremities, or upper limbs, include the shoulders, upper arms, forearms, wrists and hands. The upper arm bone is the humerus, and the two bones in the forearm are the radius and the ulna. The upper extremities are attached to the trunk at the shoulder girdle, made up of the clavicle (collarbone) and scapula (shoulder blade).

- **Lower extremities:** The lower extremities, or lower limbs, consist of the hips, upper and lower legs, ankles and feet. They are attached to the trunk at the hip joints. The upper bone is the femur or thighbone, and the bones in the lower leg are the tibia and fibula. The kneecap is a small triangular-shaped bone, also called the patella.

- **Joints:** Joints are the places where bones connect to each other (Figure 4-10). Strong, tough bands called ligaments hold the bones at a joint together. Most joints allow movement but some are immovable, as in the skull, and others allow only slight movement, as in the spine. All joints have a normal range of motion—an area in which they can move freely without too much stress or strain.

The most common types of movable joints are the ball-and-socket joint, such as the hip and shoulder, and the hinged joint, such as the elbow, knee and finger joints. Different types of joints allow different degrees of flexibility and movement. Some other joint types include pivot joints (some vertebrae), gliding joints (some bones in the feet and hands), saddle joints (ankle) and condyloid joints (wrist) (Figure 4-11).

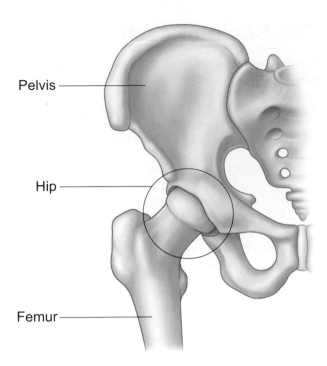

Figure 4-10. Joints are the places where bones connect to each other.

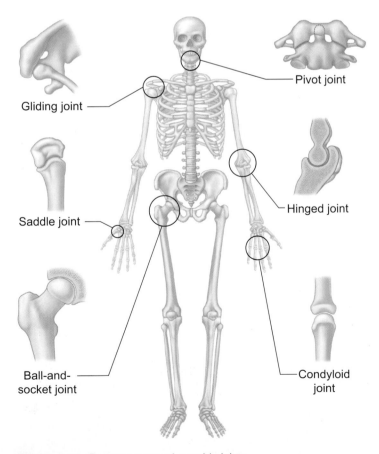

Figure 4-11. Common types of movable joints.

The Respiratory System

The body can only store enough oxygen to last for a few minutes. The simple acts of inhalation and exhalation in a healthy person are sufficient to supply normal oxygen needs. If for some reason the oxygen supply is cut off, brain cells will begin to die in about 4 to 6 minutes with permanent damage occurring within 8 to 10 minutes. The **respiratory system** delivers oxygen to the body, and removes carbon dioxide from it, in a process called respiration.

Anatomy of the Respiratory System

Upper Airway

The upper airway includes the nose, mouth and teeth, tongue and jaw, pharynx (throat), larynx (voice box) and epiglottis (Figure 4-12). During inspiration (breathing in), air enters the body through the nose and mouth, where it is warmed and moistened. Air entering through the nose passes through the nasopharynx (part of the throat posterior to the nose), and air entering by the mouth travels through the oropharynx. The air then continues down through the larynx, which houses the vocal cords. The epiglottis, a leaf-shaped structure, folds down over the top of the trachea during swallowing to prevent foreign objects from entering the trachea.

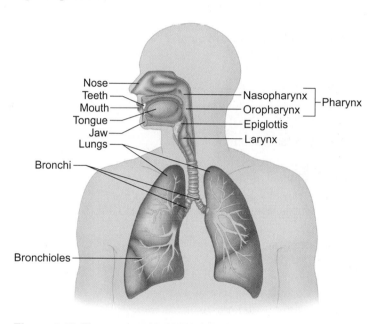

Figure 4-12. The upper and lower airways.

Lower Airway

The lower airway consists of the trachea (windpipe), bronchi, lungs, bronchioles and alveoli (Figure 4-12). Once the air passes through the larynx, it travels down the trachea, the passageway to the lungs. The trachea is made up of rings of cartilage and is the part that can be felt at the front of the neck. Once air travels down the trachea, it reaches the two bronchi, which branch off, one to each lung. These two bronchi continue to branch off into smaller and smaller passages called bronchioles, like the branches of a tree.

At the ends of each bronchiole are tiny air sacs called alveoli, each surrounded by capillaries (tiny blood vessels). These are the site of carbon dioxide and oxygen exchange in the blood. The lungs are the principal organs of respiration and house millions of tiny alveolar sacs.

The structures involved in respiration in children and infants differ from those of adults (Table 4-2). The structures are usually smaller or less developed in children and infants. Some of these differences are important when giving care. Because the structures, including the mouth and nose, are smaller, they are obstructed more easily by small objects, blood, fluids or swelling. It is important to pay special attention to a child or an infant to make sure the airway stays open.

Table 4-2. **Pediatric Considerations in the Respiratory System**

Anatomical Differences in Children and Infants as Compared with Adults	Physiological Differences and Impact on Care
Structures are smaller.	Mouth and nose are more easily obstructed by small objects, blood or swelling.
Primarily breathe through nose (especially infants).	Airway is more easily blocked.
Tongue takes up proportionately more space in the pharynx.	Tongue can block airway more easily.
Presence of "baby teeth."	Teeth can be dislodged and enter airway.
Face shape and nose are flatter.	Can make it difficult to obtain a good seal of airway with resuscitation mask.
Trachea is narrower, softer and more flexible.	Trachea can close off if the head is tipped back too far or is allowed to fall forward.
Have more secretions.	Secretions can block airway.
Use abdominal muscles to breathe.	This makes it more difficult to assess breathing.
Chest wall is softer.	Tend to rely more heavily on diaphragm for breathing.
More flexible ribs.	Lungs are more susceptible to damage. Injuries may not be as obvious.
Breathe faster.	Can fatigue more quickly, leading to respiratory distress.

Physiology of the Respiratory System

External respiration, or ventilation, is the mechanical process of moving air in and out of the lungs to exchange oxygen and carbon dioxide between body tissues and the environment. It is influenced primarily by changes in pressure inside the chest that cause air to flow into or out of the lungs. The body's chemical controls of breathing are dependent on the level of carbon dioxide in the blood. If carbon dioxide levels increase, the respiration rate increases automatically so that twice the amount of air is taken in until the carbon dioxide is eliminated. It is not the lack of oxygen but the excess carbon dioxide that causes this increase in respiratory rate. Hyperventilation may result from this condition. Internal respiration, or cellular respiration, refers to respiration at the cellular level. These metabolic processes at the cellular level, either within the cell or across the cell membrane, are carried out to obtain energy. This occurs by reacting oxygen with glucose to produce water, carbon dioxide and ATP (energy).

What if… *The person I am helping is having trouble breathing? Is it OK to loosen their clothing?*

Yes, loosening restrictive clothing such as a belt, tie or shirt collar is an appropriate step that may aid in breathing. Essentially, breathing consists of two actions: inhalation and exhalation. During inhalation, the diaphragm contracts and is drawn downward, increasing the volume of the chest cavity. At the same time the muscles of the chest cavity move the ribs upward and outward, also causing the chest cavity and lungs to expand so air can rush into the lungs. Loosening restrictive clothing may aid in freeing up the movement of the chest cavity to assist in breathing.

Structures That Support Ventilation

During inspiration, the thoracic muscles contract, and this moves the ribs outward and upward. At the same time, the diaphragm contracts and pushes down, allowing the chest cavity to expand and the lungs to fill with air. The intercostal muscles, the muscles between the ribs, then contract. During expiration (breathing out), the opposite occurs: the chest wall muscles relax, the ribs move inward, and the diaphragm relaxes and moves up. This compresses the lungs, causing the air to flow out. Accessory muscles are secondary muscles of ventilation and are used only when breathing requires increased effort. Limited use can occur during normal strenuous activity, such as exercising, but pronounced use of accessory muscles is a sign of respiratory disease or distress. These muscles include the spinal and neck muscles. The abdominal muscles may also be used for more forceful exhalations. Use of abdominal muscles represents abnormal or labored breathing and is also a sign of respiratory distress.

Vascular Structures That Support Respiration

Oxygen and carbon dioxide are exchanged in the lungs through the walls of the alveoli and capillaries. In this exchange, oxygen-rich air enters the alveoli during each inspiration and passes through the capillary walls into the bloodstream. On each exhalation, carbon dioxide and other waste gases pass through the capillary walls into the alveoli to be exhaled.

The Circulatory System

The circulatory system consists of the heart, blood and blood vessels. It is responsible for delivering oxygen, nutrients and other essential chemical elements to the body's tissue cells, and removing carbon dioxide and other waste products via the bloodstream (Figure 4-13).

Anatomy of the Circulatory System

The heart is a highly efficient, muscular organ that pumps blood through the body. It is about the size of a closed fist and is found in the thoracic cavity, between the two lungs, behind the sternum and slightly to the left of the midline.

The heart is divided into four chambers: right and left upper chambers called atria, and right and left lower chambers called ventricles (Figure 4-14). The right atrium receives oxygen-depleted blood from the veins of the body and, through valves, delivers it to the right ventricle, which in turn pumps the blood to the lungs for oxygenation. The left atrium receives this oxygen-rich blood from the lungs and delivers it to the left ventricle, to be

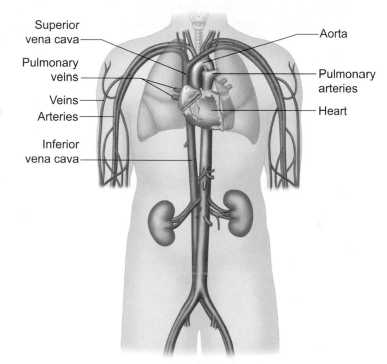

Figure 4-13. The circulatory system consists of the heart, blood and blood vessels.

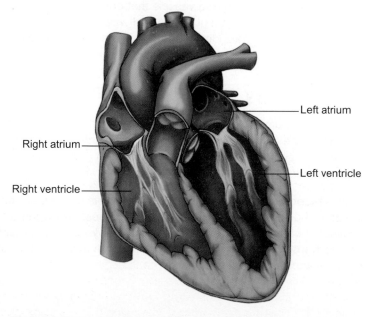

Figure 4-14. The heart's four chambers.

pumped to the body through the arteries. There are arteries throughout the body, including the blood vessels that supply the heart itself, which are the coronary arteries.

There are four main components of blood: red blood cells, white blood cells, platelets and plasma. The red blood cells carry oxygen to the cells of the body and take carbon dioxide away. This is carried out by hemoglobin, on the surface of the cells. Red blood cells give blood its red color. White blood cells are part of the body's immune system and help to defend the body against infection. There are several types of white blood cells. Platelets are a solid component of blood used by the body to form blood clots when there is bleeding. Plasma is the straw-colored or clear liquid component of blood that carries the blood cells and nutrients to the tissues, as well as waste products away to the organs involved in excretion.

There are different types of blood vessels—arteries, veins and capillaries—that serve different purposes. Arteries carry blood away from the heart, mostly oxygenated blood. The exception is the arteries that carry blood to the lungs for oxygenation, the pulmonary arteries. The aorta is the major artery that leaves the heart. It supplies all other arteries with blood. As arteries travel farther from the heart, they branch into increasingly smaller vessels called arterioles. These narrow vessels carry blood from the arteries into capillaries (Figure 4-15).

The venous system includes veins and venules. Veins carry deoxygenated blood back to the heart. The one exception is the pulmonary veins, which carry oxygenated blood away from the lungs. The superior and inferior vena cavae are the large veins that carry the oxygen-depleted blood back into the heart. Like arteries, veins also branch into smaller vessels the farther away they are from the heart. Venules are the smallest branches and are connected to capillaries. Unlike arterial blood, which is moved through the arteries by pressure from the pumping of the heart, veins have valves that prevent blood from flowing backward and help move it through the blood vessels.

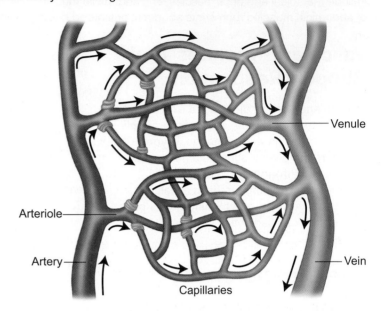

Figure 4-15. As blood flows through the body, it moves through arteries, arterioles, capillaries, venules and veins.

Capillaries are the tiny blood vessels that connect the systems of arteries and veins. Capillary walls allow for the exchange of gases, nutrients and waste products between the two systems. In the lungs, there is exchange of carbon dioxide and oxygen in the pulmonary capillaries. Throughout the body, there is exchange of gases and nutrients and waste at the cellular level.

Physiology of the Circulatory System

As the heart pumps blood from the left ventricle to the body, this causes a wave of pressure we refer to as the pulse. We can feel this pulse at several points throughout the body. These "pulse points" occur where the arteries are close to the surface of the skin (e.g., carotid pulse point in the neck) and over a bone (e.g., brachial pulse point on the inside of the upper arm).

As the blood flows through the arteries, it exerts a certain force that we call blood pressure (BP). BP is described using two measures, the systolic pressure (when the left ventricle contracts) and the diastolic pressure (when the left ventricle is at rest). Oxygen and nutrients are delivered to cells throughout the body, and carbon dioxide and other wastes are taken away, all through the delivery of blood. This continuous process is called perfusion.

The primary gases exchanged in perfusion are oxygen and carbon dioxide. All cells require oxygen to function. Most of the oxygen is transported to the cells attached to the hemoglobin, but a tiny amount is also dissolved in the liquid component of the blood, the plasma. The major waste product in the blood, carbon dioxide, is transported mostly in the blood as bicarbonate and transported by the hemoglobin molecule. A tiny amount of carbon dioxide is dissolved in the plasma.

The Nervous System

The *nervous system* is the most complex and delicate of all the body systems. The center of the nervous system, the brain, is the master organ of the body and regulates all body functions. The primary functions of the brain are the sensory functions, motor functions and the integrated functions of consciousness, memory, emotions and language.

Anatomy of the Nervous System

The nervous system can be divided into two main anatomical systems: the central nervous system and the peripheral nervous system (Figure 4-16). The central nervous system consists of the brain and spinal cord. Both are encased in bone (the brain within the cranium and the spinal cord within the spinal column), are covered in several protective layers called meninges and are surrounded by cerebrospinal fluid.

The brain itself can be further subdivided into the cerebrum, the largest and outermost structure; the cerebellum, also called "the small brain," which is responsible for coordinating movement; and the brainstem, which joins the rest of the brain with the spinal cord. The brainstem is the control center for several vital functions including respiration, cardiac function and vasomotor control (dilation and constriction of the blood vessels), and is the place of origin for most of the cranial nerves (Figure 4-17).

The peripheral nervous system is the portion of the nervous system located outside the brain and spinal cord, which includes the nerves to and from the spinal cord. These nerves carry sensory information from the body to the spinal cord and brain, and motor information from the spinal cord and brain to the body.

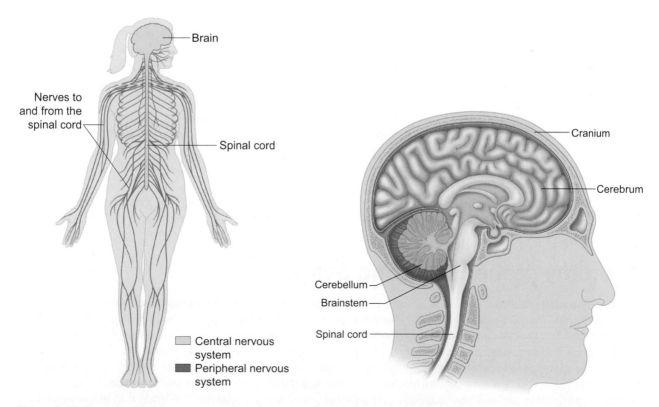

Figure 4-16. The nervous system.

Figure 4-17. The brain.

Physiology of the Nervous System

The nervous system can also be divided into two functional systems, the voluntary and autonomic systems. The voluntary system controls movement of the muscles and sensation from the sensory organs. The autonomic system is involuntary and controls the involuntary muscles of the organs and glands. It can be divided into two systems: the sympathetic and parasympathetic systems. The sympathetic system controls the body's response to stressors such as pain, fear or a sudden loss of blood. These actions are sometimes referred to as the "fight-or-flight" response. The parasympathetic system works in balance with the sympathetic system by controlling the body's return to a normal state.

The Integumentary System

The **integumentary system** consists of the skin, hair, nails, sweat glands and oil glands. The skin separates our tissues, organs and other systems from the outside world.

The skin is the body's largest organ. It has three major layers, each consisting of other layers (Figure 4-18). The epidermis, or outer layer, contains the skin's pigmentation, or melanin. The dermis, or second layer, contains the blood vessels that supply the skin, hair, glands and nerves, and is what contributes to the skin's elasticity and strength. The deepest layer, the subcutaneous layer, is made up of fatty tissue and may be of varying thicknesses depending on its positioning on the body.

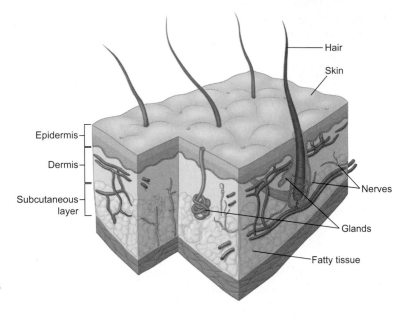

Figure 4-18. The skin's major layers are the epidermis, the dermis and the subcutaneous layer.

The skin serves to protect the body from injury and from invasion by bacteria and other disease-producing pathogens. It helps regulate fluid balance and body temperature. The skin also produces vitamin D and stores minerals. Blood supplies the skin with nutrients and helps provide its color. When blood vessels dilate (become wider), the blood circulates close to the skin's surface, making some people's skin appear flushed or red and making the skin feel warm. Reddening or flushing may not appear in darker skin tones. When blood vessels constrict (become narrower), not as much blood is close to the skin's surface, causing the skin to turn ashen, appear pale and/or feel cool. In people with darker skin tones, this pallor can be found on the palms of the hands.

The Endocrine System

The **endocrine system** is one of the body's regulatory systems and is made up of ductless glands. These glands secrete hormones, which are chemical substances that enter the bloodstream and influence activity in different parts of the body (e.g., strength, stature, hair growth and behavior).

Anatomy of the Endocrine System

There are several important glands within the body (Figure 4-19). The hypothalamus and pituitary glands are in the brain. The pituitary gland, also referred to as the "master gland," regulates growth as well as many other glands. The hypothalamus secretes hormones that act on the pituitary gland. The thyroid gland is in the anterior neck and regulates metabolism, growth and development. It also regulates nervous system activity. The adrenal glands are located on the top of the kidneys and secrete several hormones, including epinephrine (adrenalin) and norepinephrine (noradrenaline). The gonads (ovaries and testes) produce hormones that control reproduction and sex characteristics. The pineal gland is a tiny gland in the brain that helps regulate wake/sleep patterns.

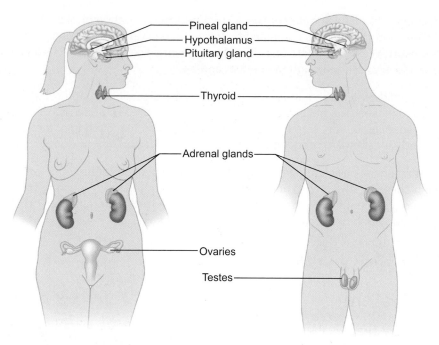

Figure 4-19. The endocrine system in females and males.

Physiology of the Endocrine System

One of the critical functions controlled by the body's endocrine system is the control of blood glucose levels. The Islet of Langerhans cells, located in the pancreas, make and secrete insulin, which controls the level of glucose in the blood and permits cells to use glucose and glucagon (a pancreatic hormone), which raises the level of glucose in the blood.

The sympathetic nervous system is also regulated through the endocrine system. Adrenaline and noradrenaline, produced by the adrenal glands, cause multiple effects on the sympathetic nervous system. Effects include vasoconstriction (constricting of vessels), increased heart rate and dilation of smooth muscles, including those that control respiration.

The adrenal glands and pituitary gland are also involved in kidney function, and regulate water and salt balance. The body works to keep water and levels of electrolytes in the body in balance.

The Digestive System

The **digestive system,** or gastrointestinal system, consists of the organs that work together to break down food, absorb nutrients and eliminate waste. It is composed of the alimentary tract (food passageway) and the accessory organs that help prepare food for the digestive process (Figure 4-20).

Food enters the digestive system through the mouth and then the esophagus, the passageway to the stomach. The stomach and other major organs involved in this system are contained in the abdominal cavity. The stomach is the major organ of the digestive system and the location where the majority of digestion, or breaking down, takes place. Food travels from the stomach into the small intestine,

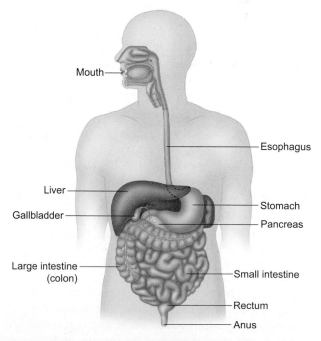

Figure 4-20. The digestive system.

where further digestion takes place and nutrients are absorbed. The hepatic portal system collects blood from the small intestine, and transfers its nutrients and toxins to the liver for absorption and processing before continuing on to the heart. Waste products pass into the large intestine, or colon, where water is absorbed and the remaining waste is passed through the rectum and anus.

The liver is the largest solid organ in the abdomen and aids in the digestion of fat through the production of bile, among other processes. The gallbladder serves to store the bile. The pancreas secretes pancreatic juices that aid in the digestion of fats, starches and proteins. It is also the location of the Islet of Langerhans cells, where insulin and glucagon are produced.

Digestion occurs both mechanically and chemically. Mechanical digestion refers to the breaking down of food that begins with chewing, swallowing and moving the food through the alimentary tract, and ends in defecation. Chemical digestion refers to the chemical process involved when enzymes break foods down into components the body can absorb, such as fatty acids and amino acids.

The Genitourinary System

The Urinary System

Part of the *genitourinary system,* the **urinary system** consists of organs involved in the elimination of waste products that are filtered and excreted from the blood. It consists of the kidneys, ureters, urethra and urinary bladder (Figure 4-21).

The kidneys are located in the lumbar region behind the abdominal cavity in the **retroperitoneal space** just beneath the chest, one on each side. The kidneys filter wastes from the circulating blood to form urine. The ureters carry the urine from the kidneys to the bladder. The bladder is a small, muscular sac that stores the urine until it is ready to be excreted. The urethra carries the urine from the bladder and out of the body.

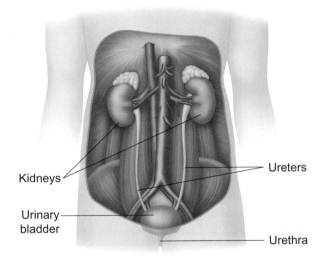

Figure 4-21. The urinary system.

The urinary system removes wastes from the circulating blood, thereby filtering it. The system helps the body maintain fluid and electrolyte balance. This is achieved through buffers, which control the pH (amount of acid or alkaline) in the urine.

The Reproductive System

Part of the genitourinary system, the **reproductive system** of both men and women includes the organs for sexual reproduction.

The male reproductive organs are located outside of the pelvis and are more vulnerable to injury than those of the female. They include the testicles, a duct system and the penis (Figure 4-22, A). Puberty usually begins between the ages of 10 and 14 and is controlled by hormones secreted by the pituitary gland in the brain. The testes produce sperm and testosterone, the primary male sex hormone. The urethra is part of the urinary system and transports urine from the bladder; it is also part of the reproductive system through which semen is ejaculated. The sperm contributes half the genetic material to an offspring.

The female reproductive system consists of the ovaries, fallopian tubes, uterus and vagina, and is protected by the pelvic bones (Figure 4-22, B). Glands in the body, including the hypothalamus and pituitary glands in the brain, and the adrenal glands on the kidneys, interact with the reproductive system by releasing hormones that control and coordinate the development and functioning of the reproductive system. The menstrual cycle is approximately 28 days in length. Approximately midway through the cycle, usually a single egg **(ovum)** is released; if united with a sperm, this egg will attach to the lining of the uterus, beginning pregnancy. The female's egg contributes half the genetic material to the characteristics of a fetus.

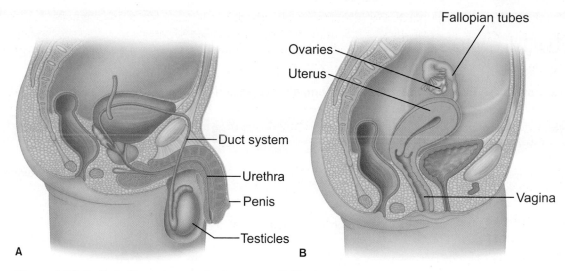

Figure 4-22, A–B. A, The male reproductive system. **B,** The female reproductive system.

Interrelationships of Body Systems

Each body system plays a vital role in survival. All body systems work together to help the body maintain a constant healthy state. When the environment changes, body systems adapt to these new conditions. For example, the musculoskeletal system works harder during exercise; the respiratory and circulatory systems must also work harder to meet the body's increased oxygen demands. Body systems also react to the stresses caused by emotion, injury or illness.

Body systems do not work independently. The impact of an injury or a disease is rarely restricted to one body system. For example, a broken bone may result in nerve damage that will impair movement and feeling. Injuries to the ribs can make breathing difficult. If the heart stops beating for any reason, breathing will also stop.

In any significant injury or illness, body systems may be seriously affected. This may result in a progressive failure of body systems called **shock.** Shock results from the inability of the circulatory system to provide oxygenated blood to all parts of the body, especially the vital organs. Shock is covered in more detail in Chapter 9.

Generally, the more body systems involved in an emergency, the more serious the emergency is. Body systems depend on each other for survival. In serious injury or illness, the body may not be able to keep functioning. In these cases, regardless of your best efforts, the person may die.

Summary

By having a fundamental understanding of body systems and how they function and interact, coupled with knowledge of basic anatomical terms, you will be more likely to accurately identify and describe injuries and illnesses. Fortunately, basic care is usually all you need to provide support for injured body systems until more advanced care is available. By learning the basic principles of care described in later chapters, you may be able to make the difference between life and death.

READY TO RESPOND? >

Think back to Jim's injury in the opening scenario, and use what you have learned to respond to these questions:

1. Why did the call taker tell you to watch Jim's breathing?

2. Which body systems appear to have been affected by Jim's fall?

Study Questions

1. Complete the box with the correct system, structures or function(s).

Systems	Structures	Function
a.	b.	Supplies the body with the oxygen it needs through breathing
c.	Heart, blood and blood vessels	d.
Integumentary	e.	f.
Musculoskeletal	g.	h.
i.	j.	Regulates all body functions; a communication network

2. Match each term with the correct definition.

a. Anatomy   c. Cell   e. Tissue   g. Vital organs

b. Organ   d. Body system   f. Physiology

_____ Organs whose functions are essential to life, including the brain, heart and lungs

_____ A collection of similar cells that perform a specific function

_____ How living organisms function

_____ The basic unit of living tissue

_____ A group of organs and other structures that works together to carry out specific functions

_____ The study of body structures

_____ A collection of similar tissues acting together to perform a specific body function

In questions 3 through 9, circle the letter of the correct answer.

3. Which structure is not located in or part of the thoracic cavity?

a. The liver   b. The rib cage   c. The heart   d. The lungs

4. The two body systems that work together to provide oxygen to the body cells are—

a. Musculoskeletal and integumentary.   b. Circulatory and musculoskeletal.   c. Respiratory and circulatory.   d. Endocrine and nervous.

(Continued)

Study Questions continued

5. One of the main functions of the integumentary system is to—

   a. Transmit information to the brain.

   b. Produce blood cells.

   c. Prevent infection.

   d. Secrete hormones.

6. The function of the digestive system is to—

   a. Perform the process of reproduction.

   b. Transport nutrients and oxygen to body cells.

   c. Break down food into a form the body can use for energy.

   d. All of the above.

7. Which structure in the airway prevents food and liquid from entering the lungs?

   a. The trachea

   b. The epiglottis

   c. The esophagus

   d. The bronchi

8. If a person's use of language suddenly becomes impaired, which body system might be injured?

   a. The musculoskeletal system

   b. The nervous system

   c. The integumentary system

   d. The circulatory system

9. Which two body systems will react initially to alert a person to a severe cut?

   a. Circulatory, respiratory

   b. Respiratory, musculoskeletal

   c. Nervous, respiratory

   d. Circulatory, nervous

Answers are listed in the Appendix.

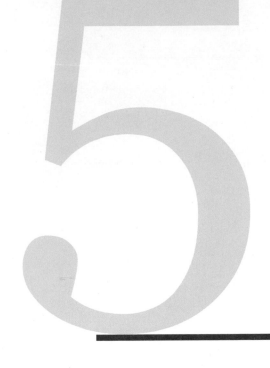

5 CHECKING THE PERSON

You are riding along the bike trail. As you round a sharp curve, you abruptly swerve to avoid two cyclists who are sitting on the side of the trail. One of the cyclists appears hurt, so you stop your bike to help. You are going to have to figure out what kind of help the person needs.

Learn and Respond

After reading this chapter, you should be able to:

- Describe how to check for life-threatening conditions for an adult, child and infant.

- Identify and explain the SAMPLE questions you should ask the person or bystanders in an interview.

- Describe how to check for non-life-threatening conditions for an adult, child and infant.

After reading this chapter and completing the class activities, you should be able to:

- Demonstrate how to check a responsive and an unresponsive adult, child and infant.

KEY TERMS

Agonal breathing: Irregular or gasping breaths.

Aspiration: Inhalation of blood, vomit, saliva or other foreign material into the lungs.

Introduction

In earlier chapters, you learned that as a trained lay responder, you can make a difference in an emergency—you may even save a life. You learned how to recognize an emergency and to follow the emergency action steps: **CHECK—CALL—CARE.** More importantly, you learned that your decision to act can have a significant impact on the person's chance of survival. You can always do something to help, even if it is only calling 9-1-1 or the designated emergency number.

In this chapter, you will learn more about how to check an injured or ill person for life-threatening conditions. You will also learn how to interview a person who is awake and any bystanders, check for non-life-threatening conditions and give basic care in any emergency until emergency medical services (EMS) personnel arrive.

Checking for Life-Threatening Conditions

After checking the scene by performing a scene size-up, you should then check the person for life-threatening conditions. Life-threatening conditions include:

- Unresponsiveness (unconsciousness).

- Trouble breathing.

- Absence of breathing.

- Severe, life-threatening bleeding.

The actions you will take depend on the conditions you find.

Refer to Placing a Person in a Recovery Position, below, for more information on what to do if you need to leave an unresponsive person who is breathing normally in order to call 9-1-1 or the designated emergency number. For a responsive or an unresponsive person who is breathing normally, after calling 9-1-1 or the designated emergency number, return to the person, complete the head-to-toe check as described later in this chapter and give care until EMS personnel arrive.

Breathing

While checking for responsiveness, look at the person's face and chest for signs of normal breathing. Normal breathing is regular, quiet and effortless. A person does not appear to be working hard or struggling when breathing normally. This means that the person is not making noise when breathing, breaths are not fast (although it should be noted that normal breathing rates in children and infants are faster than normal breathing rates in adults), and breathing does not cause discomfort or pain.

In an unresponsive adult, you may detect an irregular or gasping breath. This is known as **agonal breathing.** Do not confuse this for normal breathing. Care for the person as if there is no breathing at all.

■ If the person you are checking *is* breathing normally, their heart is beating and is circulating blood containing oxygen. In this case, continue to look for other life-threatening conditions.

■ If an unresponsive person is *not* breathing, or has irregular or gasping breaths (agonal breathing), assume cardiac arrest. Immediately begin CPR, starting with chest compressions. You will learn about CPR in Chapter 6.

> **What if...** *I am giving care to an unresponsive adult who over the course of time becomes responsive and requests that I stop giving care?*
>
> *As you learned in Chapter 3, an adult who is responsive and understands the implications of a decision has the right to refuse all or part of the care given to them by another person during an emergency. If this happens, remain at the scene and try to make sure (either by yourself or via a family member or friend) the person understands the benefits of continued care and the risks of refusing care. If the person still chooses to refuse care, remember that failure to discontinue care would be considered battery or the unlawful touching of a person without that person's permission, so you must stop giving care.*

Placing a Person in a Recovery Position

If the person responds (such as by moving, opening their eyes or moaning) and is breathing normally, the person is responsive but may not be fully awake. If the person is not fully awake but appears to be breathing normally or the person is unresponsive but breathing normally, send someone to call 9-1-1 or the designated emergency number and to obtain an automated external defibrillator (AED) and first aid kit. Gather more information by interviewing bystanders (using SAMPLE as a guide; see Figure 5-1 and Skill Sheet 5-1) and doing a head-to-toe check. Then roll the person onto their side into the recovery position (Box 5-1).

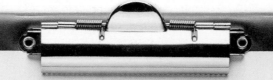

Using SAMPLE To Gather More Information

S = Signs and symptoms.

Signs are clues to the person's condition that you can observe for yourself, using one of your senses. For example, you may see that the person is sweating heavily, hear wheezing when the person is breathing, or feel that the person's skin is cool and moist. Symptoms are clues to the person's condition that only the person can describe to you, so you need to ask the person what he or she is feeling or experiencing. For example, the person may tell you that he or she is in pain, feeling nauseous, has a headache, or feels dizzy. Ask follow-up questions as needed. For example, if the person reports pain, ask the person where the pain is located, when the pain started and what the pain feels like (e.g., "crushing," "stabbing," "throbbing").

A = Allergies.

Ask the person if he or she is allergic to any foods, medications or things found in the environment (such as bees). If the person does report an allergy, ask what type of reaction the person had in the past when exposed to the allergen, and what care the person received.

M = Medications.

Ask the person if he or she is taking any prescription or over-the-counter medications. If the person is taking medication, ask the person what the medication is and when he or she last took it. Even if the person does not know the exact name or dose of the medication, he or she may still be able to tell you the purpose of the medication (for example, "I take blood pressure medication.")

P = Pertinent medical history.

Ask the person whether he or she has any medical conditions.

L = Last food or drink.

Ask the person when he or she last had something to eat or drink, what he or she ate or drank, and the amount.

E = Events leading up to the incident.

Ask the person what was happening and what he or she was doing just prior to when he or she began to feel ill or was injured.

Figure 5-1. The mnemonic SAMPLE can help you remember what to ask the injured or ill person.

Checking a Responsive Person

After sizing up the scene, if your initial check of the person reveals that they are responsive and awake, start by introducing yourself and getting consent to give care. If the person does not have any immediately obvious life-threatening conditions, begin to gather additional information about the nature of the person's injury or illness by interviewing the person and checking them from head to toe (Skill Sheet 5-1). Tailor your approach to the age of the person, as well as to any special circumstances (Box 5-2).

Box 5-1. **Recovery Positions**

When a person is responsive but not fully awake or unresponsive, but breathing normally, put the person in a recovery position if the person has no obvious signs of injury. The recovery position helps to lower the person's risk for choking and **aspiration** (the inhalation of foreign matter, such as saliva or vomit, into the lungs). You should also use the recovery position if a person with an injury begins to vomit, or if it is necessary to leave the person alone to call 9-1-1 or the designated emergency number.

To place an adult or child in a recovery position:

- Extend the person's arm that is closest to you above the person's head.

- Roll the person toward yourself onto their side, so that the person's head rests on their extended arm.

- Bend both of the person's knees to stabilize the body.

For an infant:

- You can place an infant on their side as you would an older child, or you can hold the infant in a recovery position by positioning the infant face-down along your forearm, supporting the infant's head and neck while keeping their mouth and nose clear. Keep the head and neck slightly lower than the chest.

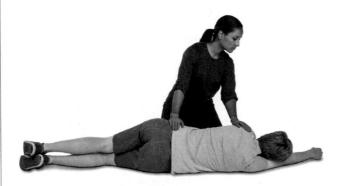

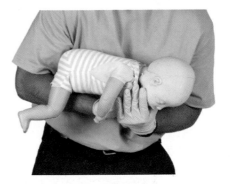

Box 5-2. **Strategies for Gathering Information Effectively**

Being able to communicate and interact effectively with the person who is injured or ill can increase the person's comfort level with you, and makes it more likely that you will be able to get the information you need in order to give appropriate care.

When the Injured or Ill Person Is a Child

- If the child's parent or guardian is present, remember to get the parent's or guardian's consent to give care.

- Be aware that children often take emotional cues from the adults around them. If the child sees that adults are upset, the child's anxiety and panic may increase. Stay calm, and encourage the child's parent or guardian to do the same.

- The child's parent or guardian can be a valuable source of information if the child is not able to speak for themself. However, if the child is old enough to understand and answer your questions, speak directly to the child using age-appropriate language, rather than addressing your questions to the parent or guardian.

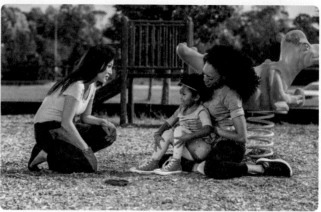

- If the care you need to give will cause discomfort or pain, describe what the child can expect to feel in terms the child can understand. Never make promises or statements that you cannot support (e.g., do not say that something will not hurt if it will).

- Take into consideration the child's developmental stage.

  - **Infants (birth to 1 year).** Infants older than 6 months often show "stranger anxiety." They may turn away from you, cry, and cling to their parent or guardian. If possible, check the infant while they are held or seated in the parent's or guardian's lap.

  - **Toddlers (1 to 3 years).** A toddler may also become anxious if separated from their parent or guardian. If possible, give the toddler a few minutes to get used to you before attempting to check them, and check the toddler while they are seated in the parent's or guardian's lap. Allowing the toddler to hold a special toy or blanket can be comforting.

  - **Preschoolers (3 to 5 years).** Preschoolers are naturally curious. Allowing the child to examine items, such as bandages, can distract the child while you are checking them and giving care. It time permits, showing the child what you are going to do on a stuffed animal or doll can help the child understand how you will care for them. Preschoolers often have a fear of body mutilation and may become very upset if they can see the results of an injury (e.g., a bleeding wound or a deformed broken limb).

  - **School-age children (5 to 12 years).** Children of this age are usually comfortable speaking with adults. They are able to understand what is happening and follow directions. Answer the child's questions honestly, and let the child know if you are going to do anything that might cause pain.

  - **Adolescents (12 to 20 years).** Adolescents may feel embarrassed and self-conscious about their changing bodies. Respect their modesty and ask if they would prefer to be checked by a male or female.

(Continued)

Box 5-2. continued

When the Injured or Ill Person Is an Older Adult

- Pay attention to how the person introduces themself. If the person gives a last name, consider addressing the person more formally (e.g., "Mr. Johnson" rather than "Bill") as a sign of respect.

- A family member, caregiver or other person who knows the older adult well can be a valuable source of information if the older adult is not able to speak for themself. However, if the older adult is able to understand and answer your questions, speak directly to them, rather than addressing your questions to others who might be present.

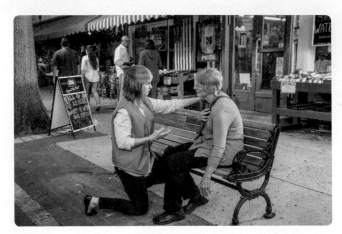

- Speak clearly and loudly enough for the person to hear you, but do not shout. If the person does not seem to understand what you are saying, change your words, not the volume of your voice, unless you spoke too softly.

- When interviewing the person, avoid rushing. Allow the person enough time to process your questions and respond.

- Be aware that in older people, the signs and symptoms of a medical emergency may be very general and nonspecific, and they may not even be noticeable to someone who does not know the person well. General signs and symptoms that could indicate a medical emergency in an older adult include headache, a change in the person's usual level of activity, a change in mental status (such as agitation, the new onset of confusion or increased confusion in a person who is already confused), lethargy (extreme drowsiness or sleepiness) and difficulty sleeping.

- Many older adults have impaired hearing, vision or both. If the person seems confused, make sure the "confusion" is not just the result of being unable to hear you or see you clearly. If the person normally wears a hearing aid, make sure it is in place and turned on. If the person usually wears glasses, make sure they have them on.

When the Injured or Ill Person Has a Disability

- A family member, caregiver or other person who knows the injured or ill person well can be a valuable source of information if the person is not able to speak for themself. However, if the person is able to understand and answer your questions, speak directly to them, rather than addressing your questions to others who might be present.

- A person with a disability may use a service animal. Be aware that service animals are trained to protect their owners, and both the service animal and the person may become anxious if they are separated. Allow the service animal to stay with the person if possible.

- If the person wears an assistive device (e.g., a leg brace), do not remove the device when you are examining the person.

- If the person has an intellectual disability:

  ○ Address the person as you would any other person in their age group. If the person does not seem to understand you, rephrase your statement or question in simpler terms.

  ○ Be aware that being injured or becoming suddenly ill may make the person very upset, anxious or fearful. Take time to explain who you are and what you intend to do, and reassure the person.

(Continued)

Box 5-2. continued

- If the person has impaired hearing:

  ○ Approach the person from the front.

  ○ Position yourself so that the person can see your mouth and facial expressions. Hearing-impaired people who know how to read lips rely on watching your mouth move. Pronounce your words slowly and clearly, and speak in short sentences.

  ○ If the person does not seem to understand what you are saying, change your words, not the volume of your voice, unless you spoke too softly. Shouting sometimes causes the person more distress, and they still may not understand what you are trying to say.

  ○ Use gestures or written messages as necessary to make your meaning clear.

- If the person has impaired vision:

  ○ Speak in a normal voice. It is not necessary to shout.

  ○ As you give care, describe what you are doing.

When the Injured or Ill Person Speaks a Different Language

- Speak in a normal voice. It is not necessary to shout.

- Find out if any bystanders speak the person's language and can assist by translating.

- Do your best to communicate nonverbally, using gestures and facial expressions.

- When you call 9-1-1 or the designated emergency number, explain that you are having difficulty communicating with the person, and tell the dispatcher which language you believe the person speaks. The dispatcher may have someone available who can help with communication.

Interviewing the Person

Begin by asking the person's name, and use it when you speak to the person. Position yourself at eye level with the person and speak clearly, calmly and in a friendly manner, using age-appropriate language. Try to provide as much privacy as possible for the person while you are conducting the interview, and keep the interview brief. The mnemonic SAMPLE (Figure 5-1) can help you remember what you should ask about. If possible, write down the information you learn during the interview or, preferably, have someone else write it down for you. Be sure to give the information to EMS personnel when they arrive. It may help them determine the type of medical care that the person should receive.

Other people at the scene may be able to provide useful information as well. They may have witnessed what happened. If there are people at the scene who know the injured or ill person well (such as family members or friends), they may also be able to provide information about the person's medical history, if the injured or ill person was not able to do so (for example, because of the effects of the injury or illness).

Checking the Person from Head to Toe

Next, check the person from head to toe. Before beginning the check, tell the person what you are going to do. Then check the person in a methodical way. Check one part of the body at a time, moving straight down the body from head to toe, and then checking the arms.

As you check, take note of any medical identification tags, such as a bracelet or sports band, on the person's wrist or ankle, or a necklace around the person's neck. Look and gently feel for signs of injury, such as bleeding, cuts, burns, bruising, swelling or deformities. Think of how the body usually looks. If you are unsure if a body part or limb looks injured, check it against the opposite limb or the other side of the body. Watch the person's face for expressions of discomfort or pain as you check for injuries.

If you detect signs or symptoms of injury or illness:

- Determine whether to call 9-1-1 or the designated emergency number (see Chapter 2, Box 2-2).

- Help the person rest in a comfortable position.

- Reassure the person by telling them that you will help and that EMS personnel have been called (if appropriate).

- Give care according to the conditions that you find and your level of knowledge and training.

- Be alert to signs that the person's condition is worsening, such as changes in level of consciousness, changes in breathing, changes in skin color or restlessness. These could be signs of shock, a life-threatening condition. You will learn more about shock in Chapter 9.

If the person has no apparent signs or symptoms of injury or illness and can move without pain, have them rest in a comfortable position. Continue to watch for changes in the person's condition. When the person feels ready, help them to stand up. Determine what additional care is needed and whether to call 9-1-1 or the designated emergency number.

In a young or frightened child who does not appear to have a life-threatening injury or illness, do the reverse—check from toe to head. Checking in this order gives the child a chance to get used to the process and allows the child to see what is going on.

Safety First! Sometimes people who have been injured or become suddenly ill may act strangely; be uncooperative; or become violent, angry or aggressive. This behavior can be the result of the injury or illness or other factors, such as the effects of drugs, alcohol or medications. Do not take this behavior personally. If you feel threatened by the person's behavior, move away from the person to safety and call 9-1-1 or the designated emergency number, if you have not already done so.

What if... *I am trying to help a person who does not speak the same language that I do? How can I get their consent or figure out what is wrong?*

Good communication is necessary when assessing and giving care to a person of any age or ethnicity. When a language barrier exists, however, communication becomes challenging and can hamper care. When dealing with a person who does not speak your language, remember to be aware of your own cultural biases and preconceptions, and respect the person's cultural beliefs. Other strategies include trying to find a friend, family member or bystander who can serve as an interpreter; or when an interpreter is not present, speaking slowly and carefully in terms as simple as possible, using simple illustrations or gestures to allow the person to describe their situation, and using your own body to demonstrate the care you'd like to give. Keep in mind that certain gestures used in your own culture may have different meanings in other cultures.

What if... *I am checking a person who reports no pain, but is unwilling to move any of their joints?*

A person who is unwilling to move a joint should not be forced to move the joint, regardless of whether they report any pain. The person likely has a reason for not moving the joint even if they cannot express it. In this case, consider the possibility of broken bones or other injuries, and call 9-1-1 or the designated emergency number.

Care for a Responsive Person

Once you complete the head-to-toe check, give care for any specific injuries you find. To give care for the person until EMS personnel arrive, follow these general guidelines:

- *Do no* further harm.

- Monitor the person's level of consciousness and breathing. A change in the person's condition may be a sign of a more serious injury or illness. A condition that may not appear serious at first may become serious over time.

- Help the person rest in the most comfortable position.

- Keep the person from getting chilled or overheated.

- Comfort and reassure the person, but do not provide false hope.

- Give any specific care as needed.

Checking for Shock

When someone is injured or becomes suddenly ill, normal body functions may be interrupted. In cases of minor injury or illness, the interruption is brief and the body is able to compensate quickly. With more severe injuries or illness, however, the body is unable to meet its demand for oxygen. The condition in which the body fails to circulate oxygen-rich blood to all the parts of the body is known as shock. If left untreated, shock can lead to death. Always look for the signs and symptoms of shock whenever you are giving care. These signs and symptoms include:

- Restlessness or irritability.

- Altered level of consciousness.

- Nausea or vomiting.

- Pale, ashen or grayish, cool, moist skin.

- Rapid breathing and pulse.

- Excessive thirst.

Be aware that the early signs and symptoms of shock may not be present in young children and infants. However, because children are smaller than adults, they are more susceptible to shock. You will learn more about how to recognize and treat a person for shock in Chapter 9.

Summary

Many variables affect dealing with emergencies. By following the emergency action steps, **CHECK—CALL—CARE,** you can ensure that the person receives the best possible care.

Check the person in the position they are found, if possible. Determine whether the person has any life-threatening conditions. Life-threatening conditions include unresponsiveness, trouble breathing, absence of breathing and severe, life-threatening bleeding. Call 9-1-1 or the designated emergency number if the person appears to have any of these signs and symptoms.

If you find no life-threatening conditions, interview the person and any bystanders and then perform a head-to-toe check (toe-to-head for a child or infant) to find and care for any injuries or signs of illness. If you do not give care, these conditions could become life threatening.

READY TO RESPOND? ▶

Think back to the incident encountered in the opening scenario, and use what you have learned to respond to these questions:

1. What might you do to make the scene safe for you to check the person?

2. If the person on the trail is awake, breathing and has no severe, life-threatening bleeding, what should you do next?

3. If the person becomes unresponsive after your check, what would your next step be?

Study Questions

1. List four life-threatening conditions.

Use the following scenario to answer questions 2 and 3.

Several people are clustered in the middle of a street. A car is stopped in the right lane. As you approach the group, you can see a mangled bicycle lying on the pavement. You see your neighbor sitting next to it. No one seems to be doing anything. You approach your neighbor and kneel next to them.

2. What type of dangers could be present at the scene? What could you do to make the scene safer?

3. You determine that your neighbor has no life-threatening emergencies. What should you do next?

Use the following scenario to answer question 4.

You walk into your boss's office for a meeting. You see a cup of coffee spilled on the desk. Your boss is lying on the floor, motionless.

4. Based on the scenario above, number the following actions in order:

_____ Control any severe, life-threatening bleeding.

_____ Check the scene by performing a scene size-up.

_____ Check for responsiveness and breathing.

_____ Perform a SAMPLE interview.

_____ Call 9-1-1 or the designated emergency number.

In questions 5 through 9, circle the letter of the correct answer.

5. What is the purpose of your initial check of the person?

a. To check for minor injuries

b. To determine whether any life-threatening conditions are present

c. To get consent from the person before giving care

d. To ask for information about the cause of the injury or illness

(Continued)

Study Questions continued

6. Once you determine the person has no life-threatening conditions, you should—

a. Call 9-1-1 or the designated emergency number.

b. Transport the person to the nearest hospital.

c. Check for other injuries or conditions that could become life threatening if not cared for.

d. Check for responsiveness.

7. Before beginning a check for life-threatening conditions, you should first—

a. Move the person to a convenient location for care.

b. Check the scene.

c. Call 9-1-1 or the designated emergency number.

d. a and b

8. If the person you are checking is unresponsive but breathing normally, what should be your next action?

a. Have a bystander call 9-1-1 or the designated emergency number.

b. Put the person in a recovery position.

c. Check for severe bleeding.

d. Begin a check for non-life-threatening conditions.

9. If the person you are checking is unresponsive and not breathing normally, what should be your next action?

a. Conduct a SAMPLE history.

b. Begin CPR.

c. Place the person in a recovery position.

d. Check for medical identification tags.

Answers are listed in the Appendix.

Checking a Responsive Person

1. Interview the person (or bystanders, if necessary) using SAMPLE to get a better understanding of the situation and the nature of the person's injury or illness.

    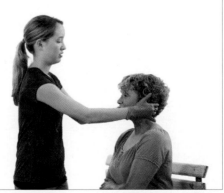

    - *S* = **Signs and symptoms.** Take note of signs (which you can observe for yourself, using your senses) and ask the person about symptoms (feelings that only the person can describe to you, such as pain, shortness of breath or nausea).

    - *A* = **Allergies.** Ask the person about allergies, noting causes of allergic reactions in the past and whether the allergic reaction was severe or life threatening.

    - *M* = **Medications.** Ask the person about over-the-counter and prescription medications that they are taking. Ask about the name of the medication and when the person last took it.

    - *P* = **Pertinent medical history.** Ask the person whether they have any medical conditions.

    - *L* = **Last food or drink.** Ask the person when they last had something to eat or drink, what the person ate or drank, and how much.

    - *E* = **Events leading up to the incident.** Ask the person what was happening and what they were doing just prior to when they began to feel ill or were injured.

2. Check each part of the body in a systematic manner from head to toe. As you check each part of the body, look and feel for signs of injury, including bleeding, cuts, burns, bruising, swelling or deformities. Note if the person has pain or discomfort, or is unable or unwilling to move the body part. Also notice how the person's skin looks and feels. Is the skin pale, ashen or flushed? Does it feel moist or dry, cool or hot?

    Note: Do not ask the person to move if you suspect a head, neck or spinal injury. Do not ask the person to move any area of the body that causes discomfort or pain.

    Note: As you check the person, take note of any medical identification tags (typically worn around the neck, wrist or ankle).

    - **Head and neck.** Check the scalp, face, ears, eyes, nose, mouth and neck for signs of injury.

    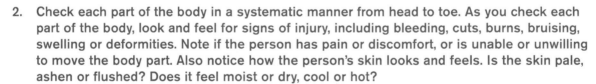

(Continued)

Checking a Responsive Person *Continued*

- ■ **Shoulders.** Check the shoulders for signs of injury.

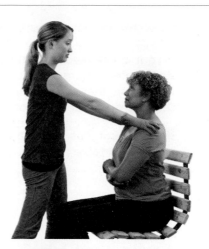

- ■ **Chest and abdomen.** Check the chest and abdomen for signs of injury. Ask the person to take a deep breath and blow the air out. Look for trouble breathing or changes in breathing. Ask the person if they are experiencing pain during breathing.

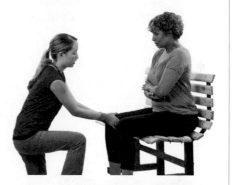

- ■ **Hips.** Check the hips for signs of injury. Ask the person if they are experiencing hip pain.

- ■ **Legs and feet.** Check each leg and foot, one at a time, for signs of injury. Ask the person to wiggle their toes and feet.

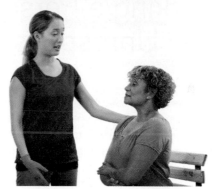

- ■ **Arms and hands.** Check each arm and hand, one at a time, for signs of injury. Ask the person to wiggle their fingers and hands.

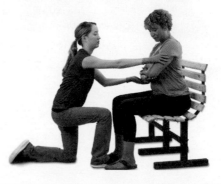

(Continued)

Checking a Responsive Person *Continued*

3. Give care for any conditions found.

- If your check reveals signs or symptoms of an injury or illness, call 9-1-1 or the designated emergency number (if necessary) and give care according to the conditions that you find and your level of knowledge and training. Be alert to signs that the person's condition is worsening.

- If the person has no apparent signs or symptoms of injury or illness, have them rest in a comfortable position. Continue to watch for changes in the person's condition.

Skill Sheet 5-2

Checking a Person Who Appears to Be Unresponsive

1. **Check for responsiveness and breathing.** Shout to get the person's attention, using the person's name if you know it. If there is no response, tap the person's shoulder (if the person is an adult or child) or the bottom of the person's foot (if the person is an infant), and shout again while checking for normal breathing.

    - Check for responsiveness and breathing for no more than 5 to 10 seconds.

    - Isolated or infrequent gasping is not normal breathing.

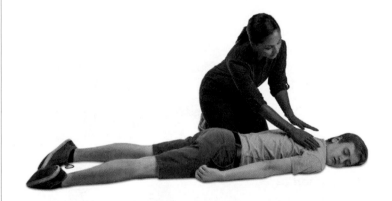
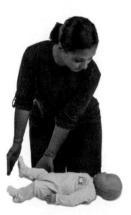

(Continued)

Checking a Person Who Appears to Be Unresponsive *Continued*

2. **If the person responds and is breathing normally but is not fully awake:**

   ■ Send someone to call 9-1-1 or the designated emergency number and to obtain an AED and first aid kit.

   ■ Interview bystanders (using SAMPLE as a guide) and do a head-to-toe check to gather more information.

   ■ Place the person into the recovery position by rolling the person onto their side.

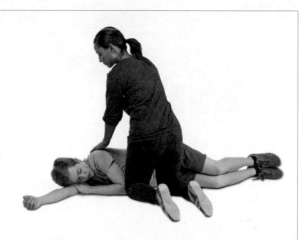

3. **If the person does not respond and is not breathing or is only gasping:**

   ■ Send someone to call 9-1-1 or the designated emergency number and to obtain an AED and first aid kit (or, if you are alone, complete these actions yourself).

   ■ If the person is face-down, carefully roll the person onto their back. If necessary, move the person to a firm, flat surface.

   ■ Immediately begin CPR (starting with compressions) and use an AED as soon as possible.

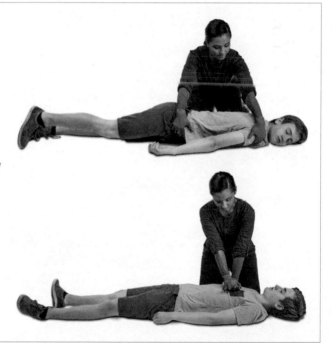

PART THREE

Life-Threatening Emergencies

CARDIAC EMERGENCIES

As you come out of your house to run a quick errand one hot summer afternoon, you see your neighbor, Mr. Getz, cheerfully mowing the lawn. Mr. Getz has been ill lately, so you are glad to see him out and about. When you return a half-hour later, however, you notice Mr. Getz sprawled face-down on the grass. You run over to help.

Learn and Respond ▶

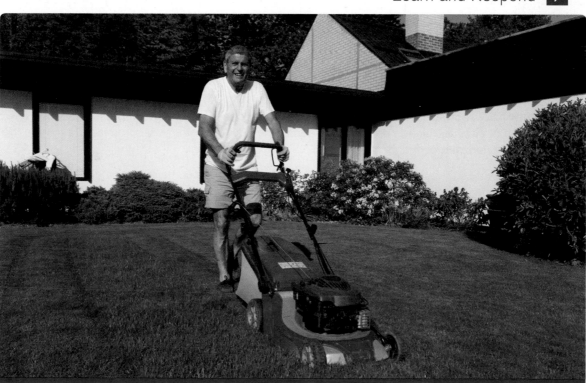

After reading this chapter, you should be able to:

- List the signs and symptoms of a heart attack for both men and women.
- Describe the care for a person having a heart attack.
- Identify the five links in the Adult Cardiac Chain of Survival.
- Identify the five links in the Pediatric Cardiac Chain of Survival.
- Describe the difference between a heart attack and cardiac arrest.
- Describe the role of CPR in cardiac arrest.
- Describe defibrillation and how it works.
- Describe the general steps for the use of an AED.
- List the precautions for the use of an AED.

After reading this chapter and completing the class activities, you should be able to:

- Demonstrate how to perform CPR for an adult, child and infant in cardiac arrest.
- Demonstrate how to use an AED to care for an adult, child and infant in cardiac arrest.

KEY TERMS

Angina pectoris: Pain in the chest that comes and goes at different times; caused by a lack of oxygen reaching the heart.

Asystole: A condition in which the heart has stopped generating electrical activity.

Atherosclerosis: A condition in which deposits of plaque, including cholesterol (a fatty substance made by the liver and found in foods containing animal or animal products) build up on the inner walls of the arteries, causing them to harden and narrow, reducing the amount of blood that can flow through; develops gradually and can go undetected for many years.

Cardiac arrest: A condition in which the heart has stopped beating or beats too irregularly or weakly to pump blood effectively.

Cardiopulmonary resuscitation (CPR): A technique that combines chest compressions and rescue breaths to circulate blood containing oxygen to the brain and other vital organs for a person whose heart and normal breathing have stopped.

Cholesterol: A fatty substance made by the liver and found in foods containing animal or animal products; diets high in cholesterol contribute to the risk of heart disease.

Coronary arteries: Blood vessels that supply the heart muscle with oxygen-rich blood.

Coronary heart disease (CHD): A disease in which cholesterol and plaque build up on the inner walls of the arteries that supply blood to the heart; also called *coronary artery disease* (CAD).

Defibrillation: An electric shock that disrupts the electrical activity of the heart long enough to allow the heart to spontaneously develop an effective rhythm on its own.

Heart attack: A sudden illness involving the death of heart muscle tissue when it does not receive oxygen-rich blood; also known as *myocardial infarction.*

(Continued)

Risk factors: Conditions or behaviors that increase the chance that a person will develop a disease.

Ventricular fibrillation (V-fib): A life-threatening heart rhythm in which the heart is in a state of totally disorganized electrical activity, and does not pump blood effectively.

Ventricular tachycardia (V-tach): A life-threatening heart rhythm in which there is very rapid contraction of the ventricles (the lower chambers of the heart), causing the heart to pump blood ineffectively or not at all.

Introduction

In this chapter, you will learn how to recognize and give care for a person who is having a heart attack or who is experiencing cardiac arrest, which are among the most common cardiac emergencies. This chapter also discusses risk factors for cardiovascular disease—the leading cause of cardiac emergencies—and what you can do to control those risks.

Cardiovascular Disease

Cardiovascular disease is an abnormal condition that affects the heart and blood vessels. It is the number one killer in the United States and is a major cause of disability. Cardiovascular disease causes **coronary heart disease (CHD),** also known as coronary artery disease. People with cardiovascular disease are likely also to have disease of other blood vessels, which can cause strokes. More information about stroke is included in Chapter 15.

CHD occurs when the **coronary arteries** that supply blood to the heart muscle harden and narrow in a process called **atherosclerosis.** The damage occurs gradually, as **cholesterol** and fatty deposits called plaque build up on the inner artery walls. As this buildup worsens, the arteries become narrower. This reduces the amount of blood that can flow through the arteries, and prevents the heart from getting the blood and oxygen it needs. If the heart does not get blood containing oxygen, it will not work properly. CHD accounts for about half of the cardiovascular-disease-related deaths in adult Americans each year. Because atherosclerosis develops gradually, it can remain undetected for many years. Most people with atherosclerosis are unaware they have it. Fortunately, atherosclerosis can be slowed or stopped by taking steps to reduce **risk factors** and adopting a healthy lifestyle.

Risk Factors for Coronary Heart Disease

Many things increase a person's chances of developing CHD. These are called risk factors. Some risk factors cannot be changed. For instance, although more women than men die each year from CHD in the United States, heart disease generally affects men at younger ages than it does women. Ethnicity also plays a role in determining the risk for heart disease. African-American and Native American populations statistically have higher rates of heart disease than do other U.S. populations. A family history of heart disease also increases the risk.

The good news is that some risk factors for CHD can be reduced. Cigarette smoking, a poor diet, uncontrolled high blood cholesterol or high blood pressure, excessive weight and lack of regular exercise all increase the risk of heart disease. When individuals exhibit multiple risk factors, the risk of heart attack is much greater. Appropriate steps can be taken to control these risk factors—such as quitting smoking, eating healthier, exercising regularly and following the care prescribed by a healthcare provider—all to improve one's chances for living a long and healthy life.

Heart Attack

A **heart attack** occurs when blood flow to part of the heart muscle is blocked (e.g., as a result of coronary artery disease). Because the cells in the affected area of the heart muscle are not receiving the oxygen and nutrients they need, they die, causing permanent damage to the heart muscle (Figure 6-1). Seeking advanced medical care as soon as you recognize the signs and symptoms of a heart attack can minimize the damage to the heart and may save the person's life.

When a person is having a heart attack, every minute counts.

Signs and Symptoms of a Heart Attack

Signs and symptoms of a heart attack vary from person to person, and can be different in women than they are in men. Even people who have had a heart attack before may not experience the same signs and symptoms if they have a second heart attack. A person who is having a heart attack may show any of the following signs and symptoms:

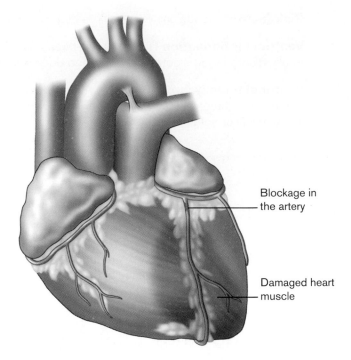

Blockage in the artery

Damaged heart muscle

Figure 6-1. A heart attack occurs when blood flow to the heart is blocked.

- Chest pain, which can range from mild to unbearable. The person may complain of pressure, squeezing, tightness, aching or heaviness in the chest. The pain or discomfort is persistent, lasting longer than 3 to 5 minutes, or going away and then coming back. It is not relieved by resting, changing position or taking medication. It may be difficult to distinguish the pain of a heart attack from the pain of indigestion, heartburn or a muscle spasm.

- Discomfort or pain that spreads to one or both arms, the back, the shoulder, the neck, the jaw or the upper part of the stomach

- Dizziness or light-headedness

- Trouble breathing, including noisy breathing, shortness of breath or breathing that is faster than normal

- Nausea or vomiting

- Pale, ashen (gray) or slightly bluish skin, especially around the face and fingers

- Sweating

- A feeling of anxiety or impending doom

- Extreme fatigue (tiredness)

- Unresponsiveness

Heart Attack

Although men often have the "classic" signs and symptoms of a heart attack, such as chest pain that radiates down one arm, women often have more subtle signs and symptoms or experience the signs and symptoms of a heart attack differently than men do (Figure 6-2). For example, in women, the "classic" signs and symptoms

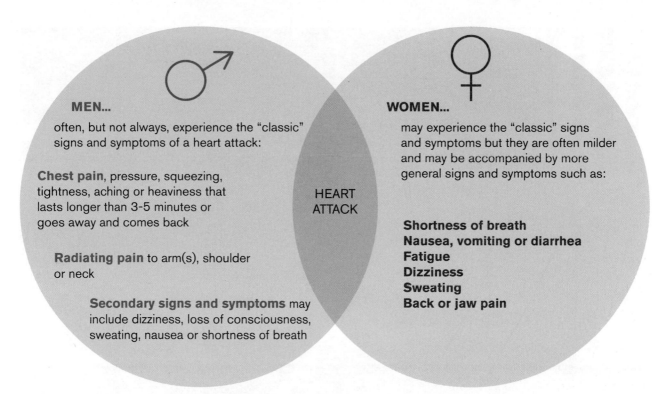

MEN...

often, but not always, experience the "classic" signs and symptoms of a heart attack:

Chest pain, pressure, squeezing, tightness, aching or heaviness that lasts longer than 3-5 minutes or goes away and comes back

Radiating pain to arm(s), shoulder or neck

Secondary signs and symptoms may include dizziness, loss of consciousness, sweating, nausea or shortness of breath

HEART ATTACK

WOMEN...

may experience the "classic" signs and symptoms but they are often milder and may be accompanied by more general signs and symptoms such as:

Shortness of breath
Nausea, vomiting or diarrhea
Fatigue
Dizziness
Sweating
Back or jaw pain

Figure 6-2. Men and women often experience heart attacks differently.

may be milder or accompanied by more general signs and symptoms such as shortness of breath, nausea or vomiting, extreme fatigue, and dizziness or light-headedness. Because these signs and symptoms are so general and nonspecific, women may experience them for hours, days or even weeks leading up to the heart attack but dismiss them as nothing out of the ordinary.

The signs and symptoms of a heart attack may also be more subtle in people with certain medical conditions such as diabetes.

First Aid Care for a Heart Attack

If you think that a person is having a heart attack, call 9-1-1 or the designated emergency number immediately. Trust your instincts. Many people who are having a heart attack delay seeking care because they hope they are experiencing signs and symptoms of a more minor condition that will go away with time, such as indigestion, heartburn, a muscle strain or the flu. People often worry about calling an ambulance and going to the emergency room for a "false alarm." However, most people who die of a heart attack die within 2 hours of first experiencing signs or symptoms. Even when a heart attack is not fatal, early advanced medical care can help to minimize the damage to the heart. Always seek advanced medical care as soon as signs and symptoms of a heart attack are noted.

If you think that someone might be having a heart attack, you should:

■ Call 9-1-1 or the designated emergency number immediately. Never try to drive a person who is experiencing signs and symptoms of a heart attack to the hospital yourself. EMS personnel can transport the person to the hospital safely while initiating care.

■ Have the person stop what they are doing and rest in a comfortable position to reduce the heart's need for oxygen. Many people experiencing a heart attack find it easier to breathe while sitting (Figure 6-3).

■ Loosen any tight or uncomfortable clothing.

■ Reassure the person. Anxiety increases the person's discomfort.

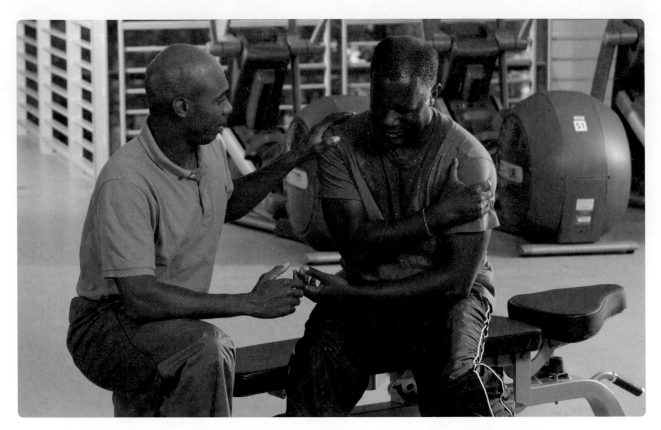

Figure 6-3. Tell a person with signs and symptoms of a heart attack to stop and rest. Many people find breathing easier while sitting.

- If the person has a history of heart disease and takes a prescribed medication to relieve chest pain (e.g., nitroglycerin), offer to locate the medication and help the person to take it.

- If the person is responsive, able to chew and swallow, and allowed to have aspirin, you may offer two low-dose (81-mg) aspirin tablets or one 5-grain (325-mg) regular-strength aspirin tablet (Box 6-1).

- Closely monitor the person's condition until EMS personnel arrive and take over. Notice any changes in the person's appearance or behavior.

- If you are trained in giving CPR and using an automated external defibrillator (AED), be prepared to give CPR and use an AED if the person becomes unresponsive.

Angina Pectoris

Some people with narrowed arteries may experience chest pain or pressure that comes and goes at different times (i.e., intermittent chest pain or pressure). This type of pain is called ***angina pectoris,*** which is a medical term for pain in the chest. Angina pectoris, often referred to simply as angina, develops when the heart needs more oxygen than it is getting. When the coronary arteries are narrow and the heart needs more oxygen, such as during physical activity or emotional stress, heart muscle tissue may not get enough oxygen. This lack of oxygen can cause a constricting chest pain that may spread to the neck, jaw and arms. Pain associated with angina seldom lasts longer than 3 to 5 minutes.

A person who knows that they have a history of angina may tell you they have a prescribed medication, such as nitroglycerin, that will temporarily widen (i.e., vasodilate) the arteries and therefore help relieve the pain. **Nitroglycerin** is commonly prescribed as a small tablet that dissolves under the tongue or as an oral spray. Sometimes nitroglycerin patches or paste are placed on the chest and the medication is absorbed transdermally (i.e., through the skin) into the bloodstream. Once absorbed into the body, nitroglycerin dilates the blood vessels to make it easier for blood to reach heart muscle tissue, thus relieving the chest pain.

Box 6-1. **Aspirin for a Heart Attack**

You may be able to help a person who is showing early signs and symptoms of a heart attack by offering the person an appropriate dose of aspirin. Aspirin can help to prevent blood clotting and is most effective when given soon after the onset of signs and symptoms of a heart attack. However, you should never delay calling 9-1-1 or the designated emergency number to find or offer aspirin.

Before offering aspirin, make sure the person is responsive, able to chew and swallow, and allowed to have aspirin. Ask the person:

- Are you allergic to aspirin?

- Do you have a stomach ulcer or stomach disease?

- Are you taking any blood thinners, such as warfarin (Coumadin™)?

- Have you ever been told by a healthcare provider to avoid taking aspirin?

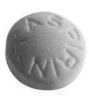

If the person answers "no" to each of these questions, you may offer the person two low-dose (81-mg) aspirin tablets or one 5-grain (325-mg) regular-strength aspirin tablet. Have the person chew the aspirin completely. Chewing the aspirin speeds its absorption into the bloodstream. Do not offer the person an aspirin-containing combination product meant to relieve multiple conditions, or another type of pain medication, such as acetaminophen (Tylenol®), ibuprofen (Motrin®, Advil®) or naproxen (Aleve®). These medications do not work the same way aspirin does and are not beneficial for a person who is experiencing a heart attack.

Most people with angina pectoris are advised by their doctors to take three nitroglycerin doses over a 10-minute period if they are experiencing pain or discomfort; however, it is important to remember that some doctors may prescribe nitroglycerin differently. Since these areas of narrowing can be the focus for clot formation and heart attack, if a person's typical pain of angina lasts longer than usual, 9-1-1 or the designated emergency number should be called. It may be that the angina has progressed to a heart attack.

Cardiac Arrest

Cardiac arrest is not the same as a heart attack. Remember, a heart attack occurs when blood flow to part of the heart muscle is blocked, causing part of the heart muscle to die. **Cardiac arrest,** on the other hand, occurs when the heart stops beating or beats too ineffectively to circulate blood to the brain and other vital organs. A network of special cells in the heart muscle conducts electrical impulses that coordinate contraction, causing the heart to beat rhythmically. In cardiac arrest, the electrical impulses become abnormal and chaotic or may even become absent. This causes the heart to lose the ability to beat rhythmically, or to stop beating altogether (Figure 6-4).

Cardiovascular disease and certain congenital heart conditions (conditions that a person is born with) can increase a person's risk for cardiac arrest. Breathing emergencies, such as choking or drowning, can also lead to cardiac arrest because if the body's supply of oxygen is interrupted, the heart soon stops beating. Every organ in

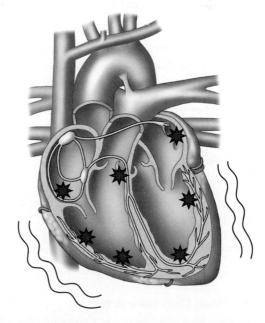

Figure 6-4. Cardiac arrest occurs when the electrical impulses that control the heartbeat become abnormal and chaotic or even absent.

the body needs a steady supply of oxygen in order to work properly, and the heart is no exception. Severe trauma, electric shock and drug overdose are other potential causes of cardiac arrest. Although cardiac arrest is more common in adults, it does occur in young people as well. The most common causes of cardiac arrest in children and infants are breathing emergencies, congenital heart disorders and trauma.

When the heart stops beating properly, the body cannot survive for long. Breathing will soon stop, and the body's organs will no longer receive the oxygen they need to function. Without oxygen, brain damage can begin in about 4 to 6 minutes, and the damage can become irreversible after about 8 to 10 minutes (Figure 6-5). Death occurs within a matter of minutes if the person does not receive immediate care.

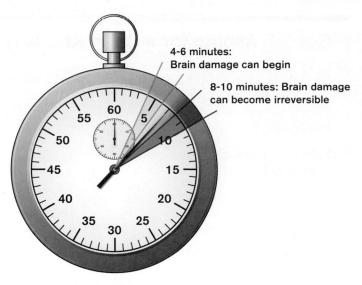

4-6 minutes:
Brain damage can begin

8-10 minutes: Brain damage can become irreversible

Figure 6-5. Every minute counts in cardiac arrest.

Signs and Symptoms of Cardiac Arrest

When a person experiences cardiac arrest, you may see the person suddenly collapse. When you check the person, you will find that the person is not responsive and not breathing, or only gasping. (In an unresponsive person, isolated or infrequent gasping in the absence of normal breathing may be **agonal breaths,** which can occur even after the heart has stopped beating. Agonal breaths are not breathing and are a sign of cardiac arrest.) The person has no heartbeat.

Cardiac arrest can happen suddenly and without any warning signs. When this occurs, the person is said to have experienced **sudden cardiac arrest.** People who have a history of cardiovascular disease or a congenital heart disorder are at higher risk for sudden cardiac arrest. However, sudden cardiac arrest can happen in people who appear healthy and have no known heart disease or other risk factors for the condition. A person who experiences sudden cardiac arrest is at very high risk for dying and needs immediate care.

First Aid Care for Cardiac Arrest

When a person experiences cardiac arrest, quick action on the part of those who witness the arrest is crucial and gives the person the greatest chance for survival. The **Cardiac Chain of Survival** describes five actions that, when performed in rapid succession, increase the person's likelihood of surviving cardiac arrest (Box 6-2). In the Cardiac Chain of Survival, each link of the chain depends on, and is connected to, the other links.

Four out of every five cardiac arrests in the United States occur outside of the hospital. That means trained lay responders like you are often responsible for initiating the Cardiac Chain of Survival. When you complete the first three links in the Cardiac Chain of Survival—recognizing cardiac arrest and activating the EMS system, immediately beginning CPR and using an AED as soon as possible—you give the person the best chance for surviving the incident.

For each minute that CPR and use of an AED are delayed, the person's chance for survival is reduced by about 10 percent.

If you think that a person is in cardiac arrest:

■   Have someone call 9-1-1 or the designated emergency number immediately.

■   Begin CPR immediately.

■   Use an AED as soon as possible.

Box 6-2. **The Cardiac Chain of Survival**

Adult Cardiac Chain of Survival

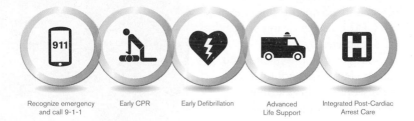

Recognize emergency and call 9-1-1   Early CPR   Early Defibrillation   Advanced Life Support   Integrated Post-Cardiac Arrest Care

■ **Recognition of cardiac arrest and activation of the emergency medical services (EMS) system.** The sooner someone recognizes that a person is in cardiac arrest and calls 9-1-1 or the designated emergency number, the sooner people capable of providing advanced life support will arrive on the scene.

■ **Early CPR.** CPR circulates oxygen-containing blood to the brain and other vital organs, helping to prevent brain damage and death.

■ **Early *defibrillation.*** Defibrillation (delivery of an electrical shock using an AED) may restore an effective heart rhythm, significantly increasing the person's chances for survival.

■ **Early advanced life support.** Provided by EMS personnel at the scene and en route to the hospital, early advanced life support gives the person access to emergency medical care delivered by trained professionals.

■ **Integrated post-cardiac arrest care.** After the person is resuscitated, an interdisciplinary team of medical professionals works to stabilize the person's medical condition, minimize complications, and diagnose and treat the underlying cause of the cardiac arrest to improve survival outcomes.

Pediatric Cardiac Chain of Survival

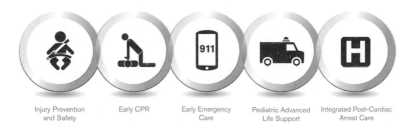

Injury Prevention and Safety   Early CPR   Early Emergency Care   Pediatric Advanced Life Support   Integrated Post-Cardiac Arrest Care

■ **Prevention.** Because cardiac arrest in children often occurs as the result of a preventable injury (such as trauma, drowning, choking or electrocution), the Pediatric Cardiac Chain of Survival has "prevention" as the first link.

■ **Early CPR.** CPR circulates oxygen-containing blood to the brain and other vital organs, helping to prevent brain damage and death.

■ **Activation of the emergency medical services (EMS) system.** The sooner someone recognizes that a person is in cardiac arrest and calls 9-1-1 or the designated emergency number, the sooner people capable of providing advanced life support will arrive on the scene.

■ **Early advanced life support.** Provided by EMS personnel at the scene and en route to the hospital, early advanced life support gives the person access to emergency medical care delivered by trained professionals.

■ **Integrated post-cardiac arrest care.** After the person is resuscitated, an interdisciplinary team of medical professionals works to stabilize the person's medical condition, minimize complications, and diagnose and treat the underlying cause of the cardiac arrest to improve survival outcomes.

CPR

CPR, or *cardiopulmonary resuscitation,* is a skill that is used when a person is in cardiac arrest to keep oxygenated blood moving to the brain and other vital organs until advanced medical help arrives (Figure 6-6). CPR involves giving sets of 30 chest compressions followed by sets of 2 rescue breaths. When you give compressions, you press down on the person's chest. This squeezes (compresses) the heart between the breastbone (sternum) and spine, moving blood out of the heart and to the brain and other vital organs. After each compression, you must let the chest return to its normal position. This allows blood to flow back into the heart. The rescue breaths you give after each set of 30 compressions deliver a fresh supply of oxygen into the person's lungs. When you give CPR, you help to keep oxygenated blood moving throughout the body, which can buy the person some time until advanced medical help arrives.

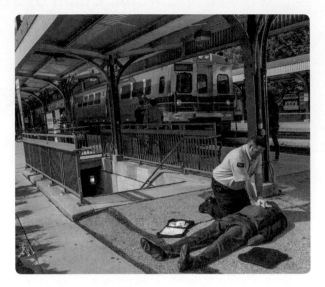

Figure 6-6. CPR keeps oxygen-containing blood circulating to the brain and other vital organs.

Although full CPR (compressions and rescue breaths) is preferred, if you are unable or unwilling for any reason to give full CPR, you can give **compression-only CPR** instead. In compression-only CPR, you give continuous chest compressions, with no rescue breaths. After checking the scene and the person and calling 9-1-1 or the designated emergency number, give chest compressions without stopping until another trained responder or EMS personnel take over or you notice an obvious sign of life.

Many lay responders worry about hurting the person (for example, by breaking the person's ribs or breastbone) while giving CPR, but a person who is in need of CPR is clinically dead (i.e., the person has no heartbeat and is not breathing). It is very unlikely that you will injure the person while giving CPR, but even if you do, consider this: any injury you may cause is secondary when compared with the person's current circumstances, and the injury will heal with medical care and time. Remember: the worst thing to do is nothing!

AED

While CPR can help to prevent brain damage and death by keeping oxygenated blood moving throughout the body, an AED can correct the underlying problem for some people who go into sudden cardiac arrest. Two abnormal heart rhythms in particular, ***ventricular fibrillation (V-fib)*** and ***ventricular tachycardia (V-tach),*** can lead to sudden cardiac arrest. Both abnormal rhythms impair the heart's ability to pump and circulate blood throughout the body and are life threatening (for more information, see When the Heart Fails later in this chapter). However, in many cases, V-fib and V-tach can be corrected by an electrical shock delivered by an AED. This shock disrupts the heart's electrical activity long enough to allow the heart to spontaneously develop an effective rhythm on its own. Starting CPR immediately and using an AED as soon as possible gives the person the best chance for surviving cardiac arrest (Figure 6-7).

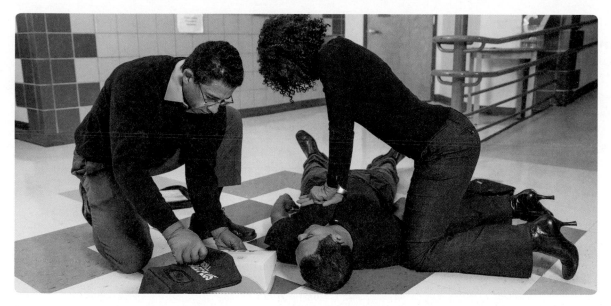

Figure 6-7. Immediately beginning CPR and using an AED as soon as possible gives the person the best chance for survival.

Caring for Cardiac Arrest

If you check a person and find that they are unresponsive and not breathing or only gasping, begin CPR immediately, starting with chest compressions. Proper technique is important. Skill sheets 6-1, 6-2 and 6-3 describe step by step how to give CPR to an adult, child and infant, respectively. Table 6-1 summarizes the key differences in giving CPR to an adult, child or infant. See also Smart Moves: Improving CPR Techniques.

Giving CPR to an Adult

First, make sure the person is lying face-up on a firm, flat surface. For example, if the person is on a soft surface like a sofa or bed, quickly move them to the floor before you begin. Kneel beside the person.

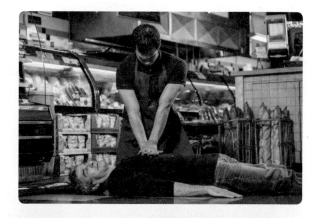

- **Position your hands.** Place the heel of one hand in the center of the person's chest on the person's breastbone (sternum). If you feel the notch at the end of the breastbone, move your hand slightly toward the person's head. Place your other hand on top of your first hand and interlace your fingers or hold them up so that your fingers are not on the person's chest. If you have arthritis in your hands, you can grasp the wrist of the hand positioned on the chest with your other hand instead. The person's clothing should not interfere with finding the proper hand position or your ability to give effective compressions. If it does, loosen or remove enough clothing to allow deep compressions in the center of the person's chest.

- **Give a set of 30 compressions.** Position your body so that your shoulders are directly over your hands. This will let you push on the chest using a straight down-and-up motion, which moves the most blood with each push and is also less tiring. Keeping

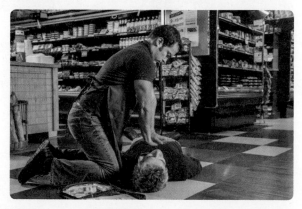

Table 6-1. Comparison of CPR Technique in Adults, Children and Infants

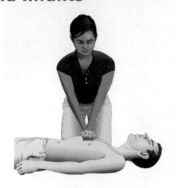

Adult
About age 12 years or older

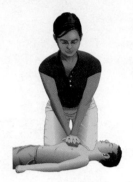

Child
Between the ages of 1 and 12 years

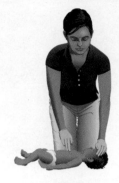

Infant
Younger than 1 year

Hand Position

Adult	Child	Infant
Two hands in center of chest	Two hands in center of chest	Two fingers on center of chest, just below the nipple line

Chest Compressions

Adult	Child	Infant
Compress **at least 2** inches Rate: 100 to 120 compressions/minute	Compress **about 2** inches Rate: 100 to 120 compressions/minute	Compress **about 1½** inches Rate: 100 to 120 compressions/minute

Rescue Breaths

Adult	Child	Infant
Tilt head to **past-neutral position;** pinch nose shut and form seal over mouth	Tilt head to **slightly past-neutral position;** pinch nose shut and form seal over mouth	Tilt head to **neutral position;** form seal over mouth and nose

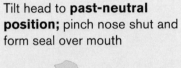
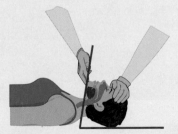
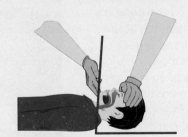
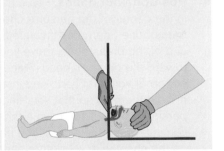

Sets

Adult	Child	Infant
30 chest compressions and 2 rescue breaths	30 chest compressions and 2 rescue breaths	30 chest compressions and 2 rescue breaths

your arms straight, push down at least 2 inches, and then let the chest completely return to its normal position. Push hard and push fast! You want to go at a rate of between 100 and 120 compressions per minute. As you give compressions, count out loud up to 30. Maintain a smooth, steady down-and-up rhythm and do not pause between compressions.

- **Give a set of 2 rescue breaths.** Once you have given 30 compressions, give 2 rescue breaths. First, open the airway using the **head-tilt/chin-lift maneuver.** Place one of your hands on the person's forehead and two fingers of your other hand on the bony part of the person's chin. Tilt the person's head back and lift the chin. For an adult, tilt the head to a past-neutral position (see Table 6-1). If possible, use a CPR breathing barrier when you are giving rescue breaths, but do not delay rescue breaths to find a breathing barrier or learn how to use it. Pinch the person's nose shut. Take a normal breath, make

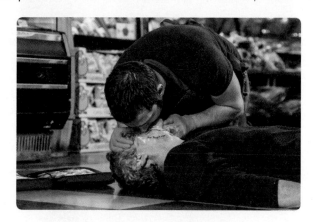

a complete seal over the person's mouth with your mouth, and blow into the person's mouth to give the first rescue breath. Take another breath, make a seal and give the second rescue breath. Each rescue breath should last about 1 second and make the person's chest rise. After you finish giving 2 rescue breaths, return to giving compressions as quickly as possible. The process of giving 2 rescue breaths and getting back to compressions should take less than 10 seconds. Never give more than 2 rescue breaths per set. Table 6-2 describes how to troubleshoot special situations when giving rescue breaths.

Once you begin CPR, continue giving sets of 30 chest compressions and 2 rescue breaths until:

- You notice an obvious sign of life, such as movement. (If the person shows an obvious sign of life, stop CPR, place the person in the recovery position and continue to monitor the person's condition until EMS personnel take over.)

- An AED is ready to use and no other trained responders are available to assist you with the AED.

SMART MOVES > IMPROVING CPR TECHNIQUES

Counting out loud as you give compressions can help you to keep a steady, even rhythm. For compressions 1 through 12, say "1 and 2 and 3 and 4 and 5 and 6 and…" up to 12. When you get to 13, just say the number: "13, 14, 15, 16…" up to 30. Push down as you say the number and come up as you say "and" (or the second syllable of the number). This will help you to keep a steady, even rhythm.

Incorrect technique or body position can cause your arms and shoulders to tire quickly when you are giving compressions. Use the weight of your upper body, not your arm muscles, to compress the chest. Avoid rocking back and forth, because rocking makes your compressions less effective and wastes your energy. Also avoid leaning on the chest, because leaning prevents the chest from returning to its normal position after each compression, limiting the amount of blood that can return to the heart.

When giving rescue breaths, keep the person's head tilted back and avoid taking too large of a breath or blowing too forcefully. Failing to keep the person's head tilted back, taking too large of a breath or blowing too forcefully can force air into the person's stomach instead of into their lungs, which can make the person vomit and cause other complications. Remember: Keep the head tilted back, take a normal breath and blow just enough to make the chest rise.

Table 6-2. **Special Situations: Rescue Breathing**

Special Situation	Solution
The breaths do not make the chest rise. 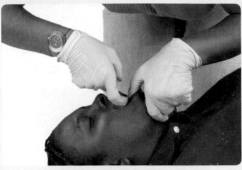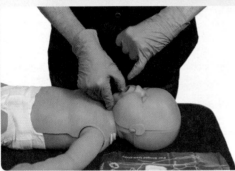	Never give more than 2 rescue breaths per set. If the first rescue breath does not cause the chest to rise, retilt the head to ensure that the airway is properly opened and ensure that the person's nose and mouth are properly sealed before giving the second rescue breath. If the second breath does not make the chest rise, an object may be blocking the person's airway. Give CPR with one modification: after each set of compressions and before giving rescue breaths, open the mouth, look for an object in the person's mouth and, if you see it, remove it.
The person vomits or there is fluid in the mouth. 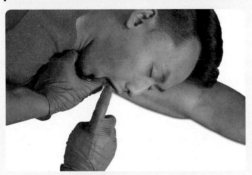	Roll the person onto their side and clear the mouth of fluid using a gloved finger or a piece of gauze. Then roll the person onto their back and resume giving care.
You are unable to form a tight seal over the person's mouth (e.g., due to an injury). 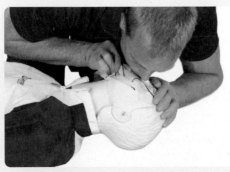	Use mouth-to-nose breathing instead. With the person's head tilted back, close the person's mouth by pushing on the person's chin. Make a complete seal over the person's nose with your mouth and blow in for 1 second to make the chest rise.

(Continued)

Table 6-2. continued

Special Situation	Solution
The person has a **tracheostomy** or **"stoma,"** a surgically created opening in the front of the neck that opens into the trachea (windpipe) to form an alternate route for breathing when the upper airway is blocked or damaged.	Use mouth-to-stoma breathing instead. Expose the person's neck down to the breastbone and remove anything covering the stoma (e.g., a filter or stoma cover). Wipe away any secretions from the stoma. Make a complete seal over the person's stoma or tracheostomy tube with your mouth and blow in for 1 second to make the chest rise. ■ If the chest does not rise, the tracheostomy tube may be blocked. Remove the inner tube and try rescue breaths again. ■ If you hear or feel air escaping from the person's mouth or nose, the person is a partial neck breather (i.e., there is still a connection between the trachea and the upper airway, and although the person breathes mainly through the stoma, they are also able to breathe to some extent through the mouth and nose). Seal the person's mouth and nose with your hand or a tight-fitting mask so that air does not escape out of the mouth or nose when you give rescue breaths into the stoma.

What if... *I am giving chest compressions to a person in cardiac arrest and I hear a rib crack?*

In the adult population, particularly among older adults, rib and sternal (breastbone) fractures can be a complication of CPR. Making sure you use proper hand placement can minimize this risk. If you do hear a cracking sound and begin to feel crepitus (grinding) while compressing the chest, reassess your hand position and correct it as needed. Try to also remember that the potential benefits of CPR—namely, saving a life—outweigh the unpleasantness of a broken rib, which in most cases is not a life-threatening injury.

What if... *During CPR I lose count of the number of chest compressions I am performing and do more or less than the recommended 30 compressions?*

While 30 compressions is the recommended amount, performing 28 chest compressions in one cycle and 32 chest compressions in another cycle is not going to hurt the person's chances of survival. Rather, what is important are the chest compression rate and depth, which, for an adult, should be between 100 and 120 compressions per minute and at least 2 inches deep, while minimizing any interruptions.

Giving CPR to a Child

Giving CPR to a child is very similar to giving CPR to an adult. However, in a child, you open the airway by tilting the head to a slightly past-neutral position, rather than to a past-neutral position (see Table 6-1). Rather than compressing the chest to a depth of *at least* 2 inches as you would for an adult, you compress the chest to a depth of *about* 2 inches for a child. Also, for a small child you may only need to give compressions with one hand, instead of two. The rate of chest compressions for a child is the same as it is for an adult—between 100 and 120 compressions per minute.

Giving CPR to an Infant

The general principles of giving CPR to an infant are the same as they are for children and adults. However, because the infant's body is smaller, you will position your hands differently to deliver compressions. Place the pads of two fingers on the center of the infant's chest, just below the nipple line. If you feel the notch at the end of the infant's breastbone, move your fingers slightly toward the infant's head. Place your other hand on the infant's forehead. Give compressions by using the pads of your fingers to compress the chest about 1½ inches at the same rate as you would for an adult or a child—between 100 and 120 compressions per minute.

When you give rescue breaths, open the airway by tilting the head to a neutral position (see Table 6-1). Instead of pinching the nose shut and covering the mouth with your mouth, cover the infant's nose and mouth with your mouth to form a seal.

When to Stop CPR

Once you begin CPR on an adult, child or infant, do not stop except in one of these situations:

- You notice an obvious sign of life, such as normal breathing.

- An AED becomes available and is ready to use.

- Another trained responder or EMS personnel arrive and take over.

- You are too exhausted to continue.

- The scene becomes unsafe.

If at any time the adult, child or infant begins to breathe normally or show another sign of life, stop CPR, place the person in the recovery position (see Chapter 5) and closely monitor breathing and any changes in the person's condition until EMS personnel take over.

The Heart's Electrical System

The heart's electrical system controls its pumping action. In normal conditions, specialized cells of the heart initiate and transmit electrical impulses. These cells make up the conduction system. Electrical impulses travel through the upper chambers of the heart, called the atria, to the lower chambers of the heart, called the ventricles (Figure 6-8).

The normal point of origin of the electrical impulse is the sinoatrial (SA) node above the atria. This impulse travels to a point midway between the atria and ventricles called the atrioventricular (AV) node. The pathway divides after the AV node into two branches, the right and left ventricles. These right and left branches become a network of fibers, called Purkinje fibers, which spread electrical impulses across the heart. Under normal conditions, this impulse reaches the muscular walls of the ventricles and causes the ventricles to contract.

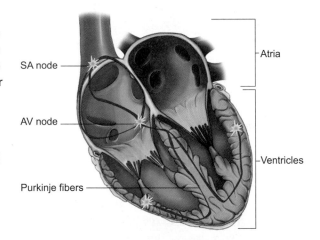

Figure 6-8. The heart's electrical system.

This contraction forces blood out of the heart to circulate through the body. The contraction of the left ventricle results in a pulse. The pauses between the pulse beats are the periods between contractions. When the heart muscles relax, blood refills the chambers.

Electrical activity of the heart can be evaluated with a cardiac monitor or electrocardiograph. Electrodes attached to an electrocardiograph pick up electrical impulses and transmit them to a monitor. This graphic record is referred to as an electrocardiogram (EKG). Heart rhythms appear on an EKG as a series of peaks and valleys.

When the Heart Fails

Any damage to the heart from disease or injury can disrupt the heart's electrical system. This disruption can result in an abnormal heart rhythm that can stop circulation. The two most common abnormal rhythms leading to cardiac arrest are ventricular fibrillation (V-fib) and ventricular tachycardia (V-tach).

V-fib is a state of totally disorganized electrical activity in the heart. It results in fibrillation, or quivering, of the ventricles. In V-fib, the electrical impulses fire at random, creating chaos and preventing the heart from pumping and circulating blood. A person with V-fib will suddenly collapse and stop breathing normally (occasional gasping breaths, or agonal breathing, may be observed for a period of time, but these gasps are not normal breathing).

V-tach refers to a very rapid contraction of the ventricles. Although there is electrical activity resulting in a regular rhythm, the rate is often so fast that the heart is unable to pump blood properly. As with V-fib, the person with V-tach may collapse, become unresponsive and stop breathing normally.

Defibrillation

In many cases, V-fib and V-tach rhythms can be corrected by early defibrillation. Delivering an electrical shock with an AED disrupts the electrical activity of V-fib and V-tach long enough to allow the heart to spontaneously develop an effective rhythm on its own. If V-fib or V-tach is not interrupted, all electrical activity will eventually cease, a condition called **asystole.** Asystole cannot be corrected by defibrillation. Remember that you cannot tell what rhythm, if any, the heart has by checking for signs of life. CPR, started immediately and continued until defibrillation, helps maintain a low level of circulation in the body until the abnormal rhythm can be corrected by defibrillation.

The Amazing Heart

Too often, we take our hearts for granted. The heart beats about 70 times each minute or more than 100,000 times a day. During an average lifetime, the heart will beat nearly 3 billion times. The heart circulates about a gallon of blood per minute or about 40 million gallons in an average lifetime. The heart circulates blood through about 60,000 miles of blood vessels.

What if... *I accidentally deliver an unnecessary shock while using an AED?*

An AED is designed to allow the responder to deliver a shock only when the AED has detected the presence of a life-threatening arrhythmia (e.g., V-fib or V-tach). If the device does not detect a shockable rhythm, it will instruct you to perform CPR.

Using an AED

Different types of AEDs are available, but all are similar to operate and use visual displays, voice prompts or both to guide the responder. If your place of employment has an AED on site, know where it is located, how to operate it and how to maintain it (Box 6-3). Also take note of the location of AEDs in public places that you frequent, such as shopping centers, airports, recreation centers and sports arenas.

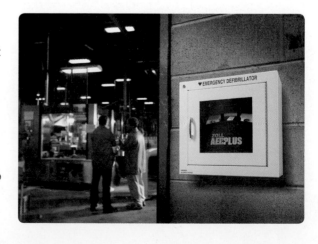

When a person is in cardiac arrest, use an AED as soon as possible. Skill Sheet 6-4 describes how to use an AED step by step. Environmental and person-specific considerations for safe and effective AED use are given in Box 6-4.

Box 6-3. **AED Maintenance**

AEDs require minimal maintenance, but it is important to check them regularly according to the manufacturer's instructions or your employer's policy to ensure that they are in good working order and ready for use whenever they are needed.

- Familiarize yourself with the owner's manual and follow the manufacturer's instructions for maintaining the equipment.

- Familiarize yourself with the method the AED uses to indicate the status of the device. Many AEDs have a status indicator that displays a symbol or illuminates to indicate that the AED is in proper working order and ready to respond. The status indicator may also display symbols indicating that routine maintenance (e.g., a battery change) is needed or that a problem with the device has been detected. Some AEDs have a warning indicator that will illuminate or beep if the AED is not in proper working order and ready to respond.

- Check to make sure the battery is properly installed and within its expiration date.

- Make sure AED pads are adequately stocked, stored in a sealed package and within their expiration date.

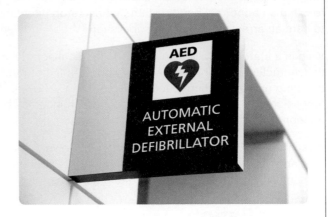

- After using the AED, make sure that all supplies are restocked and that the device is in proper working order.

- If at any time the AED fails to work properly or warning indicators illuminate, take the AED out of service and contact the manufacturer or the appropriate person at your place of employment, according to your employer's policy. You may need to return the AED to the manufacturer for service. If the AED stops working during an emergency, continue giving CPR until EMS personnel take over.

Box 6-4. **Considerations for Safe and Effective AED Use**

Environmental Considerations

- **Flammable or combustible materials.** Do not use an AED around flammable or combustible materials, such as gasoline or free-flowing oxygen.

- **Metal surfaces.** It is safe to use an AED when the person is lying on a metal surface, as long as appropriate precautions are taken. Do not allow the AED pads to contact the metal surface, and ensure that no one is touching the person when the shock is delivered.

- **Water.** If the person is in water, remove them from the water before using the AED. Once you have removed the person from the water, be sure there are no puddles of water around you, the person or the AED.

- **Inclement weather.** It is safe to use AEDs in all weather conditions, including rain and snow. Provide a dry environment if possible (for example, by sheltering the person with umbrellas), but do not delay defibrillation to do so. Remove wet clothing and wipe the person's chest dry before placing the AED pads. Avoid getting the AED or AED pads wet.

(Continued)

Box 6-4. continued

Person-Specific Considerations

- **Pregnancy.** It is safe to use an AED on a woman who is pregnant.

- **Pacemakers and implantable cardioverter-defibrillators (ICDs).** A person who has a known arrhythmia (irregular heartbeat) may have a pacemaker or an ICD. These are small devices that are surgically implanted under the skin to automatically prevent or correct an irregular heartbeat. You may be able to see or feel the outline of the pacemaker or ICD in the area below the person's collarbone, or the person may wear a medical identification tag indicating that they have a pacemaker or ICD. If the implanted device is visible or you know that the person has a pacemaker or ICD, adjust pad placement as necessary to avoid placing the AED pads directly over the device because doing so may interfere with the delivery of the shock. However, if you are not sure whether the person has an implanted device, place the pads as you normally would.

- **Transdermal medication patches.** Some types of medications, including nitroglycerin (used to relieve chest pain caused by cardiovascular disease) and smoking-cessation medications, are delivered through patches applied to the skin. Remove any medication patches that you see before applying AED pads and using an AED. Wear disposable latex-free gloves to prevent absorption of the drug through your own skin.

- **Chest hair.** Time is critical in a cardiac arrest situation, and chest hair rarely interferes with pad adhesion, so in most cases you should proceed as you normally would—attach the AED pads, pressing firmly to attach them. However, if the person has a great deal of thick chest hair and it seems like the chest hair could interfere with pad-to-skin contact, quickly shave the areas where the pads will be placed and then attach the pads.

- **Jewelry and body piercings.** You do not need to remove the person's jewelry or body piercings before using an AED, but you should avoid placing the AED pads directly over any metallic jewelry or piercings. Adjust pad placement if necessary.

Using an AED on an Adult

To use an AED, first turn the device on. Remove or cut away clothing and undergarments to expose the person's chest. If the person's chest is wet, dry it using a towel or gauze pad. Dry skin helps the AED pads to stick properly. Do not use an alcohol wipe to dry the skin because alcohol is flammable. Next, apply the AED pads. Peel the backing off the pads as directed, one at a time, to expose the adhesive. Place one pad on the upper right side of the person's chest and the other pad on the lower left side of the person's chest below the armpit, pressing firmly to adhere (Figure 6-9). Plug the connector cable into the AED (if necessary) and follow the device's directions. Most AEDs will begin to analyze the heart rhythm automatically, but some may require you to push an "analyze" button to start this process. No one should touch the person while the AED is analyzing the heart rhythm because this could result in a faulty reading.

Next, the AED will tell you to push the "shock" button if a shock is advised. Again, avoid touching the person, because anyone who is touching the person while the device is delivering a

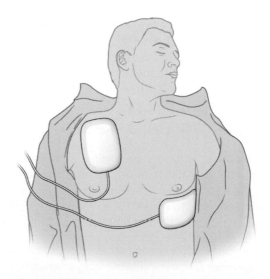

Figure 6-9. Place one AED pad on the upper right side of the chest and the other on the lower left side of the chest, below the armpit.

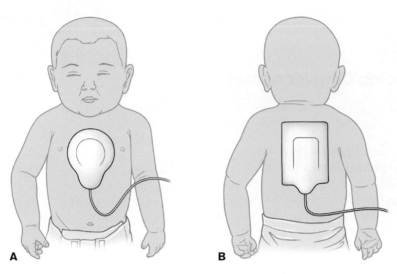

Figure 6-10, A–B. If the person is too small to place both AED pads on the front of the chest without the pads touching, place one on the middle of the chest, **A,** and the other on the back between the shoulder blades, **B.**

shock is at risk for receiving a shock as well. After a shock is delivered (or if the AED determines that no shock is necessary), immediately resume CPR, starting with compressions. The AED will continue to check the heart rhythm every 2 minutes. Listen for prompts from the AED and continue giving CPR and using the AED until you notice an obvious sign of life or EMS personnel arrive. If you notice an obvious sign of life, stop CPR but leave the AED turned on and the pads in place on the person's chest, and continue to follow the AED's prompts.

Using an AED on a Child or Infant

The procedure for using an AED on a child or infant is the same as the procedure for using an AED on an adult. Some AEDs come with pediatric AED pads that are smaller and designed specifically to analyze a child's heart rhythm and deliver a lower level of energy. These pads should be used on children up to 8 years of age or weighing less than 55 pounds. Other AEDs have a key or switch that configures the AED for use on a child up to 8 years of age or weighing less than 55 pounds. If pediatric AED pads are not available or the AED does not have a pediatric setting, it is safe to use adult AED pads and adult levels of energy on a child or infant. (Note that the opposite is not true—you should not use pediatric AED pads or the pediatric setting on an adult because the shock delivered will not be sufficient if the person is older than 8 years of age or weighs more than 55 pounds.)

Just as when you are using an AED on an adult, apply the AED pads to the child's bare, dry chest, placing one pad on the upper right chest and the other pad on the lower left side of the chest below the armpit. If you cannot position the pads this way without them touching (as in the case of an infant or a small child), position one pad in the middle of the chest and the other pad on the back between the shoulder blades (Figure 6-10, A–B). Then follow the standard procedure for using an AED.

Working as a Team

Remember, when you are giving CPR, you want to give high-quality compressions at the appropriate depth and rate. You also want to minimize interruptions to chest compressions. If you are the only trained responder at the scene, you will begin to tire as you give CPR, and the quality of your compressions will diminish. You will also need to stop CPR to ready the AED for use when it arrives, which means that during that time, there is no oxygenated blood moving through the person's body.

Working as a team can lead to a better chance of survival for the person in cardiac arrest, by reducing responder fatigue and minimizing interruptions to chest compressions. Trained responders can share the responsibility for giving compressions, switching off every 2 minutes, which reduces fatigue and leads to better-quality compressions. Having two or more trained responders at the scene also minimizes interruptions to chest compressions when the AED arrives.

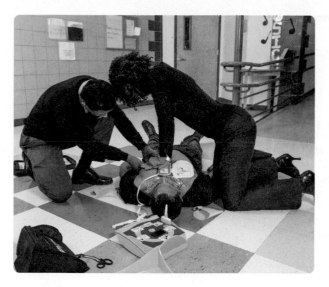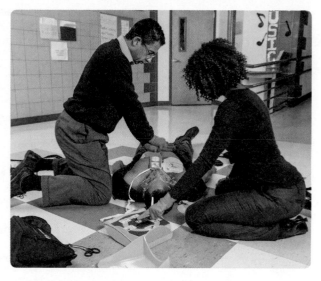

Figure 6-11. Working as a team can lead to a better chance of survival for the person in cardiac arrest.

When two or more responders trained in CPR and using an AED are at the scene, all should identify themselves as being trained. The first responder should begin CPR while the second responder calls 9-1-1 or the designated emergency number, obtains the AED and readies the AED for use by turning the device on, applying the pads to the person's chest and plugging in the connector cable, if necessary (Figure 6-11). The first responder should not pause CPR until the device is ready to analyze the person's heart rhythm and the second responder tells everyone to stand clear. While the AED is analyzing, the responders should switch roles so that the second responder can take over giving chest compressions. The responder who is taking over compressions should hover with their hands positioned just above the person's chest so that they can immediately start compressions as soon as the AED prompts that a shock was delivered or that no shock was advised. The responders then switch roles every time the AED analyzes the person's heart rhythm, which occurs every 2 minutes.

Summary

Cardiac emergencies present a major health threat to our communities. Heart attack and cardiac arrest are the two common cardiac emergencies. Learning to recognize the signs and symptoms of a heart attack and responding immediately can reduce the risk of complications and help prevent cardiac arrest. If a person experiences cardiac arrest, the greatest chance of survival occurs when the Cardiac Chain of Survival happens as rapidly as possible. By learning to recognize the signs and symptoms of cardiac emergencies and how to give care, you can make a difference.

READY TO RESPOND? >

Think back to Mr. Getz in the opening scenario, and use what you have learned to respond to these questions:

1. Could atherosclerosis have led to Mr. Getz's collapse?

2. If Mr. Getz had experienced chest pain, how might stopping and resting have prevented his collapse?

3. Why is it important to know whether Mr. Getz may be suffering cardiac arrest?

4. If Mr. Getz is in cardiac arrest, why will CPR alone not sustain his life?

Study Questions

1. **Match each term with the correct definition.**

   a. Cardiac arrest   c. Cholesterol   e. Heart attack

   b. CPR   d. Coronary arteries   f. Angina pectoris

   ____ A fatty substance that contributes to the risk for heart disease

   ____ Temporary chest pain caused by a lack of oxygen to the heart

   ____ Blood vessels that supply the heart with oxygen-rich blood

   ____ A combination of chest compressions and rescue breaths

   ____ Condition that results when the heart stops beating or beats too irregularly or weakly to circulate blood

   ____ A sudden illness involving the death of heart muscle tissue caused when it does not receive oxygen-rich blood

2. **Identify the signs and symptoms of cardiac arrest.**

3. **List the situations in which a trained lay responder may stop CPR.**

4. **Describe the conditions that most often cause cardiac arrest in children and infants.**

In questions 5 through 12, circle the letter of the correct answer.

5. **Which is the most common sign or symptom of a heart attack?**

   a. Profuse sweating   b. Persistent chest pain, discomfort or pressure   c. Pale skin   d. Trouble breathing

6. **Which of the following best describes the chest pain associated with heart attack?**

   a. An uncomfortable pressure   b. Persistent pain that may spread to the shoulder, arm, neck or jaw   c. Throbbing pain in the legs   d. a and b

(Continued)

Study Questions continued

7. What may happen as a result of a heart attack?

a. The heart functions inadequately.

b. The heart may stop.

c. Some heart muscle tissue dies from lack of oxygen.

d. All of the above

8. Which should you do first to care effectively for a person having a heart attack?

a. Position the person for CPR.

b. Begin giving rescue breaths.

c. Call 9-1-1 or the designated emergency number.

d. Call the person's physician.

9. How can you know whether a person's heart is beating?

a. The person is breathing.

b. The person shows another sign of life.

c. The person is responsive.

d. Any or all of the above

10. When is CPR needed for an adult?

a. When the person is responsive

b. For every person having a heart attack

c. When the person is unresponsive and not breathing normally

d. When the person who is having a heart attack becomes unresponsive but is breathing normally

11. Which is the purpose of CPR?

a. To keep a person's airway open

b. To identify any immediate threats to life

c. To supply the vital organs with blood containing oxygen

d. To reverse the effects of a heart attack

12. CPR artificially takes over the functions of which two body systems?

a. Nervous and respiratory systems

b. Respiratory and circulatory systems

c. Circulatory and nervous systems

d. Circulatory and musculoskeletal systems

Use the following scenario to answer questions 13 and 14.

It is Saturday afternoon. You and your mother are at home watching a tennis match on television. At the commercial break, your mother mumbles something about indigestion and heads to the medicine cabinet to get an antacid. Twenty minutes later, you notice that your mom does not respond to a great play made by her favorite player. You ask what is wrong, and she complains that the antacid has not worked. She states that her chest and shoulder hurt. She is sweating heavily. You notice that she is breathing fast and she looks ill.

(Continued)

Study Questions continued

13. List the signs and symptoms of a heart attack that you find in this scenario.

14. Your mother suddenly becomes unresponsive. Number in order the following actions you would now take.

____ Ensure she is on a firm, flat surface.

____ Call 9-1-1 or the designated emergency number.

____ Check for responsiveness and breathing. *(She does not respond and is not breathing normally.)*

____ Correctly position your hands.

____ Give cycles of 30 compressions and 2 rescue breaths.

In questions 15 through 17, circle the letter of the correct answer.

15. If during an analysis an AED prompts, "no shock advised," you should—

a. Check pad placement on the person's chest.

b. Reset the AED by turning it off for 10 seconds.

c. Immediately resume CPR until the AED reanalyzes or you notice an obvious sign of life.

d. Unplug the connector from the machine.

16. While the AED analyzes the heart rhythm, you should—

a. Ensure that no one, including you, is touching the person.

b. Make sure that the person's airway is maintained.

c. Finish a cycle of CPR.

d. None of the above

17. If the AED pads risk touching each other, such as with a small child or infant, you should—

a. Place the pads as usual. It does not matter if they touch each other.

b. Place one pad on the stomach and one pad on the chest.

c. Reverse the position of the pads on the chest.

d. Place one pad in the middle of the chest, and the other on the back between the shoulder blades.

Answers are listed in the Appendix.

Giving CPR to an Adult

1. Verify that the person is unresponsive and not breathing.

   ■ Shout to get the person's attention, using the person's name if you know it. If the person does not respond, tap the person's shoulder and shout again while checking for normal breathing.

   ■ If the person does not respond and is not breathing or only gasping, continue to step 2.

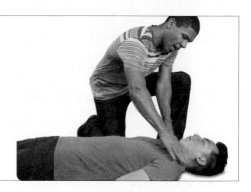

2. Place the person on their back on a firm, flat surface. Kneel beside the person.

3. Give **30 chest compressions.**

   ■ Place the heel of one hand in the center of the person's chest, with your other hand on top. Position your body so that your shoulders are directly over your hands.

   ■ Keeping your arms straight, push down at least 2 inches, and then let the chest return to its normal position.

   ■ Push hard and push fast! Give compressions at a rate of between 100 and 120 compressions per minute.

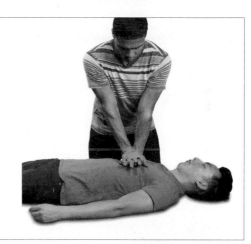

4. Give **2 rescue breaths.**

   ■ Place the breathing barrier over the person's nose and mouth.

   ■ Open the airway. (Put one hand on the forehead and two fingers on the bony part of the chin and tilt the head back to a past-neutral position.)

   ■ Pinch the nose shut and make a complete seal over the person's mouth with your mouth.

   ■ Take a normal breath and blow into the person's mouth for about 1 second, looking to see that the chest rises.

   ■ Take another breath, make a seal, then give the second rescue breath.

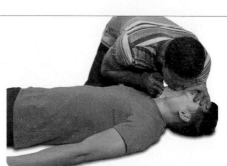

Note: *If the first rescue breath does not cause the chest to rise, retilt the head and ensure a proper seal before giving the second rescue breath. If the second breath does not make the chest rise, an object may be blocking the airway. After the next set of chest compressions and before attempting rescue breaths, open the mouth, look for an object and, if seen, remove it using a finger sweep. Continue to check the person's mouth for an object after each set of compressions until the rescue breaths go in.*

(Continued)

Giving CPR to an Adult *Continued*

5. Continue giving sets of **30** chest compressions and **2** rescue breaths until:

   - You notice an obvious sign of life.

   - An AED is ready to use, and no other trained responders are available to assist you with the AED.

   - You have performed approximately 2 minutes of CPR (5 sets of 30:2), and another trained responder is available to take over compressions.

   - EMS personnel take over.

   - You are alone and too tired to continue.

   - The scene becomes unsafe.

Skill Sheet 6-2

Giving CPR to a Child

1. Verify that the child is unresponsive and not breathing.

   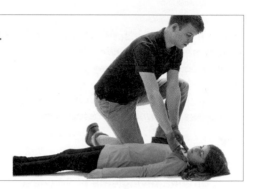

   ■ Shout to get the child's attention, using the child's name if you know it. If the child does not respond, tap the child's shoulder and shout again while checking for normal breathing.

   ■ If the child does not respond and is not breathing or only gasping, continue to step 2.

2. Place the child on their back on a firm, flat surface. Kneel beside the child.

3. Give **30 chest compressions.**

   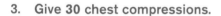

   ■ Place the heel of one hand in the center of the child's chest, with your other hand on top. Position your body so that your shoulders are directly over your hands. (Alternatively, in a small child, you can use a one-handed CPR technique: place the heel of one hand in the center of the child's chest.)

   ■ Keeping your arms straight, push down about 2 inches, and then let the chest return to its normal position.

   ■ Push hard and push fast! Give compressions at a rate of between 100 and 120 compressions per minute.

4. Give **2 rescue breaths.**

   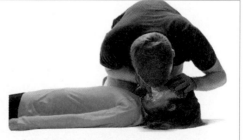

   ■ Place the breathing barrier over the child's nose and mouth.

   ■ Open the airway. (Put one hand on the forehead and two fingers on the bony part of the chin and tilt the head back to a slightly past-neutral position.)

   ■ Pinch the nose shut and make a complete seal over the child's mouth with your mouth.

   ■ Take a normal breath and blow into the child's mouth for about 1 second, looking to see that the chest rises.

   ■ Take another breath, make a seal, then give the second rescue breath.

   (Continued)

Giving CPR to a Child *Continued*

Note: *If the first rescue breath does not cause the chest to rise, retilt the head and ensure a proper seal before giving the second rescue breath. If the second breath does not make the chest rise, an object may be blocking the airway. After the next set of chest compressions and before attempting rescue breaths, open the mouth, look for an object and, if seen, remove it using a finger sweep. Continue to check the child's mouth for an object after each set of compressions until the rescue breaths go in.*

5. Continue giving sets of **30** chest compressions and **2** rescue breaths until:

   ■ You notice an obvious sign of life.

   ■ An AED is ready to use, and no other trained responders are available to assist you with the AED.

   ■ You have performed approximately 2 minutes of CPR (5 sets of 30:2), and another trained responder is available to take over compressions.

   ■ You have performed approximately 2 minutes of CPR (5 sets of 30:2), you are alone and caring for a child, and you need to call 9-1-1 or the designated emergency number.

   ■ EMS personnel take over.

   ■ You are alone and too tired to continue.

   ■ The scene becomes unsafe.

Giving CPR to an Infant

1. Verify that the infant is unresponsive and not breathing.

   - Shout to get the infant's attention, using the infant's name if you know it. If the infant does not respond, tap the bottom of the infant's foot and shout again while checking for normal breathing.

   - If the infant does not respond and is not breathing or only gasping, continue to step 2.

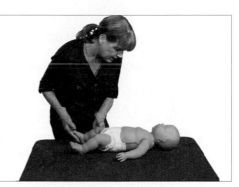

2. Place the infant on their back on a firm, flat surface. Stand or kneel next to the infant.

3. Give 30 chest compressions.

   - Place one hand on the infant's forehead.

   - Place the pad of two fingers on the center of the infant's chest, just below the nipple line.

   - Compress the chest about 1½ inches, and then let the chest return to its normal position.

   - Push hard and push fast! Give compressions at a rate of between 100 and 120 compressions per minute.

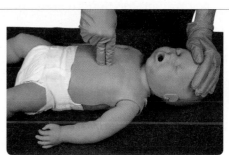

4. Give 2 rescue breaths.

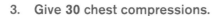

   - Place the breathing barrier over the infant's nose and mouth.

   - Open the airway. (Put one hand on the forehead and two fingers on the bony part of the chin and tilt the head back to a neutral position.)

   - Make a complete seal over the infant's nose and mouth with your mouth.

   - Take a normal breath and blow into the infant's nose and mouth for about 1 second, looking to see that the chest rises.

   - Take another breath, make a seal, then give the second rescue breath.

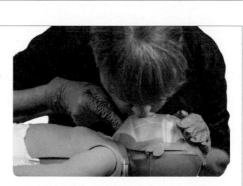

Note: *If the first rescue breath does not cause the chest to rise, retilt the head and ensure a proper seal before giving the second rescue breath. If the second breath does not make the chest rise, an object may be blocking the airway. After the next set of chest compressions and before attempting rescue breaths, open the mouth, look for an object and, if seen, remove it using a finger sweep. Continue to check the infant's mouth for an object after each set of compressions until the rescue breaths go in.*

(Continued)

Giving CPR to an Infant *Continued*

5. Continue giving sets of **30** chest compressions and **2** rescue breaths until:

   ■ You notice an obvious sign of life.

   ■ An AED is ready to use and no other trained responders are available to assist you with the AED.

   ■ You have performed approximately 2 minutes of CPR (5 sets of 30:2) and another trained responder is available to take over compressions.

   ■ You have performed approximately 2 minutes of CPR (5 sets of 30:2), you are alone and caring for an infant, and you need to call 9-1-1 or the designated emergency number.

   ■ EMS personnel take over.

   ■ You are too tired to continue.

   ■ The scene becomes unsafe.

Using an AED

Note: *Do not use pediatric AED pads on an adult or on a child older than 8 years of age or weighing more than 55 pounds. However, adult AED pads can be used on a child younger than 8 years of age or weighing less than 55 pounds if pediatric AED pads are not available.*

---

1. Turn on the AED and follow the voice prompts.

---

2. Remove all clothing covering the chest and, if necessary, wipe the chest dry.

---

3. Place the pads.

   ■ Place one pad on the upper right side of the chest and the other on the lower left side of the chest below the armpit.

   ■ If the pads may touch (e.g., on an infant or small child), place one pad in the middle of the chest and the other pad on the back between the shoulder blades.

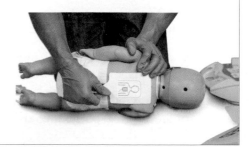

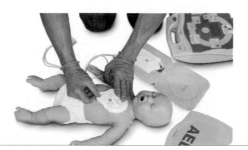

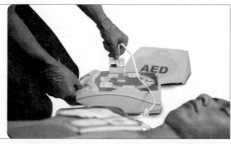

---

4. Plug the connector cable into the AED, if necessary.

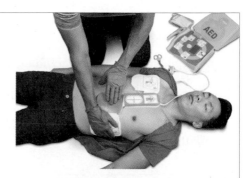

(Continued)

Using an AED *Continued*

5. Prepare to let the AED analyze the heart's rhythm.

   ■ Make sure no one, including you, is touching the person. Say, "EVERYONE CLEAR!" in a loud, commanding voice.

   ■ If the AED tells you to, push the "analyze" button to start this process.

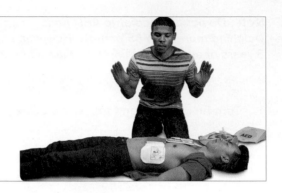

6. Deliver a shock, if the AED determines one is needed.

   ■ Make sure no one, including you, is touching the person. Say, "EVERYONE CLEAR!" in a loud, commanding voice.

   ■ Push the "shock" button to deliver the shock.

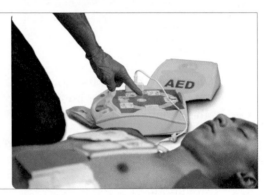

7. After the AED delivers the shock, or if no shock is advised:

   ■ Immediately begin CPR, starting with compressions. Continue giving CPR (about 2 minutes, or 5 sets of 30:2) until prompted by the AED.

   ■ Continue giving CPR and following the AED's prompts until you see an obvious sign of life or EMS personnel arrive.

7
BREATHING EMERGENCIES

You and your friends are at a local coffee shop, having a late-morning snack and catching up. Someone relates a funny story about what happened in one of their classes and you are all laughing hard. Suddenly, one of your friends, James, jumps up in a panic. Your friend seems to be choking on a piece of his bagel.

Learn and Respond ▶

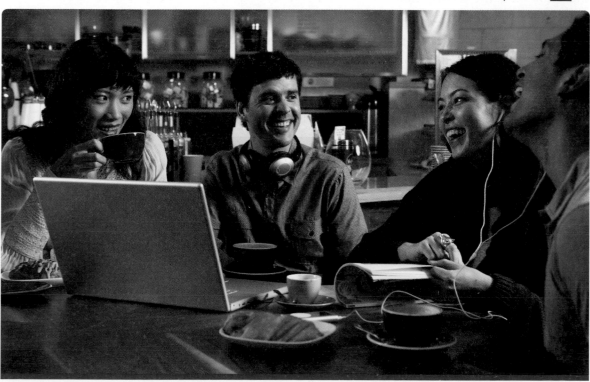

OBJECTIVES

After reading this chapter, you should be able to:

- Identify the causes of breathing emergencies.
- Identify conditions that cause respiratory distress.
- Identify signs and symptoms of respiratory distress.
- Describe the care for a person in respiratory distress.
- Identify signs and symptoms of asthma.
- Describe the care for a person having an asthma attack.
- Identify common causes of choking for adults, children and infants.
- Describe the care for a choking adult, child and infant who is awake.
- Describe the care for a choking adult, child and infant who becomes unresponsive.

After reading this chapter and completing the class activities, you should be able to:

- Demonstrate how to assist a person with an asthma inhaler.
- Demonstrate how to give care for a choking adult, child and infant who is awake.

KEY TERMS

Airway obstruction: Complete or partial blockage of the airway, which prevents air from reaching a person's lungs; a common cause of respiratory emergencies.

Anatomical airway obstruction: Complete or partial blockage of the airway by the tongue or swollen tissues of the mouth, throat or other airway structures.

Cyanotic: Bluish discoloration of the skin around the mouth or the fingertips resulting from a lack of oxygen in the blood.

Hyperventilation: Breathing that is faster than normal.

Mechanical airway obstruction: Complete or partial blockage of the airway by a foreign object such as a piece of food or a small toy, or by fluids such as vomit or blood.

Respiratory arrest: A condition in which breathing has stopped but the heart is still beating.

Respiratory distress: A condition in which a person is having trouble breathing or requires extra effort to breathe.

Introduction

A **breathing emergency** is any respiratory problem that can threaten a person's life. Breathing emergencies happen when air cannot travel freely and easily into the lungs. *Respiratory distress* and *respiratory arrest* are examples of breathing emergencies, and can have a variety of causes including asthma and other illnesses.

Airway obstruction is one of the most common causes of breathing emergencies. There are two types of airway obstruction. An ***anatomical airway obstruction*** occurs when the airway is blocked by the tongue or swollen tissues of the mouth, throat or other airway structures. This type of obstruction may result from injury to the neck or a medical emergency, such as anaphylaxis. A ***mechanical airway obstruction*** occurs when the airway is partially or completely blocked by a foreign object such as a piece of food or a small toy, by fluids such as vomit or blood, or by mucus. A person with a complete mechanical airway obstruction is choking.

It is important to recognize breathing emergencies in children and infants and act before the heart stops beating. Frequently, an adult's heart stops working (known as *cardiac arrest*) because of heart disease. However, children and infants usually have healthy hearts. When the heart stops in a child or infant, it usually is the result of a breathing emergency.

No matter what the age of the person, trouble breathing can be the first sign of a more serious emergency. Recognizing the signs and symptoms of breathing problems and giving care often are the keys to preventing these problems from becoming more serious emergencies.

If the injured or ill person is awake, they may be able to indicate what is wrong by speaking or gesturing to you and may be able to answer questions. However, if you are unable to communicate with the person, it can be difficult to determine what is wrong. Therefore, it is important to recognize the signs and symptoms of breathing emergencies, know when to call 9-1-1 or the designated emergency number, and know what to do until help arrives.

In any breathing emergency, seconds count, so you must act immediately. This chapter discusses how to recognize and care for breathing emergencies.

The Breathing Process

The human body needs a constant supply of oxygen to survive. When you breathe through your mouth and nose, air travels down your throat, through your windpipe and into your lungs. This pathway from the mouth and nose to the lungs is called the airway.

As you might imagine, the airway, mouth and nose are smaller in children and infants than they are in adults (Figure 7-1, A–B). As a result, they can be blocked more easily by small objects, blood, fluids or swelling.

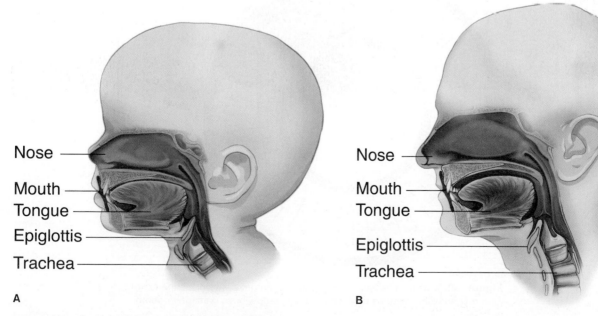

Nose
Mouth
Tongue
Epiglottis
Trachea

A

Nose
Mouth
Tongue
Epiglottis
Trachea

B

Figure 7-1, A–B. A, A child's airway. **B,** An adult's airway.

The goal in a breathing emergency is for air to reach the lungs. For any person, regardless of age, it is important to keep the airway open when giving care. Once air reaches the lungs, oxygen in the air is transferred to the blood. The heart then pumps the oxygenated blood throughout the body. The blood flows through the blood vessels, delivering oxygen to the brain, heart and all other parts of the body.

In some breathing emergencies the oxygen supply to the body is greatly reduced, whereas in others the oxygen supply is cut off entirely. As a result, the heart soon stops beating and blood no longer moves throughout the body. Without oxygen, brain cells can begin to die within 4 to 6 minutes (Figure 7-2). Unless the brain receives oxygen, permanent brain damage or death will result.

Respiratory Distress and Respiratory Arrest

Respiratory distress, or difficulty breathing, is evidenced by signs and symptoms such as shortness of breath, gasping for breath, **hyperventilation** (breathing that is faster than normal), or breathing that is uncomfortable or painful. Respiratory distress can lead to respiratory arrest (absence of breathing).

Normal breathing is regular, quiet and effortless. A person does not appear to be working hard or struggling when breathing normally. This means that the person is not making noise when breathing, breaths are not fast, and breathing does not cause discomfort or pain. However, it should be noted that normal breathing rates in children and infants are faster than normal breathing rates in adults. Infants have periodic breathing, so changes in breathing patterns are normal for infants.

You usually can identify a breathing problem by watching and listening to the person's breathing and by asking the person how they feel.

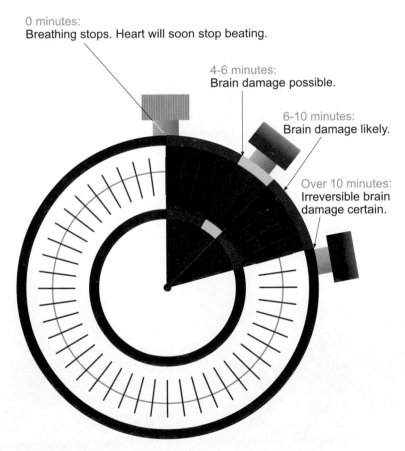

0 minutes:
Breathing stops. Heart will soon stop beating.

4-6 minutes:
Brain damage possible.

6-10 minutes:
Brain damage likely.

Over 10 minutes:
Irreversible brain damage certain.

Figure 7-2. Time is critical in life-threatening emergencies. Unless the brain gets oxygen within minutes of when breathing stops, brain damage or death will occur.

Causes of Respiratory Distress and Respiratory Arrest

A number of different conditions can cause respiratory distress, including acute flare-ups of chronic respiratory conditions such as asthma or chronic obstructive pulmonary disease (COPD); lung and respiratory tract infections (such as pneumonia or bronchitis); severe allergic reactions (anaphylaxis); heart conditions (such as a heart attack or heart failure); trauma; poisoning; drug overdose; electrocution and mental health conditions (such as panic disorder).

Infections of the respiratory system are more common in children and infants than in adults. These can range from minor infections, such as the common cold, to life-threatening infections that block the airway. Respiratory distress in children is often caused by respiratory infections, such as croup and epiglottitis.

Some of the specific causes of respiratory distress and respiratory arrest are covered in more detail in the sections that follow.

Chronic Obstructive Pulmonary Disease

Chronic obstructive pulmonary disease (COPD) is a long-term lung disease encompassing both chronic bronchitis and emphysema. COPD causes a person to have trouble breathing because of damage to the lungs. In a person with COPD, the airways become partly blocked and the air sacs in the lungs lose their ability to fill with air. This makes it hard to breathe in and out. There is no cure for COPD, and it worsens over time.

The most common cause of COPD is cigarette smoking, but breathing in other types of lung irritants, pollution, dust or chemicals over a long period also can cause COPD. It usually is diagnosed when a person is middle-aged or older. It is the third-ranking cause of death in the United States and a major cause of illness.

Common signs and symptoms of COPD include:

- Coughing up a large volume of mucus.

- Tendency to tire easily.

- Loss of appetite.

- Bent posture with shoulders raised and lips pursed to make breathing easier.

- A fast heartbeat.

- Round, barrel-shaped chest.

- Confusion (caused by lack of oxygen to the brain).

Emphysema

A type of COPD, **emphysema** is a disease that involves damage to the air sacs in the lungs. It is a chronic (long-lasting or frequently recurring) disease that worsens over time. The most common symptom of emphysema is shortness of breath. Exhaling is extremely difficult. In advanced cases, the affected person may feel restless, confused and weak, and may even go into respiratory or cardiac arrest.

Bronchitis

Bronchitis is an inflammation of the main air passages to the lungs. It can be acute (short lasting) or chronic. Chronic bronchitis is a type of COPD. To be diagnosed with chronic bronchitis, a person must have a cough with mucus on most days of the month for at least 3 months.

Acute bronchitis is *not* a type of COPD; it develops after a person has had a viral respiratory infection. Acute bronchitis first affects the nose, sinuses and throat, and then spreads to the lungs. Those most at risk for acute bronchitis include children, infants, older adults, people with heart or lung disease and smokers.

Signs and symptoms of both types of bronchitis include:

- Chest discomfort.
- Cough that produces mucus.
- Fatigue.

- Fever (usually low).
- Shortness of breath that worsens with activity.
- Wheezing.

Additional signs of chronic bronchitis include:

- Ankle, feet and leg swelling.
- Blue lips.

- Frequent respiratory infections, such as colds or the flu.

Hyperventilation

Hyperventilation occurs when a person's breathing is faster than normal. When this happens, the body does not take in enough oxygen to meet its demands. People who are hyperventilating feel as if they cannot get enough air. Often they are afraid and anxious or seem confused. They may say that they feel dizzy or that their fingers and toes feel numb and tingly.

Hyperventilation often results from fear or anxiety and usually occurs in people who are tense and nervous. However, it also can be caused by head injuries, severe bleeding or illnesses, such as high fever, heart failure, lung disease and diabetic emergencies. Asthma and exercise also can trigger hyperventilation.

Allergic Reactions

An allergic reaction is the response of the immune system to a foreign substance that enters the body. Common **allergens** include bee or insect venom, antibiotics, pollen, latex, animal dander, sulfa and some foods such as nuts, peanuts, shellfish, strawberries and coconut oils.

Allergic reactions can cause breathing problems. At first the reaction may appear to be just a rash and a feeling of tightness in the chest and throat, but this condition can become life threatening. The person's face, neck and tongue may swell, closing the airway.

A severe allergic reaction can cause a condition called **anaphylaxis,** also known as anaphylactic shock. During anaphylaxis, air passages swell and restrict a person's breathing. Anaphylaxis can be brought on when a person with an allergy comes in contact with allergens via insect stings, food, certain medications or other substances. Signs and symptoms of anaphylaxis include a rash, tightness in the chest and throat, and swelling of the face, neck and tongue. The person also may feel dizzy or confused. Anaphylaxis is a life-threatening emergency. You will learn more about the signs and symptoms and care of anaphylaxis in Chapter 16.

Some people know that they are allergic to certain substances or to insect stings. They may have learned to avoid these things and may carry medication, such as an epinephrine auto-injector, to reverse the allergic reaction. People who have severe allergic reactions may wear a medical identification tag, bracelet or necklace.

Croup

Croup is a common upper airway virus marked by a harsh, repetitive cough that most commonly affects children younger than 5 years of age. The airway constricts, limiting the passage of air, which causes the child to produce an unusual-sounding cough that can range from a high-pitched wheeze to a barking cough. The cough associated with croup mostly occurs during the evening and nighttime.

Most children with croup can be cared for at home using mist treatment or cool air. However, in some cases, a child with croup can progress quickly from respiratory distress to respiratory arrest.

Epiglottitis

Epiglottitis, a far less common infection than croup, causes severe swelling of the epiglottis. The epiglottis is a piece of cartilage at the back of the airway. When it swells, it can block the windpipe and lead to severe breathing problems and even death. Epiglottitis usually is caused by bacterial infection with the *Haemophilus influenzae* bacteria.

The signs and symptoms of epiglottitis may be similar to those of croup, but epiglottitis is a more serious illness and can result in death if the airway becomes blocked completely.

In the past, epiglottitis was a common illness in children between 2 and 6 years of age. However, the incidence of epiglottitis in children has decreased dramatically in the United States since the 1980s, when children began routinely receiving the *H. influenzae* type b (Hib) vaccine.

For children and adults, epiglottitis begins with a high fever and sore throat. A person with epiglottitis may need to sit up and lean forward, perhaps with the chin thrust out, in order to breathe. Other signs and symptoms include drooling, trouble swallowing, voice changes, chills, shaking and fever.

Seek medical care immediately for a person who may have epiglottitis. This condition is a true medical emergency.

Signs and Symptoms of Respiratory Distress

A person who is experiencing respiratory distress is, understandably, often very frightened. The person may feel like they cannot get enough air and may gasp for breath. Because the person is struggling to breathe, speaking in complete sentences may be difficult. You might hear wheezing, gurgling or high-pitched noises as the person tries to breathe. You may also notice that the person's breathing is unusually slow or fast, unusually deep or shallow, or irregular. The person's skin may feel moist or cool, and it may be pale, ashen (gray), bluish or flushed. Lack of oxygen can make the person feel dizzy or light-headed.

First Aid Care for Respiratory Distress

When a person is experiencing a breathing emergency, it is important to act at once. In some breathing emergencies, the oxygen supply to the body is greatly reduced, whereas in others the oxygen supply is cut off entirely. If breathing stops or is restricted long enough, the person will become unresponsive, the heart will stop beating and body systems will quickly fail. Recognizing that a person is having trouble breathing and giving appropriate first aid care can save the person's life.

You usually can identify a breathing problem by watching and listening to the person's breathing and by asking the person how they feel. If a person is having trouble breathing, do not wait to see if the person's condition improves. Call 9-1-1 or the designated emergency number and give appropriate first aid care until help arrives:

- If you know the cause of the respiratory distress (for example, an asthma attack or anaphylaxis) and the person carries medication used for the emergency treatment of the condition, offer to help the person take their medication.

- Encourage the person to sit down and lean forward. Many people find that this position helps to make breathing easier (Figure 7-3). Providing reassurance can reduce anxiety, which may also help to make breathing easier.

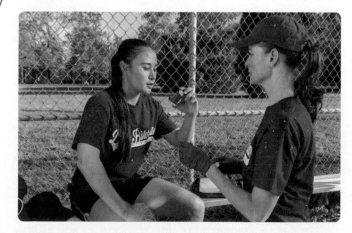

Figure 7-3. A person who is having trouble breathing may breathe more easily in a sitting position.

- If the person is responsive, gather additional information by interviewing the person and performing a head-to-toe check. Remember that a person having breathing problems may find it difficult to talk. Try phrasing your questions as "yes" or "no" questions so the person can nod or shake their head in response instead of making the effort to speak. You may also be able to ask bystanders what they know about the person's condition.

- Be prepared to give CPR and use an AED if the person becomes unresponsive.

Asthma

Many people have **asthma,** a chronic illness in which certain substances or conditions, called **triggers,** cause inflammation and narrowing of the airways, making breathing difficult. Common triggers include exercise, temperature extremes, allergies, air pollution, strong odors (such as perfume, cologne and scented cleaning products), respiratory infections, and stress or anxiety. The trigger causes inflammation and swelling, which causes the opening of the airways to become smaller and makes it harder for air to move in and out of the lungs. People who have asthma usually know what can trigger an attack and take measures to avoid these triggers.

A person who has been diagnosed with asthma may take two forms of medication. **Long-term control medications** are taken regularly, whether or not signs and symptoms of asthma are present. These medications help prevent asthma attacks by reducing inflammation and swelling and making the airways less sensitive to triggers. **Quick-relief (rescue) medications** are taken when the person is experiencing an acute asthma attack. These medications work quickly to relax the muscles that tighten around the airways, opening the airways right away so that the person can breathe more easily. Both long-term control medications and quick-relief (rescue) medications may be given through an inhaler, a nebulizer (Box 7-1) or orally.

What if... *A person is suffering from what appears to be an acute asthma attack and they do not have a prescribed bronchodilator inhaler, but I have mine? Should I let the person use it?*

No! Sharing prescribed medication is never recommended, nor is it advisable. When a bronchodilator inhaler is unavailable, make sure that someone has called 9-1-1 or the designated emergency number, or call yourself, then help the person rest in a comfortable position, calm and reassure the person, and continue to monitor the person for signs and symptoms of respiratory distress.

Signs and Symptoms of an Asthma Attack

Even when a person takes steps to manage their asthma by avoiding triggers and taking prescribed long-term control medications, they may still experience asthma attacks occasionally. Signs and symptoms of an asthma attack include:

- Wheezing or coughing.

- Rapid, shallow breathing (or trouble breathing).

- Sweating.

- Being unable to talk without stopping for a breath in between every few words.

- Feelings of tightness in the chest or being unable to get enough air into the lungs.

- Anxiety and fear.

First Aid Care for an Asthma Attack

An asthma attack can become life threatening because it affects the person's ability to breathe. If the person has an **asthma action plan** (a written plan that the person develops with their healthcare provider that details daily management of the condition as well as how to handle an asthma attack), help the person to follow that plan. Encourage the person to use their prescribed quick-relief (rescue) medication, assisting if

Box 7-1. **Asthma Inhalers and Nebulizers**

The most common way to take long-term control and quick-relief (rescue) medications is by inhaling them. Inhalation allows the medication to reach the airways faster and work quickly. There also are fewer side effects. Medications are inhaled using a metered dose inhaler (MDI), a dry powder inhaler (DPI) or a small-volume nebulizer.

Metered Dose Inhalers

An MDI delivers a measured dose of medication in mist form directly into the person's lungs. The person gently presses down the top of the inhaler. This causes a small amount of pressurized gas to push the medication out quickly. Sometimes a spacer (or chamber) is used to make it easier for the person to use the inhaler correctly. The medication goes into the spacer, and then the person inhales the medication through the mouthpiece on the spacer. For children, a spacer may be used with a face mask instead of a mouthpiece.

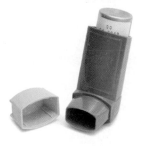

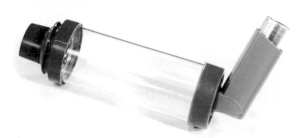

Dry Powder Inhalers

A DPI delivers a measured dose of medicine in a dry powder form directly into the person's lungs. Instead of pressing down on the top of the device to dispense the medication, the person breathes in quickly to activate the DPI and dispense the medication. Some people have difficulty using DPIs because they require the user to take in a quick, strong breath.

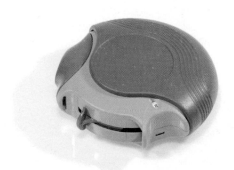

Small-Volume Nebulizers

Small-volume nebulizers convert liquid medication into a mist, which is delivered over several minutes. Nebulizers are especially helpful when the person is unable to take deep breaths, for children younger than 5 years of age and for older adults. They also are used for people who have trouble using inhalers and for those with severe asthma.

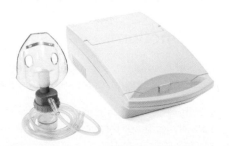

needed and if state or local regulations allow. (Skill Sheet 7-1 provides step-by-step instructions for helping a person to use an asthma inhaler.) If you have not already done so, call 9-1-1 or the designated emergency number if the person's breathing does not improve after taking the quick-relief (rescue) medication or if the person becomes unresponsive. Stay with the person and monitor their condition until the person is able to breathe normally or help arrives.

See also Smart Moves: Preventing Asthma Attacks for steps you can take to limit the effect of asthma triggers.

Remember: *The instructions for administering asthma medication found in this chapter should not be substituted for those given by a medical professional to an individual person. Nor should these instructions be substituted for directions given by a medical professional in consultation with a site where asthma medication will be administered. Consult a healthcare provider for specific advice on the use of asthma inhalers and nebulizers.*

SMART MOVES > **PREVENTING ASTHMA ATTACKS**

When it comes to asthma, prevention is key. Following these measures can help reduce a person's risk of an attack.

Limit Triggers in the Home

To reduce triggers in your home:

- Keep plants outside.

- Wash bedclothes and pajamas weekly in hot water.

- Use hypoallergenic covers on mattresses and pillows.

- Eliminate or reduce the number of carpets and rugs.

- Regularly steam clean all carpets, rugs and upholstery.

- Keep the home clean and free of dust and pests— wet dusting can be more effective than dry dusting.

- Do not allow, or be around, smoke.

- Regularly change the air filter in the central air conditioning or heating unit.

- Eliminate or minimize the number of stuffed toys.

- Use hypoallergenic health and beauty products.

- Bathe pets weekly.

- Keep pets outside the house.

Control Emotions

Certain strong emotions can trigger an asthma attack. When you feel a strong emotion, such as anger or fear, the following suggestions can reduce the chances that an asthma attack will be triggered:

- Take a long deep breath in through the nose, and slowly let it out through the mouth.

- Count to 10.

- Talk with a family member, trusted friend or healthcare provider.

- Do a relaxing activity.

(Continued)

Prevent Infections

Colds and other respiratory infections can make an asthma condition worse. One of the most common ways to catch colds is by rubbing the nose or eyes with hands contaminated with a cold virus. Contamination often occurs by touching surfaces (such as doorknobs) or objects that other people have touched. Some ways to reduce the chances of getting a cold or other respiratory infection include:

- Washing hands regularly, especially after using the restroom or shaking hands with other people and before eating.

- Cleaning environmental surfaces, such as telephones, keyboards and counters, with a virus-killing disinfectant. The viruses that cause colds can survive up to 3 hours on objects such as telephones, counters and stair railings. Disinfecting these objects regularly can help to prevent the spread of colds and viruses.

- Getting vaccinated for illnesses when a vaccine is available, such as for influenza and whooping cough (pertussis).

- Talking to your healthcare provider who might have other suggestions based on your medical history.

Reduce Environmental Triggers

Sudden changes in the weather, heavy mold or pollen content in the air, and pollution can trigger an asthma attack. To avoid attacks brought on by triggers in the environment:

- Wear the right clothing for the weather conditions.

- Stay indoors on days when there is a high risk of respiratory trouble.

- Take preventative medications, as prescribed by your healthcare provider.

- Stay away from places with high amounts of dirt, smoke and other irritants.

- Know how the weather affects your condition.

- Talk to your healthcare provider about other prevention strategies.

Exercise Carefully

Exercise-induced asthma happens during or shortly after exercise. Having this type of asthma does not mean one cannot or should not exercise or play sports. It is, however, important to know what to do to prevent an asthma attack. Things to keep in mind when you have exercise-induced asthma include the following:

- Take prescribed medications 30 to 60 minutes before exercising.

- Slowly warm up before exercising. Cool down gently after exercising.

- Make sure that you drink plenty of fluids during exercise.

- Seek and follow the advice of your healthcare provider.

- If participating in organized sports, notify the coach of your condition.

Choking

Choking is a common breathing emergency. It is especially common in young children, but a person of any age can choke. Choking occurs when the airway becomes either partially or completely blocked by a foreign object such as a piece of food or a small toy, by swelling in the mouth or throat, or by fluids such as vomit or blood. A person who is choking can quickly become unresponsive and die, so it is important to act quickly.

With a partially blocked airway, the person usually can breathe, but with some trouble. A person whose airway is completely blocked cannot cough, speak, cry or breathe at all.

Risk Factors for Choking

Certain behaviors can put a person at risk for choking, such as talking or laughing with their mouth full or eating too fast. Medical conditions (such as a neurological or muscular condition that affects the person's ability to chew, swallow or both) can increase risk for choking. So can dental problems or poorly fitting dentures that affect the person's ability to chew food properly.

Children younger than 5 years of age are at particularly high risk for choking (Box 7-2). Infants and toddlers explore by putting things in their mouths and can easily choke on them. Even some common foods can be

---

Box 7-2. **Choking Hazards**

In children younger than 4 years of age, the following foods, household objects and toys may be choking hazards:

Foods

- Nuts and seeds
- Hot dogs and sausages
- Chunks of meat or cheese
- Chunks of fruit (such as apples) and whole grapes
- Raw vegetables (such as carrots and celery)
- Popcorn
- Peanut butter

- Hard, gooey or sticky candy (such as peppermint candies, fruit strips, marshmallows, gummy bears and chewing gum)
- Large foods that break easily into small pieces (such as teething biscuits and cookies)

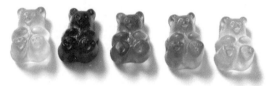

Household Objects and Toys

- Plastic bags, broken or uninflated balloons, and disposable gloves (the thin material can block the airway)
- Coins
- Buttons
- Small "button" batteries (found inside watches, car key fobs, singing greeting cards, hearing aids and other electronics)
- Magnets
- Marbles
- Beads
- Pebbles
- Pen or marker caps

- Safety pins and hairpins
- Jewelry
- Baby powder
- Vitamins
- Items from the trash (such as eggshells or the pull tabs from soda cans)
- Toys meant for older children, which may be small or have small parts*

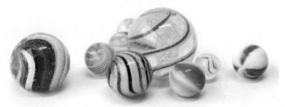

*For infants and toddlers, no toy should be smaller than 1¾ inches in diameter. If you can fit the toy through a toilet paper roll, then it is too small and not safe for a young child.

---

choking hazards in young children. For example, a young child can choke on small foods (such as nuts and seeds); round, firm foods (such as grapes, hot dogs and hard candies); and sticky foods (such as peanut butter). This is because young children do not have the skills needed to chew these foods thoroughly, so they often try to swallow them whole. Laughing, talking or running with their mouth full can also lead to choking.

See Smart Moves: Preventing Choking in Children and Infants for additional ways to prevent choking emergencies from happening.

SMART MOVES > **PREVENTING CHOKING IN CHILDREN AND INFANTS**

- Supervise mealtimes for young children and infants.

- Do not let children eat while playing or running.

- Teach children to chew and swallow food before talking or laughing.

- Do not give chewing gum to young children.

- Make sure that toys are too large to be swallowed.

- Make sure that toys have no small parts that could be pulled off.

- If you are unsure whether an object is safe for young children, test it by trying to pass it through a toilet paper roll. If it fits through the 1¾-inch diameter roll, it is not safe for young children.

Signs and Symptoms of Choking

A person who is choking typically has a panicked, confused or surprised facial expression. Some people may place one or both hands on their throat. The person may cough (either forcefully or weakly), or they may not be able to cough at all. You may hear high-pitched squeaking noises as the person tries to breathe, or nothing at all. If the airway is totally blocked, the person will not be able to speak, cry or cough. The person's skin may initially appear flushed (red), but will become pale or bluish in color as the body is deprived of oxygen.

Partial Airway Obstruction

A person with a partial airway obstruction can still move air to and from the lungs. In the case of choking, this air allows the person to cough, in an attempt to dislodge the object. The person may also be able to move air past the vocal cords to speak. The person may clutch at their throat with one or both hands as a natural reaction to choking. This action is the universal sign for choking (Figure 7-4).

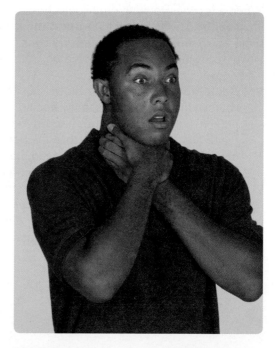

Figure 7-4. Clutching the throat with one or both hands is universally recognized as a sign for choking.

Complete Airway Obstruction

A partial airway obstruction can quickly become a complete airway obstruction. A person with a completely blocked airway is choking and is unable to cough, speak, cry or breathe, or else can only cough weakly and ineffectively or make high-pitched noises. The person may have a bluish skin color. All of these signs tell you the person is not getting enough air to sustain life. Act immediately! If a bystander is available, have them call 9-1-1 or the designated emergency number while you begin to give care.

What if... *I am trying to help a choking person who is much taller than me and I am having trouble finding the correct landmarks for back blows and abdominal thrusts?*

If the person to whom you are trying to give back blows and abdominal thrusts is much taller than you are, and they have consented to care, in a calm and reassuring voice have the person kneel down. You can then begin giving 5 back blows followed by 5 abdominal thrusts until the airway obstruction is dislodged.

First Aid for Choking

If you are with a person who starts to choke, first ask the person if they are choking, or check to see if an infant is crying or making other noises. If the person can speak or cry and is coughing forcefully, encourage them to keep coughing. A person who is getting enough air to speak, cry or cough forcefully is getting enough air to breathe. But be prepared to act if the person's condition changes.

If the person is making high-pitched noises or coughing weakly, or if the person is unable to speak or cry, the airway is blocked and the person will soon become unresponsive unless the airway is cleared. Have someone call 9-1-1 or the designated emergency number immediately while you begin to give first aid for choking.

Caring for an Adult or Child Who Is Choking

When a responsive adult or child is choking, give a combination of 5 **back blows** (blows between the shoulder blades) followed by 5 **abdominal thrusts** (inward and upward thrusts just above the navel) (Figure 7-5, A–B). The goal of giving back blows and abdominal thrusts is to force the object out of the airway, allowing the person to breathe.

- **Back blows.** To give back blows, position yourself to the side and slightly behind the person. For a child, you may need to kneel. Place one arm diagonally across the person's chest (to provide support) and bend the person forward at the waist so that the person's upper body is as close to parallel to the ground as possible. Firmly strike the person between the shoulder blades with the heel of your other hand. Each back blow should be separate from the others.

- **Abdominal thrusts.** To give abdominal thrusts, stand behind the person, with one foot in front of the other for balance and stability. If possible, place your front foot between the person's feet. Wrap your arms around the person's waist. Alternatively, if the person is a child, you can kneel behind the child, wrapping your arms around the child's waist. Find the person's navel by placing one finger on the person's navel and the adjacent finger above the first. Make a fist with your other hand and place the thumb side just above your fingers. Cover your fist with your other hand and give quick inward and upward thrusts into the person's abdomen. Each abdominal thrust should be separate from the others.

Continue giving sets of back blows and abdominal thrusts until the person can cough forcefully, speak, cry or breathe, or the person becomes unresponsive. After the choking incident is over, even if the person seems fine, they should still be evaluated by a healthcare provider to make sure there is no damage to the airway or other internal injuries.

For step-by-step instructions on giving first aid to an adult or child who is choking, see Skill Sheets 7-2 and 7-3. Table 7-1 describes how to troubleshoot special situations when an adult or child is choking.

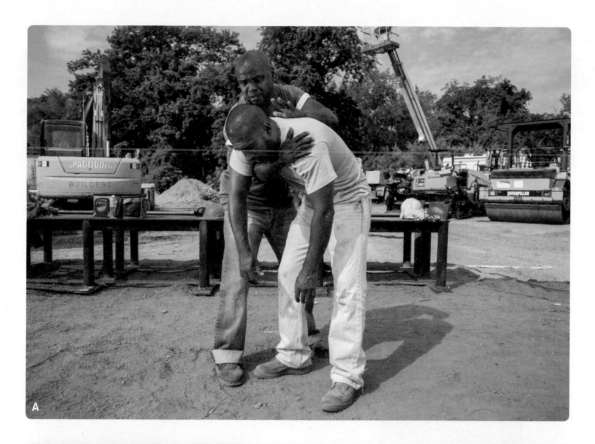

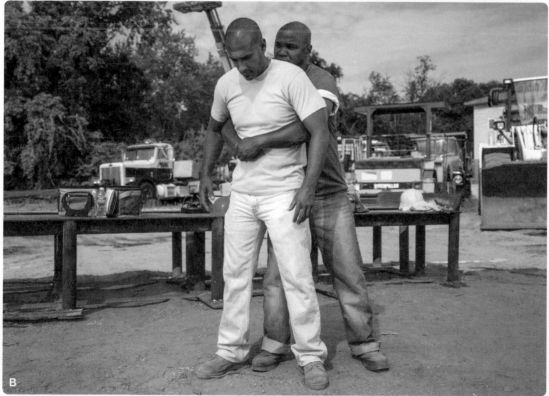

Figure 7-5, A–B. Use a combination of back blows, **A,** and abdominal thrusts, **B,** when an adult or child is choking.

Table 7-1. **Special Situations: Choking in an Adult or Child**

Special Situation	Solution
The person is too large for you to wrap your arms around to give abdominal thrusts. 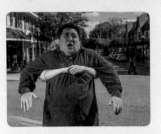	Give chest thrusts instead of abdominal thrusts. To give chest thrusts, position yourself behind the person as you would for abdominal thrusts. Place the thumb side of your fist against the center of the person's breastbone. Then cover your fist with your other hand and pull straight back, giving a quick inward thrust into the person's chest.
The person is obviously pregnant or known to be pregnant. 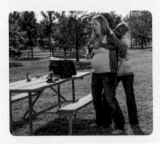	Give chest thrusts instead of abdominal thrusts.
The person is in a wheelchair. 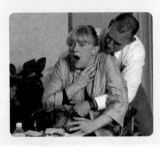	Give abdominal thrusts in the same way that you would for a person who is standing. It may be necessary to kneel behind the wheelchair. If features of the wheelchair make it difficult to give abdominal thrusts, give chest thrusts instead.
You are alone and choking. 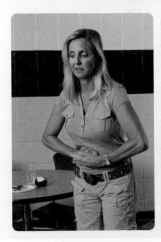 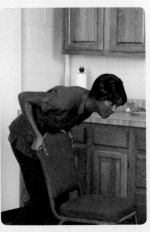	Call 9-1-1 or the designated emergency number using a landline or a GPS-enabled mobile phone. Even if you are not able to speak, the open line will cause the dispatcher to send help. Give yourself abdominal thrusts, using your hands, just as if you were giving abdominal thrusts to another person. Alternatively, bend over and press your abdomen against any firm object, such as the back of a chair or a railing. Do not bend over anything with a sharp edge or corner that might hurt you, and be careful when leaning on a railing that is elevated.

Caring for an Infant Who Is Choking

When a responsive infant is choking, give a combination of 5 back blows followed by 5 chest thrusts (instead of abdominal thrusts) (Figure 7-6, A–B). You can sit, kneel or stand to give first aid care to a choking infant, as long as you are able to support the infant on your thigh with the infant's head lower than their chest. If the infant is large or your hands are small, you may find it easiest to sit or kneel.

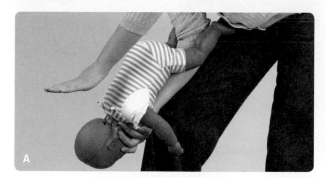 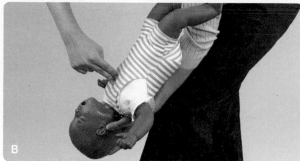

Figure 7-6, A–B. Use a combination of back blows, **A,** and chest thrusts, **B,** when an infant is choking.

- **Back blows.** First, get the infant into position for back blows. Place your forearm along the infant's back, cradling the back of the infant's head with your hand. Place your other forearm along the infant's front, supporting the infant's jaw with your thumb and fingers. (Be careful not to cover the infant's mouth with your hand while you are supporting the infant's jaw.) Turn the infant over so that they are face-down along your forearm. Lower your arm onto your thigh so that the infant's head is lower than their chest. Continue to support the infant's jaw with the thumb and fingers of one hand while you firmly strike the infant between the shoulder blades with the heel of your other hand. Keep your fingers up to avoid hitting the infant's head or neck. Each back blow should be separate from the others.

- **Chest thrusts.** Next, place one hand along the infant's back, cradling the back of the infant's head with your hand. While continuing to support the infant's jaw with the thumb and fingers of your other hand, support the infant between your forearms and turn the infant over so that they are face-up along your forearm. Lower your arm onto your thigh so that the infant's head is lower than their chest. Place the pads of two fingers in the center of the infant's chest, on the breastbone just below the nipple line. Press down about 1½ inches and then let the chest return to its normal position, keeping your fingers in contact with the breastbone. Each chest thrust should be separate from the others.

Continue sets of 5 back blows and 5 chest thrusts until the infant can cough forcefully, cry or breathe, or the infant becomes unresponsive. After the choking incident is over, even if the infant seems fine, the infant should still be evaluated by a healthcare provider to make sure there is no damage to the airway or other internal injuries.

For step-by-step instructions on giving first aid to an infant who is choking, see Skill Sheet 7-4.

If the Person Becomes Unresponsive

If a person who is choking becomes unresponsive, carefully lower them to the ground and begin CPR, starting with chest compressions. After each set of chest compressions and before attempting rescue breaths, open the person's mouth and look for the object. If you see an object in the person's mouth, remove it using your finger (Figure 7-7, A–B). Never put your finger in the person's mouth unless you actually see the object. If you cannot see the object and you put your finger in the person's mouth, you might accidentally push the object deeper into the person's throat.

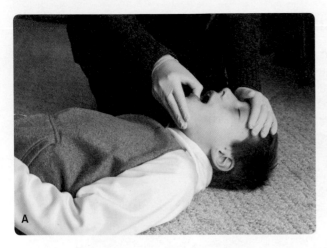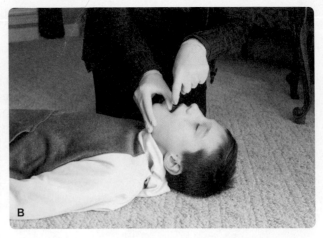

Figure 7-7, A–B. If the person becomes unresponsive, after giving 30 compressions, look for the object in the person's mouth, **A,** and if you see it, use a finger sweep to remove it, **B.**

> **What if...** *I am giving back blows to an adult with a complete airway obstruction who is very heavy and the person becomes unresponsive. Do I let the person fall to the ground?*
>
> *While giving care to a choking adult, child or infant who is awake, you should always anticipate that the person may become unresponsive. Maintaining proper body positioning while giving care will help prepare you if the person becomes unresponsive and starts to fall. If this does occur, every attempt should be made to lower the person to the floor safely using proper body mechanics (e.g., lifting with your legs, not your back), which will help prevent injuries to both you and the person. If at any point you fear the risk of injury to yourself, do your best to safely lower the person, but your priority is to protect yourself, because an injured first aid provider is of limited use.*

After Giving Care to a Choking Person

A person who has choked and has been given back blows, abdominal thrusts and/or chest thrusts to clear the airway requires a medical evaluation. Internal injuries and damage to the airway may not be evident immediately.

Summary

Breathing emergencies, including respiratory distress, respiratory arrest and choking, are life-threatening conditions. Respiratory distress is a condition in which breathing becomes difficult. Respiratory arrest occurs when breathing stops. Airway obstruction such as choking is one of the most common causes of breathing emergencies. As a trained lay responder, your role is to recognize the signs and symptoms of a breathing emergency, call 9-1-1 or the designated emergency number and give appropriate care.

READY TO RESPOND? >

Think back to James in the opening scenario, and use what you have learned to respond to these questions:

1. How would you know that James's airway is partially blocked?

2. How would the actions you take differ if James's airway was partially blocked versus completely blocked?

3. If James became unresponsive while giving care, what would your next step be?

Study Questions

1. **Match each term with the correct definition.**

   a. Airway   b. Respiratory   c. Anatomical   d. Respiratory   e. Cyanotic
      obstruction   arrest   airway   distress
                                                  obstruction

   ____ Blockage of the airway that prevents air from reaching a person's lungs

   ____ Condition in which breathing stops

   ____ Condition in which breathing becomes difficult

   ____ Bluish discoloration of the skin around the mouth or the fingertips

   ____ Occurs when the airway is blocked by the tongue or swollen tissues of the mouth and throat

2. **Circle four signs and symptoms associated with respiratory distress that you find in the following scenario.**

   When Rita walked into Mr. Boyd's office, she found him collapsed across his desk. His eyes were closed but she could hear him breathing, making a high whistling noise. He was flushed, sweating and seemed to be trembling uncontrollably. When he heard Rita, he raised his head a little. "My chest hurts," he gasped, "and I feel dizzy and can't seem to catch my breath." He looked frightened.

3. **List three causes of choking in adults.**

4. **Match each type of care with its purpose.**

   a. Give back blows and   b. Recognize and care for   c. Start with chest
      abdominal thrusts   respiratory distress   compressions, then do
                                                                      foreign object check/
                                                                      removal and rescue breaths

   ____ CPR technique for a choking person who becomes unresponsive

   ____ Force a foreign object out of the airway

   ____ May prevent respiratory arrest from occurring

   In questions 5 through 11, circle the letter of the correct answer.

5. **Which of the following is a sign of respiratory distress?**

   a. Gasping for air   b. Breathing that   c. Wheezing   d. All of the above
                                is slower than
                                normal

(Continued)

Study Questions continued

6. How are asthma, hyperventilation and anaphylactic shock alike?

a. They require rescue breaths.

b. They are forms of respiratory distress.

c. They are all always life threatening.

d. They occur only in children and infants.

7. Care for people in respiratory distress always includes which of the following?

a. Encouraging the person to sit down and lean forward

b. Giving the person water to drink

c. Giving rescue breaths

d. Delivering abdominal thrusts

8. While eating dinner, a friend suddenly grabs their throat and appears to be trying to cough without success. What should you do after getting consent?

a. Lower the person to the floor, check for and remove an object if it is visible at the back of the throat, give 2 breaths and up to 5 abdominal thrusts.

b. Give back blows and abdominal thrusts until the object is dislodged or the person becomes unresponsive.

c. Encourage the person to continue coughing to try to dislodge the object.

d. Open the airway using the head-tilt/chin-lift maneuver.

9. A woman is choking on a piece of candy but is awake and coughing forcefully. What should you do?

a. Slap the woman on the back until the object is coughed up.

b. Give abdominal thrusts.

c. Encourage the woman to continue coughing.

d. Perform a check at the back of the throat.

10. What should you do for an infant who is awake and choking but who cannot cry, cough or breathe?

a. Give back blows and chest thrusts.

b. Give 1 rescue breath.

c. Give abdominal thrusts.

d. Lower the infant to the floor and open the airway.

11. Number in order the following actions for giving care to a choking infant who suddenly becomes unresponsive.

____ Give 30 chest compressions.

____ Check for an object.

____ Open the airway using the head-tilt/chin-lift maneuver.

____ Give 2 rescue breaths.

____ Remove an object if you see one.

Answers are listed in the Appendix.

Assisting with an Asthma Inhaler

Note: *The instructions for assisting a person with an asthma inhaler found on this skill sheet should not be substituted for those given by the manufacturer and the person's healthcare provider. Read and follow all instructions printed on the inhaler prior to assisting the person with administering the medication, and consult the person's asthma control plan.*

---

1. Help the person to sit up and lean slightly forward to make breathing easier.

---

2. Verify with the person that the medication is for "quick relief" or "acute attacks." Also check the expiration date on the inhaler.

    ■ If the medication is not for "quick relief" or "acute attacks," do not use it.

    ■ If the medication is expired, do not use it.

---

3. Shake the inhaler.

---

4. Remove the mouthpiece cover. If the person uses a spacer, attach it to the mouthpiece.

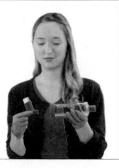

---

5. Ask the person to breathe out as much as possible through the mouth.

(Continued)

Assisting with an Asthma Inhaler *Continued*

6. Help the person to take the medication.

■ **No spacer.** Position the mouthpiece of the inhaler according to the method the person uses. Some people may close their lips tightly around the mouthpiece of the inhaler. Others may hold the mouthpiece an inch or two away from the mouth. Have the person take a long, slow breath (about 3 to 5 seconds) while pressing down on the top of the canister. Then have the person hold their breath for a count of 10.

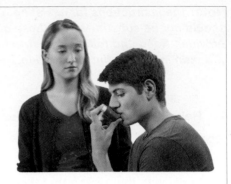

■ **Spacer.** Have the person close their lips tightly around the spacer and push the button on the top of the canister to release the medication into the spacer. Have the person take a long, slow breath (about 3 to 5 seconds) and then hold the breath for a count of 10.

■ **Spacer with mask.** Position the mask over the person's nose and mouth. Have the person push the button on the top of the canister to release the medication into the spacer. Have the person breathe in and out normally 5 or 6 times.

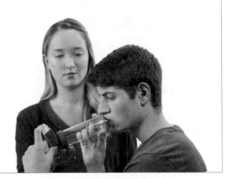

7. Note the time. The person's breathing should improve within 5 to 15 minutes. More than one dose of medication may be needed to stop the asthma attack. The label will tell you how long to wait between doses.

■ If the person's breathing does not improve or the person becomes unresponsive, call 9-1-1 or the designated emergency number.

Caring for an Adult Who Is Choking

1. Verify that the person is choking by asking the person to speak to you.

    ■ **If the person is able to speak to you or is coughing forcefully:** Encourage the person to keep coughing, but be prepared to give first aid for choking if the person's condition changes.

    ■ **If the person is unable to speak to you or is coughing weakly:** Send someone to call 9-1-1 or the designated emergency number and to obtain an AED and first aid kit. Continue to step 2 after obtaining consent.

2. Give **5** back blows.

    ■ Position yourself to the side and slightly behind the person. Place one arm diagonally across the person's chest (to provide support) and bend the person forward at the waist so that the person's upper body is as close to parallel to the ground as possible.

    ■ Firmly strike the person between the shoulder blades with the heel of your hand.

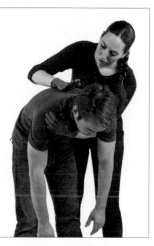

3. Give **5** abdominal thrusts.

    ■ Have the person stand up straight. Stand behind the person with one foot in front of the other for balance and wrap your arms around the person's waist.

    ■ Using two fingers of one hand, find the person's navel. With your other hand, make a fist and place the thumb side against the person's stomach, right above your fingers.

    ■ Cover the fist with your other hand.

    ■ Pull inward and upward to give an abdominal thrust.

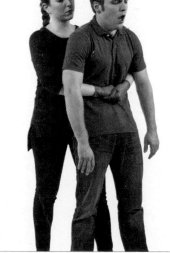

(Continued)

Caring for an Adult Who Is Choking *Continued*

4. Continue giving sets of **5** back blows and **5** abdominal thrusts until:

   ■ The person can cough forcefully, speak, cry or breathe.

   ■ The person becomes unresponsive.

Note: *If the person becomes unresponsive, gently lower the person to the floor and begin CPR if you are trained, starting with compressions. After each set of compressions and before attempting rescue breaths, open the person's mouth, look for the object and remove it if seen. Never put your finger in the person's mouth unless you actually see the object.*

Caring for a Child Who Is Choking

1. Verify that the child is choking by asking the child to speak to you.

   ■ **If the child is able to speak to you or is coughing forcefully:** Encourage the child to keep coughing, but be prepared to give first aid for choking if the child's condition changes.

   ■ **If the child is unable to speak to you or is coughing weakly:** Send someone to call 9-1-1 or the designated emergency number and to obtain an AED and first aid kit. Continue to step 2 after obtaining consent.

2. Give **5 back blows.**

   ■ Position yourself to the side and slightly behind the child. Place one arm diagonally across the child's chest (to provide support) and bend the child forward at the waist so that the child's upper body is as close to parallel to the ground as possible. Depending on the child's size, you may need to kneel.

   ■ Firmly strike the child between the shoulder blades with the heel of your hand.

   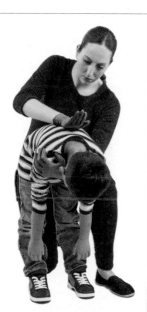

3. Give **5 abdominal thrusts.**

   ■ Have the child stand up straight. Stand behind the child with one foot in front of the other for balance (or kneel) and wrap your arms around the child's waist.

   ■ Using two fingers of one hand, find the child's navel. With your other hand, make a fist and place the thumb side against the child's stomach, right above your fingers.

   ■ Cover the fist with your other hand.

   ■ Pull inward and upward to give an abdominal thrust.

   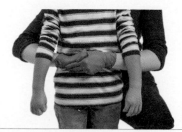

   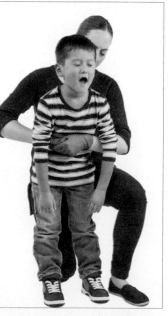

(Continued)

Caring for a Child Who Is Choking *Continued*

4. Continue giving sets of **5** back blows and **5** abdominal thrusts until:

   ■ The child can cough forcefully, speak, cry or breathe.

   ■ The child becomes unresponsive.

Note: *If the child becomes unresponsive, gently lower the child to the floor and begin CPR if you are trained, starting with compressions. After each set of compressions and before attempting rescue breaths, open the child's mouth, look for the object and remove it if seen. Never put your finger in the child's mouth unless you actually see the object.*

Caring for an Infant Who Is Choking

1. Verify that the infant is choking by checking to see if the infant is crying or coughing forcefully.

    ■ **If the infant is crying or coughing forcefully:** Allow the infant to keep coughing, but be prepared to give first aid for choking if the infant's condition changes.

    ■ **If the infant is unable to cry or is coughing weakly:** Send someone to call 9-1-1 or the designated emergency number and to obtain an AED and first aid kit. Continue to step 2 after obtaining consent.

2. Position the infant.

    ■ Place your forearm along the infant's back, cradling the back of the infant's head with your hand.

    ■ Place your other forearm along the infant's front, supporting the infant's jaw with your thumb and fingers.

    ■ Turn the infant over so that the infant is face-down along your forearm.

    ■ Lower your arm onto your thigh so that the infant's head is lower than their chest.

    Note: *Always support the infant's head, neck and back while giving back blows and chest thrusts.*

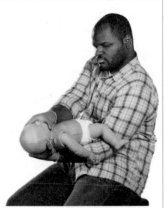

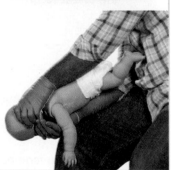

3. Give **5 back blows.**

    ■ Firmly strike the infant between the shoulder blades with the heel of your hand. Keep your fingers up to avoid hitting the infant's head or neck.

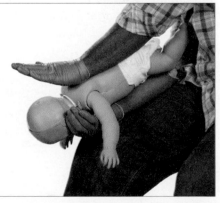

(Continued)

Caring for an Infant Who Is Choking *Continued*

4. Reposition the infant.

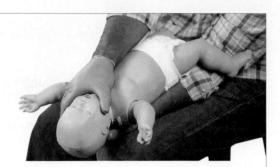

- Place one hand along the infant's back, cradling the back of the infant's head with your hand.

- While continuing to support the infant's jaw with the thumb and fingers of your other hand, support the infant between your forearms and turn the infant over so that they are face-up along your forearm.

- Lower your arm onto your other thigh so that the infant's head is lower than their chest.

5. Give **5 chest thrusts.**

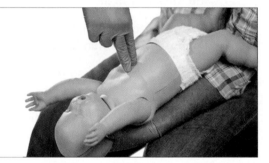

- Place the pads of two fingers in the center of the infant's chest on the breastbone, just below the nipple line.

- Press down about 1½ inches and then let the chest return to its normal position.

6. Continue giving sets of **5 back blows** and **5 chest thrusts** until:

- The infant can cough forcefully, cry or breathe.

- The infant becomes unresponsive.

Note: *If the infant becomes unresponsive, lower the infant to a firm, flat surface and begin CPR if you are trained, starting with compressions. After each set of compressions and before attempting rescue breaths, open the infant's mouth, look for the object and remove it if seen. Never put your finger in the infant's mouth unless you actually see the object.*

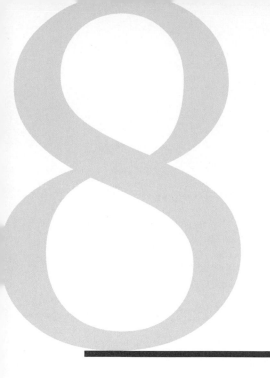

8 BLEEDING

You are on a camping trip, and your friend Joe is starting to clean a fish that was caught for dinner. Suddenly, the knife slips and cuts Joe's left arm deeply. While the blood does not come gushing out, the blood does start to flow steadily from the wound. You are bothered a bit by the sight of it, but you know you need to help. You take a deep breath, control your emotions and go to Joe's side.

Learn and Respond ▶

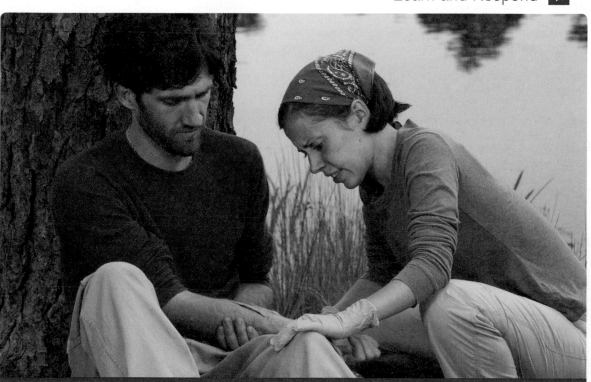

After reading this chapter, you should be able to:

- Explain why severe bleeding must be controlled immediately.

- Identify two signs of severe, life-threatening external bleeding.

- Describe when to consider the use of a tourniquet or a hemostatic dressing for severe, life-threatening bleeding.

- Describe the first aid care for external bleeding.

- Describe how to minimize the risk of disease transmission when giving care in a situation that involves visible blood.

- Identify the signs and symptoms of severe internal bleeding.

- Describe the care for minor internal bleeding.

After reading this chapter and completing the class activities, you should be able to:

- Demonstrate how to control minor and severe, life-threatening external bleeding.

- Demonstrate how to use a commercially manufactured tourniquet.

KEY TERMS

Arteries: Large blood vessels that carry oxygen-rich blood from the heart to all parts of the body, except for the pulmonary arteries, which carry oxygen-poor blood from the heart to the lungs.

Bandage: Material used to wrap or cover a part of the body; commonly used to hold a dressing or splint in place.

Blood volume: The total amount of blood circulating within the body.

Capillaries: Tiny blood vessels linking arteries and veins; they transfer oxygen and other nutrients from the blood to all body cells and remove waste products.

Clotting: The process by which blood thickens at a wound site to seal an opening in a blood vessel and stop bleeding.

Direct pressure: Pressure applied on a wound to control bleeding.

Dressing: A pad placed directly over a wound to absorb blood and other body fluids and to prevent infection.

External bleeding: Bleeding on the outside of the body; often, visible bleeding.

Internal bleeding: Bleeding inside the body.

Pressure bandage: A bandage applied snugly to create pressure on a wound to aid in controlling bleeding.

Severe, life-threatening bleeding: Profuse bleeding from a wound that is a potential threat to life.

Tourniquet: A wide band placed tightly enough around an arm or a leg to constrict blood vessels in order to stop blood flow to a wound.

Veins: Blood vessels that carry oxygen-poor blood from all parts of the body to the heart, except for the pulmonary veins, which carry oxygen-rich blood to the heart from the lungs.

Introduction

Bleeding is the escape of blood from arteries, capillaries or veins. A large amount of bleeding occurring in a short amount of time is called a **hemorrhage.** Bleeding is either external or internal. ***External bleeding,*** or bleeding you can see coming from a wound, is usually obvious because it is visible. However, ***internal bleeding,*** or bleeding inside the body, is often difficult to recognize.

Uncontrolled bleeding, whether external or internal, is a life-threatening emergency. As you learned in previous chapters, severe bleeding can result in death. In this chapter, you will learn how to recognize and give care for both external and internal bleeding.

The Blood and Blood Vessels

Blood

Blood consists of liquid and solid components and comprises approximately 7 percent of the body's total weight. The average adult (weight of 150 pounds) has a blood volume of 10 to 12 pints. Blood has three major functions:

- Transporting oxygen, nutrients and wastes

- Protecting against disease by producing antibodies and defending against pathogens

- Maintaining body temperature by circulating throughout the body

The liquid part of the blood is called **plasma.** Plasma makes up about half the total ***blood volume,*** or half of the total amount of blood that is circulating in the body. Composed mostly of water, plasma maintains the blood volume needed for normal function of the circulatory system. Plasma also contains nutrients essential for energy production, growth and cell maintenance; carries waste products for elimination; and transports the other blood components.

The solid components of blood include red and white blood cells and cell fragments called **platelets.** Red blood cells account for most of the solid components of the blood. They are produced in the marrow in the spongy center of large bones, such as the long bones of the arm (humerus) and thigh (femur). Red blood cells number nearly 260 million in each drop of blood. The red blood cells transport oxygen from the lungs to the body cells and carbon dioxide from the cells to the lungs. Red blood cells outnumber white blood cells about 1000 to 1. White blood cells are a key disease-fighting part of the immune system. They defend the body against invading microorganisms, or pathogens. They also aid in producing antibodies that help the body resist infection. Platelets are disk-shaped structures in the blood that are made up of cell fragments. Platelets are an essential part of the blood's clotting mechanism because of their tendency to bind together. Platelets help stop bleeding by promoting blood clot formation at wound sites. Until blood clots form, bleeding must be controlled artificially.

Blood Vessels

As you learned in Chapter 4, blood is channeled through blood vessels. The three major types of blood vessels are arteries, capillaries and veins (Figure 8-1). ***Arteries*** carry blood away from the heart. Arteries vary in size, with the smallest ones (arterioles) carrying blood to the capillaries. ***Capillaries*** are microscopic blood vessels linking arterioles and venules (the smallest branches of the veins). Capillaries transfer oxygen and other nutrients from the blood into the surrounding tissue and pick up waste products, such as carbon dioxide, and move them into the venules. The ***veins*** carry blood back to the heart. The veins also carry waste products from the cells to the kidneys, liver, intestines and lungs, where waste products are processed and eliminated.

Because the blood in the arteries is closer to the pumping action of the heart, blood in the arteries travels faster and under greater pressure than blood in the capillaries or veins. Blood flow in the arteries pulses with the heartbeat; blood in the veins flows more slowly and evenly.

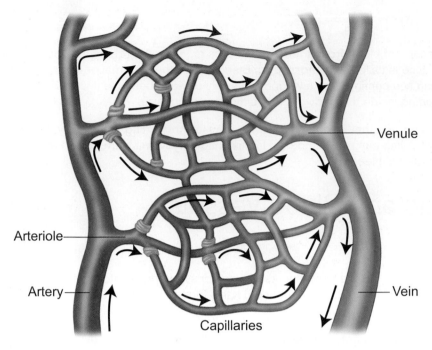

Figure 8-1. Blood flows through the three major types of blood vessels: arteries, capillaries and veins.

When Severe Bleeding Occurs

When severe bleeding occurs, a complex chain of events is triggered in the body. The brain, heart and lungs immediately attempt to compensate for blood loss to maintain the flow of oxygen-rich blood to the body tissues, particularly to the vital organs. The brain, recognizing a blood shortage, signals the heart to circulate more blood and to constrict blood vessels in the extremities. The brain signals the lungs to work harder, providing more oxygen.

Other important reactions to bleeding occur on a microscopic level. Platelets collect at the wound site in an effort to stop blood loss through the process of ***clotting.*** White blood cells prevent infection by attacking microorganisms that enter through breaks in the skin. Over time, the body manufactures extra red blood cells to help transport more oxygen to the cells.

Blood volume is also affected by bleeding. Normally, excess fluid is absorbed from the bloodstream by the kidneys, lungs, intestines and skin. However, when bleeding occurs, this excess fluid is reabsorbed into the bloodstream as plasma. This reabsorption helps to maintain the critical balance of fluids needed by the body to keep blood volume constant. Bleeding that is severe enough to critically reduce the blood volume is life threatening because tissues will die from lack of oxygen. Life-threatening bleeding can be either external or internal.

External Bleeding

External bleeding occurs when a blood vessel is opened externally, such as through a tear in the skin. Each type of blood vessel bleeds differently. Arterial bleeding (bleeding from an artery) is often rapid and severe, and is at highest risk to be life threatening (Figure 8-2, A). Because arterial blood is under more pressure, it often spurts from the wound, making it difficult for clots to form. As a result, arterial bleeding is harder to stop. The high concentration of oxygen gives arterial blood a bright red color.

Venous bleeding (bleeding from a vein) is generally easier to control than arterial bleeding (Figure 8-2, B). Veins are damaged more often than arteries because veins are closer to the skin's surface. Venous blood is under less pressure than arterial blood and flows steadily from a wound without spurting. Only damage to veins deep in the body, such as those in the trunk or thigh, produces severe bleeding that is difficult to control. Large wounds with tissue loss may also have severe bleeding that is mostly venous. Because it is oxygen poor, venous blood is dark red or maroon.

Capillary bleeding, the most common type of bleeding, is usually slower because the vessels are small and the blood is under low pressure (Figure 8-2, C). It is often described as oozing from the wound. Clotting occurs easily with capillary bleeding.

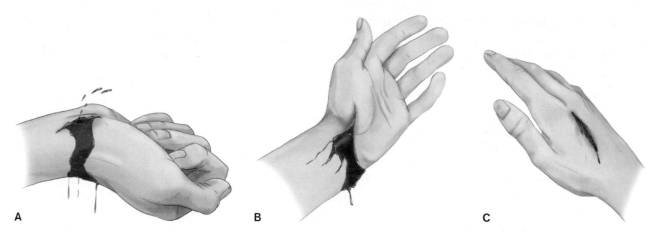

A   B   C

Figure 8-2, A–C. A, Arterial bleeding is the most serious type of bleeding, followed by **B,** venous bleeding. **C,** Capillary bleeding is not usually a concern in healthy people.

First Aid Care for Open Wounds

Many open wounds are minor and can be cared for effectively using first aid. However, if the wound is deep or extensive, bleeding heavily or uncontrollably, or carries a high risk for infection (e.g., a puncture wound), medical care will be needed.

Minor Open Wounds

To care for a minor open wound, put on disposable latex-free gloves and other personal protective equipment (PPE) as necessary. Apply **direct pressure** with a gauze pad to stop the bleeding. It may take several minutes for the bleeding to stop. After the bleeding stops, wash the area with soap and warm water. Rinse under warm running water for about 5 minutes until the wound appears clean and free of debris, and then dry the area. Apply a small amount of antibiotic ointment, cream or gel to the wound if the person has no known allergies or sensitivities to the ingredients. Then cover the area with a sterile gauze pad and a bandage, or apply an adhesive bandage. When you are finished giving care, wash your hands with soap and water, even if you wore gloves.

> **Myth-Information.** *Myth: Use hydrogen peroxide to clean a wound and prevent infection; the bubbles mean it is working to kill germs.* Although applying hydrogen peroxide to a wound will kill germs, it also can harm the tissue and delay healing. The best way to clean a wound is with soap and warm running water or saline.

> **Myth-Information.** *Myth: Letting a wound "breathe" by exposing it to air helps it to heal.* A better strategy to promote wound healing is to keep the wound moist (with an antibiotic ointment, cream or gel) and covered (under a dressing and bandage).

Major Open Wounds

A major open wound (for example, one that involves extensive tissue damage or is bleeding heavily or uncontrollably) requires prompt action. Call 9-1-1 or the designated emergency number immediately and then take steps to control the bleeding until help arrives.

Applying Direct Pressure

Put on disposable latex-free gloves and other PPE as necessary (for example, if blood is spurting, you may need to wear eye and face protection). Cover the area with a sterile gauze pad or other clean dressing (Box 8-1) and apply direct pressure with your gloved hand until the bleeding stops. This may take as long as 15 minutes. If blood soaks through the first dressing, place another dressing on top of the first and apply additional direct pressure (press harder than you did before, if possible). Repeat with additional dressings as needed, always maintaining direct pressure. Do not remove the blood-soaked dressings because disturbing them may disrupt clot formation and restart the bleeding.

When the bleeding stops, check the skin on the side of the injury farthest away from the heart (e.g., the hand or foot) for feeling, warmth and color. Then apply a bandage over the dressing to maintain pressure on the wound and to hold the dressing in place. To apply a roller bandage, hold one end of the roller bandage in place while you wrap the other end around the wound and dressing several times, using overlapping turns. Make sure the dressing is completely covered and allow a margin of several inches on all sides. Tie or tape the bandage to secure it (Figure 8-3, A–F). The bandage should be snug but not too tight. Check for feeling, warmth and color again. If there is a change in feeling, warmth or color from your first check (for example, the skin is cooler or paler than it was before, the area is swollen, or the person complains of a numb or tingly feeling), then the bandage is too tight and needs to be loosened.

Box 8-1. **Dressings and Bandages**

Dressings and bandages are staples of any well-stocked first aid kit and have a variety of uses.

Dressings

A **dressing** is a pad that is placed directly on a wound to absorb blood and other fluids, promote clotting and prevent infection. To minimize the chance of infection, dressings should be sterile. There are many different types of dressings available. In a first aid situation, gauze pads, which are available in a variety of sizes, are most commonly used as dressings.

Bandages

A **bandage** is a strip of material used to hold the dressing in place and to control bleeding. Roller bandages, made of gauze or a gauze-like material, are frequently included in first aid kits and come in a variety of widths and lengths. Wrap the bandage around the injured body part, covering the dressing completely and allowing a margin of several inches on all sides. Then tie or tape the bandage to secure it in place. Bandage compresses, which are specially designed to control severe bleeding and usually come in sterile packages, are thick gauze dressings attached to a bandage that is tied in place.

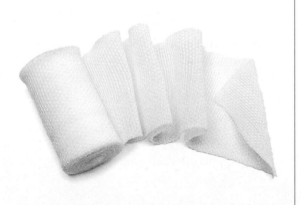

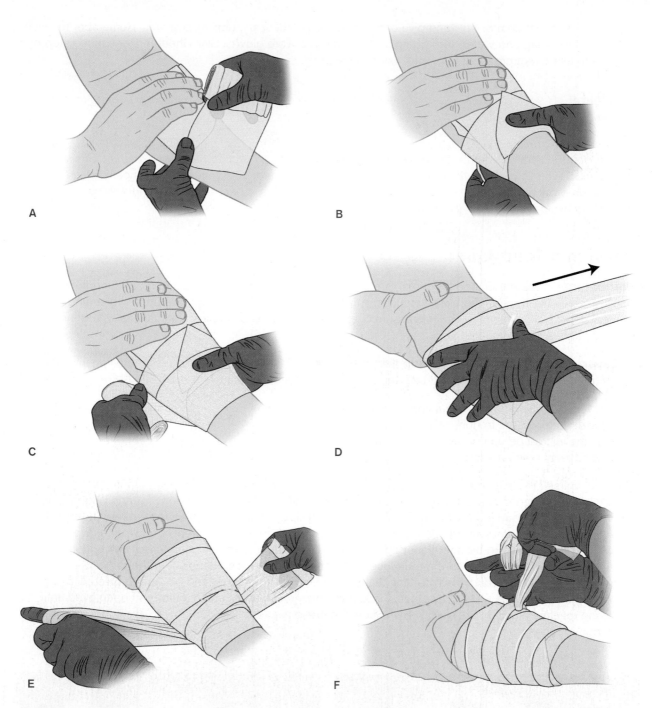

Figure 8-3, A–F. To tie a bandage: **A,** begin by placing the end of the bandage on the dressing at a 45-degree angle.
B, Wrap the bandage one full turn, and then fold the angled end of the bandage up, creating a "dog-ear." **C,** Continue
wrapping the bandage, overlaying the "dog ear" to anchor it and moving upward. **D,** Once the dressing is covered, roll
out the remaining length of bandage. **E,** While holding the bandage, use the index finger of the other hand to split the
bandage in half, moving it down and underneath the limb. **F,** Bring the two ends of the bandage up and tie them in a
bow or knot.

Have the person rest comfortably and give care for shock, if necessary, until help arrives. Remember to wash your hands with soap and water after giving care, even if you wore gloves. Skill Sheet 8-1 describes step by step how to use direct pressure to control external bleeding.

> **What if…** *I secure a pressure bandage too tightly on the arm of an unresponsive person? How will I know if I can't ask the person?*
>
> *A bandage applied too tightly can act like a tourniquet, limiting venous and/or arterial blood flow and causing the extremity to appear reddened or pale as compared to the uninjured extremity. Similarly, the skin of an extremity with a too-tight bandage will be cool or cold to the touch as compared to the uninjured extremity. If any of these signs are present, loosen the bandage and recheck for bleeding, abnormal skin color or temperature.*

Applying a Tourniquet

A **tourniquet** is a device placed around an arm or leg to constrict blood vessels and stop blood flow to a wound. In some life-threatening circumstances, you may need to use a tourniquet to control bleeding as the first step instead of maintaining direct pressure over several minutes. Examples of situations where it may be necessary to use a tourniquet include:

- **Severe, life-threatening bleeding** that cannot be controlled using direct pressure.

- A physical location that makes it impossible to apply direct pressure to control the bleeding (e.g., the injured person or the person's limb is trapped in a confined space).

- Multiple people with life-threatening injuries who need care.

- A scene that is or becomes unsafe.

If you find yourself in a situation where you need to apply a tourniquet, a commercially manufactured tourniquet is preferred over a makeshift device. Follow the manufacturer's instructions for applying the tourniquet. Although tourniquets may have slightly different designs, all are applied in generally the same way. First, place the tourniquet around the wounded extremity about 2 inches above the wound, avoiding the joint if possible. Secure the tourniquet tightly in place according to the manufacturer's instructions. Twist the rod (windlass) to tighten the tourniquet until the bleeding stops, then secure the rod in place (Figure 8-4, A–B). Note and record the time that you applied the tourniquet and be sure to give EMS personnel this information when they arrive. Once the tourniquet is applied, it should not be removed until the person reaches a healthcare facility. Skill Sheet 8-2 describes step by step how to apply a commercially manufactured tourniquet.

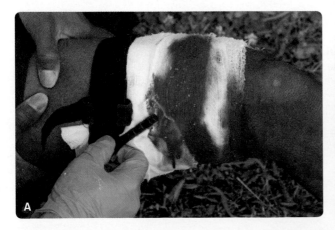 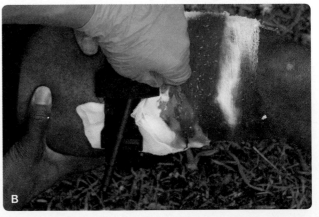

Figure 8-4, A–B. When applying a tourniquet: **A,** Twist the rod to tighten until bleeding stops. **B,** Secure the rod in place.

If it is necessary to use a tourniquet and a commercially manufactured tourniquet is not available, make a tourniquet using a strip of soft material that is 2 to 4 inches wide (such as a triangular bandage that has been folded into a tie) and a short, sturdy stick or other rigid object. Tie the stick or other rigid object into the material and twist it to tighten the makeshift tourniquet.

Tourniquets can be extremely painful. If you must apply a tourniquet, make sure the person understands the reason for the tourniquet, and warn the person that it may be painful.

Using Hemostatic Dressings

A **hemostatic dressing** is a dressing treated with a substance that speeds clot formation. As is the case with tourniquets, hemostatic dressings are used when severe life-threatening bleeding exists and standard first aid procedures fail or are not practical. Typically, hemostatic dressings are used on parts of the body where a tourniquet cannot be applied, such as the neck or torso. A hemostatic dressing can also be used to control bleeding from an open wound on an arm or a leg if a tourniquet is ineffective or not available. The hemostatic dressing is applied at the site of the bleeding (possibly inside of the wound) and is used along with direct pressure.

What if… *A bystander tells me I should be using pressure points and elevation to help control external bleeding? Are these suggestions valid?*

According to the most recent science, there is no evidence to support using elevation to control external bleeding, and there is evidence against the use of pressure points to control external bleeding. Instead, follow your training and use direct pressure, which remains the most effective method to control external bleeding!

Internal Bleeding

Internal bleeding (bleeding that occurs inside the body, into a body cavity or space) can be a consequence of traumatic injury and may be life threatening. **Blunt trauma,** which is caused by impact with a flat object or surface, is a common cause of internal bleeding. Mechanisms of injury that can lead to blunt trauma and internal bleeding include falls, being struck by a vehicle or a piece of heavy equipment, being struck by a blunt object (such as a bat) or being thrown into a blunt object (such as a steering wheel). Crushing forces (for example, when a person's body is squeezed between two hard surfaces) can also cause blunt trauma, leading to internal bleeding. **Penetrating trauma,** which occurs when the body is pierced by a sharp, narrow object (such as a knife or bullet) or impaled on a sharp object (such as a branch or piece of metal), can also lead to internal bleeding.

Internal bleeding may not be immediately obvious because the blood is contained within the body (e.g., within the abdomen, chest or skull). Often, when a person has sustained an injury that could cause internal bleeding, they will have other, more obvious injuries as well. When this is the case, medical treatment is usually sought for the more obvious injuries, and the internal bleeding is discovered while the person is being assessed by medical personnel. However, internal bleeding can also occur as a result of seemingly minor trauma, and it may reveal itself hours or days after the initial injury. When the mechanism of injury is one that could lead to internal bleeding (such as blunt or penetrating trauma), be alert to signs and symptoms that may indicate internal bleeding.

Signs and Symptoms of Internal Bleeding

As a result of the blood loss, the person may show signs and symptoms of shock, such as excessive thirst; skin that feels cool or moist and looks pale or bluish; an altered level of consciousness; and a rapid, weak heartbeat. The person may cough or vomit blood. You may also notice that the area of the body where the blood is collecting (such as the abdomen) is tender, swollen or rigid, and there may be bruising over the area. If internal bleeding is occurring in an injured limb, the limb may be blue or extremely pale, swollen and rigid.

First Aid Care for Internal Bleeding

If a person is showing signs and symptoms of internal bleeding, call 9-1-1 or the designated emergency number immediately, if you have not already done so. If necessary, give first aid care for shock until help arrives.

You will learn about specific care for closed wounds that often result in internal bleeding in Chapter 10.

Summary

One of the most important things you can do in any emergency is to recognize and control severe, life-threatening bleeding. Check for severe, life-threatening bleeding while conducting your scene size-up and forming your initial impression. If severe, life-threatening bleeding is found, control the bleeding with any resources that are immediately available.

External bleeding is easily recognized and should be cared for by using direct pressure and, once controlled, a *pressure bandage.* Consider the use of tourniquets and hemostatic dressings when there is severe, life-threatening bleeding and direct pressure is not effective or possible. Avoid contact with the injured person's blood by taking standard precautions such as using disposable latex-free gloves and washing your hands with soap and water as soon as possible after giving care.

Although internal bleeding is less obvious, it can also be life threatening. Recognize when a serious injury has occurred, and suspect internal bleeding. You may not identify internal bleeding until you check for non-life-threatening conditions. When you identify or suspect life-threatening internal bleeding, activate the EMS system immediately by calling 9-1-1 or the designated emergency number and give care until EMS personnel arrive and take over.

READY TO RESPOND? >

Think back to Joe in the opening scenario, and use what you have learned to respond to these questions:

1. From the description, would you suspect that Joe's bleeding is a result of an injury to an artery, a vein or capillaries? Why?

2. How could Joe's situation become life threatening?

3. What precautions should you use to minimize the risk of disease transmission while giving care?

Study Questions

1. **Match each term with the correct definition.**

   a. External bleeding   c. Pressure bandage   e. Arteries   g. Tourniquet

   b. Direct pressure   d. Internal bleeding   f. Veins

   ____ Using your gloved hand to apply pressure on the wound to control bleeding

   ____ Bleeding that can be seen coming from a wound

   ____ The escape of blood from an artery, vein or capillary inside the body

   ____ A tight band placed around an arm or leg to constrict blood vessels in order to stop blood flow to a wound

   ____ Blood vessels that carry blood from all parts of the body to the heart

   ____ Vessels that transport blood to the capillaries for distribution to the cells

   ____ A bandage applied snugly to maintain pressure on the wound to control bleeding

2. **List two signs and symptoms of severe, life-threatening external bleeding.**

3. **Describe how to control severe, life-threatening external bleeding.**

4. **List five signs and symptoms of severe internal bleeding.**

Use the following scenario to answer question 5.

The usual Saturday morning baseball game is in progress. A few spectators are standing around on the sidelines. As Milo takes a swing at a curve ball, he loses his grip on the bat, which flies several feet, hitting Chris hard on the thigh. Chris drops to the ground, clutching his leg. The skin where the leg was struck immediately becomes red and begins to swell.

5. **What type of bleeding do you suspect Chris has?**

For question 6, circle the letter of the correct answer.

6. **A child has a deep cut on their arm. The child's face is moist and very pale. What would you do first?**

   a. Have someone call 9-1-1 or the designated emergency number.

   b. Apply a hemostatic dressing to the wound.

   c. Place a cold pack on the affected arm.

   d. Apply pressure at the closest pressure point.

Answers are listed in the Appendix.

Using Direct Pressure to Control External Bleeding

1. Cover the wound with a sterile gauze pad and apply direct pressure until the bleeding stops.

   - If blood soaks through the first gauze pad, put another one on top and apply additional direct pressure (press harder than you did before, if possible). It may take several minutes for the bleeding to stop.

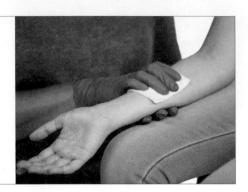

2. When the bleeding stops, check for circulation (feeling, warmth and color) beyond the injury.

3. Apply a roller bandage. Wrap the bandage around the wound several times to hold the gauze pad(s) in place.

   - Tie or tape the bandage to secure it.

   - Check for circulation (feeling, warmth and color) beyond the injury. If there is a change in feeling, warmth or color (indicating that the bandage is too tight), gently loosen it.

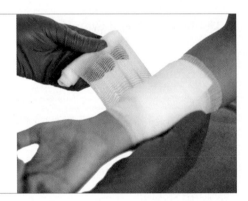

4. Remove your disposable latex-free gloves and wash your hands.

Note: *If the bleeding does not stop with the application of direct pressure, call 9-1-1 or the designated emergency number if you have not already, and give care for shock if necessary.*

Using a Commercial Tourniquet

Note: *Always follow the manufacturer's instructions when applying a tourniquet.*

1. Place the tourniquet around the limb, approximately 2 inches above the wound. Avoid placing the tourniquet over a joint.

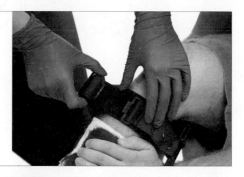

2. Secure the tourniquet tightly in place according to the manufacturer's instructions.

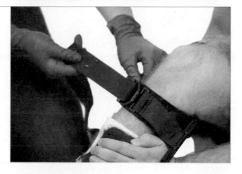

3. Tighten the tourniquet by twisting the rod until the flow of bright red blood stops.

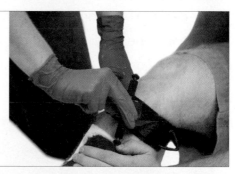

4. Secure the rod in place using the clip or holder.

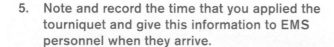

5. Note and record the time that you applied the tourniquet and give this information to EMS personnel when they arrive.

   - Once you apply a tourniquet, do not loosen or remove it.

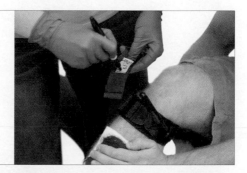

9 SHOCK

You are driving down an isolated road. As you round a curve, you are surprised to see a car that has crashed into a tree. You pull over, then carefully check the scene and approach the car. You find a woman who is awake but very anxious and in obvious pain. The woman tells you she cannot move her legs, which appear to have been crushed by the collision. You dial 9-1-1. As you wait for emergency medical services (EMS) personnel to arrive, you can see the woman's condition is changing. She is now breathing faster, looks pale and appears drowsy. As you check the woman, you touch her hand and notice that her skin feels cool and moist. A moment later, the woman becomes unresponsive.

Learn and Respond

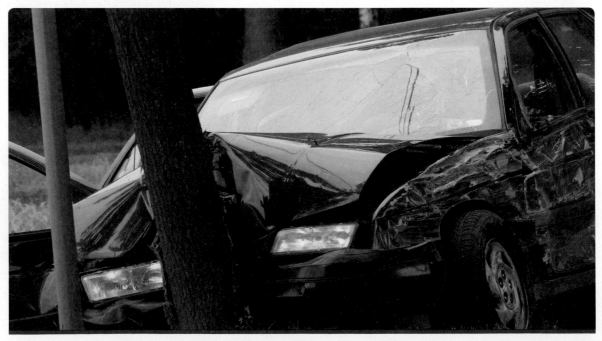

After reading this chapter, you should be able to:

- Identify the types of shock and the conditions that cause each of them.

- List the signs and symptoms of shock.

- Explain what care can be given to minimize shock.

Shock: A life-threatening condition that occurs when the circulatory system fails to provide adequate oxygenated blood to all parts of the body.

Supraventricular tachycardia (SVT): An abnormal heart rhythm resulting in a very rapid heartbeat. People with SVT often feel palpitations in their chest or their heart racing.

Introduction

Injuries and medical emergencies can become life threatening as a result of **shock.** When the body experiences injury or sudden illness, it responds in a number of ways. Survival depends on the body's ability to adapt to the physical stresses of injury or illness. When the body's measures to adapt fail, the injured or ill person can progress into a life-threatening condition called shock. Shock complicates the effects of injury or sudden illness. In this chapter, you will learn to recognize the signs and symptoms of shock and how to give care to minimize it.

Shock

Shock is a progressive, life-threatening condition in which the circulatory system fails to deliver enough oxygen-rich blood to the body's tissues and organs. As a result, organs and body systems begin to fail. Common causes of shock include severe bleeding and severe allergic reactions (anaphylaxis), but shock can develop quickly after any serious injury or illness. A person who is showing signs and symptoms of shock needs immediate medical attention.

When the body is healthy, three conditions are necessary to maintain adequate blood flow to perfuse all the body cells, tissues and organs:

- The heart must be working well.

- The blood vessels must be intact and able to adjust blood flow.

- An adequate amount of blood must be circulating in the body.

Injury or sudden illness can interrupt normal body functions. In cases of minor injury or illness, this interruption is brief because the body is able to compensate quickly. With more severe injuries or illnesses, however, the body is unable to adjust. When the body is unable to meet its demands for oxygen because the circulatory system fails to adequately circulate oxygenated blood to all parts of the body, shock occurs.

Shock is a progressive condition. When **vital organs,** such as the brain, heart and lungs, do not receive sufficient oxygenated blood, the body initiates a series of responses to protect those organs. The amount of blood circulating to the less important tissues of the arms, legs and skin is reduced so that more blood can go to the vital organs. This reduction in blood circulation to the skin causes a person in shock to appear pale or ashen (grayish) and feel cool. While this can protect the body's most crucial organs in the short term, if the situation is not treated quickly, shock can lead to death. See Shock: The Domino Effect to learn more about this progression.

Causes of Shock

There are many possible reasons for shock to occur. These include:

- Cardiogenic shock, resulting from failure of the heart to pump enough oxygened blood. If the heart rate is too slow, the rate of new oxygenated blood cells reaching each part of the body will not be enough to keep up with body's demand. Likewise, when the heart beats too rapidly (**ventricular tachycardia** or ***supraventricular tachycardia [SVT]),*** the heart is not an effective pump, and oxygenated blood is not sent throughout the body as it should be. Damage to the heart can lead to weak and ineffective contractions; this can be related to trauma, disease (e.g., diabetes or cardiovascular disease), poisoning or respiratory distress.

- Distributive shock, resulting from abnormal dilation of the blood vessels. If the blood vessels are not able to adequately constrict or become abnormally dilated, even though the **blood volume** is adequate and the heart is beating well, the vessels are not filled completely with blood. Since oxygen is absorbed into the body through the walls of the blood vessels, this condition leads to less oxygen being delivered to the body. There are several types of distributive shock based on the cause. Abnormal dilation of the blood vessels can be caused by spinal cord or brain trauma (neurogenic/vasogenic shock), by infection (septic shock) or anaphylaxis (anaphylactic shock).

- Hypovolemic shock, resulting from severe bleeding or loss of fluid from the body. Insufficient blood volume can lead to shock. Also, if the levels of some components of the blood, such as plasma or fluids, become too low, blood flow will be impaired and shock can result. Hemorrhagic shock is the most common type of hypovolemic shock. It results from blood loss, either through external or internal bleeding. Other causes include severe vomiting, diarrhea and burns.

- Other causes. Shock can also occur following any injury to the chest, obstruction of the airway or any other respiratory problem that decreases the amount of oxygen in the lungs. This means insufficient oxygen enters the bloodstream.

SHOCK: The Domino Effect

Follow the progression to see how shock can quickly become a life-threatening emergency if not treated and stopped.

- An injury causes severe bleeding.

- The heart attempts to compensate for the disruption of blood flow by beating faster.

- The person first has a rapid heartbeat. More blood is lost. As blood volume drops, the heartbeat becomes weaker and the heart's ability to effectively pump blood decreases.

- The increased workload on the heart results in an increased oxygen demand. Breathing becomes faster.

- To maintain circulation of blood to the vital organs, blood vessels constrict in the arms, legs and skin. The skin appears pale or ashen and feels cool.

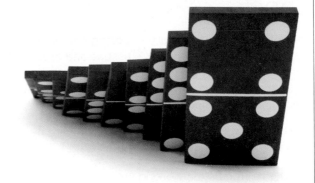

PHOTO: ©iStockphoto.com/redmal

- In response to the stress, the body perspires heavily and the skin feels moist.

- Because tissues of the arms and legs are now without oxygen, cells start to die.

- In response, the brain sends a signal to return blood to the arms and legs in an attempt to balance blood flow between these body parts and the vital organs.

(Continued)

SHOCK: The Domino Effect continued

- Vital organs now are not receiving adequate oxygen.

- The heart tries to compensate by beating even faster.

- More blood is lost and the person's condition worsens.

- Without oxygen, the vital organs fail to function properly.

- As the brain is affected, the person becomes restless, drowsy and eventually unresponsive.

- As the heart is affected, it beats irregularly. The rhythm then becomes chaotic and the heart fails to circulate blood.

- There are no longer signs of life.

- When the heart stops, breathing stops.

- The body's continuous attempt to compensate for severe blood loss eventually results in death.

Signs and Symptoms of Shock

Although you may not always be able to determine the cause of shock, remember that shock is a life-threatening condition. You should learn to recognize the signs and symptoms that indicate a person may be going into shock. These include:

- Apprehension, anxiety, restlessness or irritability.
- Altered level of consciousness.
- Nausea or vomiting.
- Pale, ashen or grayish, cool, moist skin.

- Rapid breathing.
- Rapid, weak heartbeat.
- Excessive thirst.

First Aid Care for Shock

When a person who has been injured or is ill shows signs and symptoms of shock, call 9-1-1 or the designated emergency number immediately, if you have not already done so. Shock cannot be managed effectively by first aid alone, so it is important to get the person emergency medical care as soon as possible. While you are waiting for help to arrive:

- Have the person lie flat on their back.

- Control any external bleeding.

- Cover the person with a blanket to prevent loss of body heat (Figure 9-1).

- Do not give the person anything to eat or drink, even though they may complain of thirst. Eating or drinking increases the person's risk for vomiting and aspiration (inhalation of foreign matter into the lungs). Aspiration can cause serious complications, such as pneumonia.

- Ensure the person's airway is open and clear.

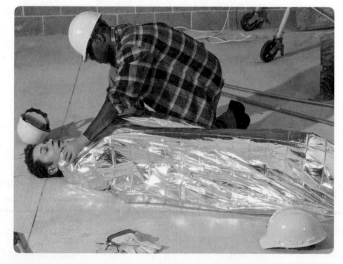

Figure 9-1. Keep a person with signs and symptoms of shock from getting chilled or overheated.

- Provide reassurance, and help the person rest comfortably. Anxiety and pain can intensify the body's stress and speed up the progression of shock.

- Continue to monitor the person's condition and watch for changes in level of consciousness.

What if... *A person with a serious injury goes into shock—I learned before that I am supposed to elevate the legs. Should I?*

Current science suggests that a seriously injured person who shows evidence of shock should lie flat on their back in a face-up position. However, when there are no suspected or obvious signs of injury, some studies suggest that elevating the legs of a person in shock may have temporary benefits, such as increasing blood pressure. Therefore, it is reasonable to consider raising the feet 6 to 12 inches as long as there is no evidence of trauma or injury, and the movement or position does not cause pain.

What if... *I recognize that a person is demonstrating the signs and symptoms of shock, but then I also notice signs of severe bleeding after I have completed the primary assessment. What should I do next?*

As soon as you notice severe bleeding, especially with signs and symptoms of shock, you must take immediate steps to control the bleeding using direct pressure and/or a pressure bandage as continued bleeding can make shock progress faster. Once the bleeding is controlled, continue to monitor the person, immobilize any broken bones or damaged joints, keep the person from becoming chilled or overheated, and talk to them in a calm and reassuring manner.

Special Considerations

Be aware that the early signs and symptoms of shock may not be present in young children and infants. However, because children are smaller than adults, they have less blood volume and are more susceptible to shock.

The signs and symptoms of shock may be harder to detect in children. Suspect that shock may develop if a child is experiencing severe vomiting or diarrhea for an extended period of time (1 day). Replacing the fluids lost through vomiting or diarrhea is critical. Do not hesitate to call 9-1-1 or the designated emergency number for a child who has developed severe vomiting or diarrhea.

Summary

Shock can be caused by loss of blood or body fluid, by the heart not pumping blood effectively, by abnormal dilation of the blood vessels, or by damage to the chest or airway. *Do not wait* for shock to develop before giving care to a person who has an injury or sudden illness. Left untreated, shock is a progressive condition that can be fatal. Always follow the general care steps for any emergency to minimize the progression of shock. Care for life-threatening conditions, such as breathing emergencies or severe external bleeding, before caring for non-life-threatening conditions by ensuring the person has an open and clear airway. Remember that the key to managing shock effectively is calling 9-1-1 or the designated emergency number and giving care as soon as possible.

READY TO RESPOND? ❯

Think back to the injured driver in the opening scenario, and use what you have learned to respond to these questions:

1. Why did the woman likely go into shock?

2. What steps could you have taken to care for shock until EMS personnel arrived?

Study Questions

For question 1, circle T if the statement is true, F if it is false.

1. Shock is a condition resulting *only* from severe blood loss.　　　T　　F

2. List the signs and symptoms of shock.

3. List two of the conditions that frequently result in shock in children.

Use the following scenario to answer question 4.

Tara saw her nephew Daren fall out of the tree he was climbing. When she reached him, he was lying on his back on the ground, awake, but in pain. One leg was strangely twisted. Tara ran into the house, called 9-1-1 and told the emergency medical dispatcher what had happened. Then she ran back to Daren, who was pale and appeared restless.

4. What can Tara do to care for Daren until EMS personnel arrive?

In questions 5 through 8, circle the letter of the correct answer.

5. Which of the following can cause shock?

   a. Bleeding　　　　b. Bee sting　　　　c. Heart attack　　　　d. All of the above

6. When shock occurs, the body prioritizes its need for blood. Where does it send blood first?

   a. The arms and legs　　b. The brain, heart and lungs　　c. The skin　　　　d. The spinal cord

7. Which of the following are included in the care for shock?

   a. Controlling external bleeding when present
   b. Having the person lie down
   c. Helping the person maintain a normal body temperature
   d. All of the above

8. Which body systems are affected by shock?

   a. Circulatory and respiratory
   b. All body systems
   c. Circulatory, respiratory and nervous
   d. Respiratory and nervous

Answers are listed in the Appendix.

PART FOUR

Injuries

10 SOFT TISSUE INJURIES

After a week of all-nighters and grueling exams, you are happy to be having some fun with your friends at a bonfire on the beach. Everyone is enjoying themselves when Jeremy gets up to get something from his bag. As he goes to sit back down, he loses his balance and falls, burning his hand badly on the hot embers at the edge of the fire. As you inspect his injury after he agrees to your help, you can see the skin is red and already beginning to form blisters.

Learn and Respond ▸

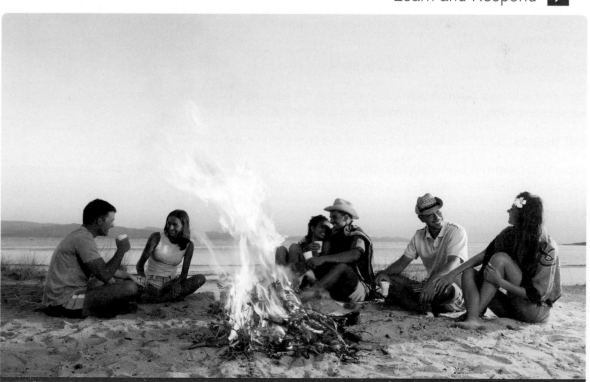

After reading this chapter, you should be able to:

- Describe the difference between a closed and open wound.

- List the signs and symptoms of a severe closed wound.

- List six main types of open wounds.

- Describe how to care for closed and open wounds.

- List the signs and symptoms of an infected wound.

- Describe how to prevent infection in an open wound.

- Describe how burns are classified.

- Describe the signs and symptoms of the different types of burns.

- Describe how to care for heat (thermal), chemical, electrical and radiation burns.

KEY TERMS

Burn: An injury to the skin or to other body tissues caused by heat, chemicals, electricity or radiation.

Closed wound: A wound in which soft tissue damage occurs beneath the skin and the skin is not broken.

Critical burn: Any burn that is potentially life threatening, disabling or disfiguring; a burn requiring advanced medical care.

Full-thickness burn: A burn injury involving all layers of skin and underlying tissues; skin may be brown or charred, and underlying tissues may appear white; formerly referred to as a third-degree burn.

Open wound: A wound with a break in the skin's surface.

Partial-thickness burn: A burn injury involving the epidermis and dermis, characterized by red, wet skin and blisters; formerly referred to as a second-degree burn.

Soft tissues: Body structures that include the layers of skin, fat and muscles.

Superficial burn: A burn injury involving only the top layer of skin, the epidermis, characterized by red, dry skin; formerly referred to as a first-degree burn.

Wound: An injury to the soft tissues.

Introduction

Soft tissue injuries happen to people of all ages. Fortunately, most soft tissue injuries are minor and will require little attention. However, some soft tissue injuries, such as those resulting from nonpenetrating or penetrating forces, may be severe or life threatening and require immediate medical attention.

Examples of minor soft tissue injuries include scrapes, bruises and mild sunburns. Examples of serious soft tissue injuries include large cuts that require stitches and partial-thickness burns. Life-threatening soft tissue injuries include stab wounds to the abdomen, lacerations that cause severe bleeding and full-thickness burns.

This chapter discusses the signs and symptoms of soft tissue injuries, including closed wounds, open wounds and burns, as well as signs and symptoms of infection. You will learn the differences between major wounds and minor wounds and between different types of burns. In addition, you will learn when to call 9-1-1 or the designated emergency number and how to give care.

The Soft Tissues

The **soft tissues** include the layers of skin, fat and muscle that protect the underlying body structures. As you learned in Chapter 4, the two primary layers of the skin are the outer layer, called the **epidermis,** that provides a barrier to bacteria and other organisms that can cause infection, and a deeper layer, called the **dermis,** that contains the nerves, sweat glands, oil glands and blood vessels. Because the skin is well supplied with blood vessels and nerves, most soft tissue injuries are likely to bleed and be painful depending on the severity of the injury.

The subcutaneous layer (also called the **hypodermis**), located beneath the epidermis and dermis, contains adipose (fat), blood vessels and connective tissues. The adipose layer insulates the body to help maintain body temperature, mechanical cushion and, most importantly, a source of energy. The amount of adipose varies among the different parts of the body and from person to person.

The muscles lie beneath the fat layer and comprise the largest segment of the body's soft tissues. Although the muscles are considered soft tissues, muscle injuries are discussed more thoroughly in Chapter 11.

Wounds

A **wound** is any physical injury involving the soft tissues. Wounds are typically classified as either closed or open. In a **closed wound,** the skin's surface is not broken; therefore, tissue damage and any bleeding occur below the surface. In an **open wound,** the skin's surface is broken, and blood may come through the break in the skin.

Fortunately, most of the bleeding you will encounter will not be serious. The trauma of an injury may cause a blood vessel to tear, causing bleeding, but the blood at the wound site usually clots quickly and stops flowing. Sometimes, however, the damaged blood vessel is too large or the pressure in the blood vessel is too great for the blood to clot. Also, many people take daily medication to thin their blood, such as aspirin or another blood thinner called warfarin, which affects the blood's ability to clot. In these cases, bleeding can be life threatening. This can happen with both closed and open wounds.

Closed Wounds

The simplest closed wound is a bruise, also called a **contusion** (Figure 10-1). Bruises result when the body is subjected to a blunt force, such as when you bump your leg on a table or chair. This bump or blow results in damage to soft tissue layers and vessels beneath the skin, causing internal bleeding. When blood and other fluids seep into the surrounding tissues, the area discolors and swells. The amount of discoloration and swelling varies depending on the severity of the injury. At first, the area may only appear red. Over time, more blood and other fluids leak into the area, causing the area to turn dark red or purple.

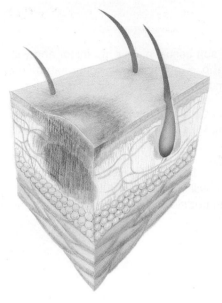
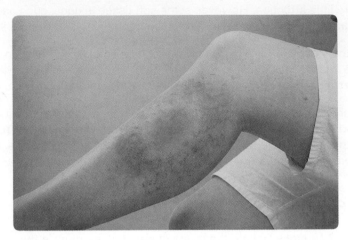

Figure 10-1. The simplest closed wound is a bruise.

A significant violent force can cause injuries involving larger blood vessels, deeper layers of muscle tissue and internal organs. These injuries can result in severe bleeding beneath the skin that may become life threatening. As you learned in Chapter 8, signs and symptoms of severe internal bleeding include:

- Signs and symptoms of shock:

  ○ Skin that feels cool or moist and looks pale or bluish

  ○ An altered level of consciousness

  ○ A rapid, weak heartbeat

  ○ Excessive thirst

- Tender, swollen or rigid areas of the body, such as the abdomen.

- Bruising over the injured area.

- Rapid breathing.

- Vomiting blood or coughing up blood.

- An injured extremity that is blue or extremely pale, swollen and rigid.

Care for Closed Wounds

Many closed wounds are minor and do not require special medical care. Applying cold, however, can be effective early on in helping control both pain and swelling (Figure 10-2). When applying cold:

- Make a cold pack by filling a sealable plastic bag with a mixture of ice and water, and then apply it to the injured area for about 20 minutes. Place a thin towel as a barrier between the cold pack and the bare skin. If an ice-and-water mixture is not available, use a bag of frozen vegetables or a chemical cold pack as an alternative. *Do not* place ice directly on a wound.

- Remove the cold pack and wait 20 minutes before reapplying a new cold pack.

- If the person is not able to tolerate a 20-minute application, limit application to 10 minutes.

- Elevating the injured part may help to reduce swelling; however, *do not* elevate the injured part if doing so causes more pain or you suspect a dislocation or fracture (see Chapter 11).

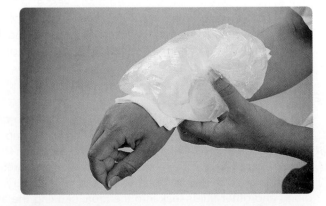

Figure 10-2. For a closed wound, apply cold to help control pain and swelling.

Do not assume that all closed wounds are minor injuries. Take the time to evaluate whether more serious injuries could be present. Call 9-1-1 or the designated emergency number immediately if:

- A person complains of severe pain or cannot move a body part without pain.

- You think the force that caused the injury was great enough to cause serious damage.

- An injured extremity is blue or extremely pale.

- The person's abdomen is tender and distended.

- The person is vomiting blood or coughing up blood.

- The person shows signs and symptoms of shock or becomes confused, drowsy or unresponsive.

With all closed wounds, help the person to rest in the most comfortable position possible. If you suspect the person may be in shock, have them lie flat on their back and care for shock as described in Chapter 9. In addition, keep the person from getting chilled or overheated. Be sure that a person with an injured lower extremity does not bear weight on it until advised to do so by a medical professional.

Open Wounds

In an open wound, the break in the skin can be as minor as a scrape of the surface layers or as severe as a deep penetration. The amount of bleeding depends on the location and severity of the injury as well as other factors, including the person's use of certain medications such as blood thinners or aspirin. The six main types of open wounds are abrasions, lacerations, avulsions, amputations, punctures/penetrations and crush injuries.

Abrasions

An **abrasion** is the most common type of open wound. It is characterized by skin that has been rubbed or scraped away, such as often occurs when a child falls and scrapes their hands or knees on a rough surface (road) (Figure 10-3). An abrasion is sometimes called a scrape, a road rash or a strawberry. It is usually painful because scraping of the outer skin layers exposes sensitive nerve endings. Bleeding is not severe and is easily controlled, since only the small capillaries are damaged. Dirt and germs frequently have been rubbed into this type of wound, which is why it is important to clean and irrigate an abrasion thoroughly as described in the section, Specific Care for Minor Open Wounds.

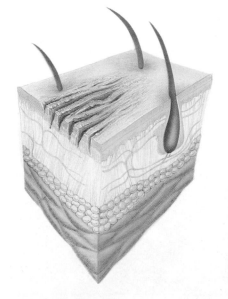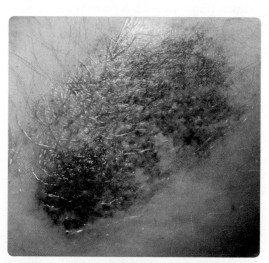

Figure 10-3. Abrasions can be painful, but bleeding is easily controlled.

Lacerations

A **laceration** is a cut, which may have either jagged or smooth edges (Figure 10-4). Lacerations are commonly caused by sharp-edged objects, such as knives, scissors or broken glass. A laceration can also result when a blunt force disrupts or splits the skin. This splitting often occurs in areas where bone lies directly underneath the skin's surface, such as the chin bone or skull. Deep lacerations can also affect the layers of adipose and muscle, as well as damaging both nerves and blood vessels. Lacerations usually bleed freely and, depending on the structures involved, can bleed heavily. Lacerations are not always painful because damaged nerves cannot transmit pain signals to the brain. Lacerations can easily become infected if not cared for properly.

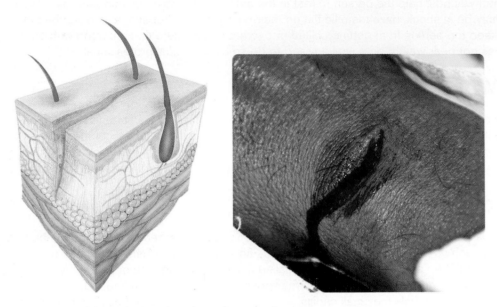

Figure 10-4. A laceration may have jagged or smooth edges.

Avulsions

An **avulsion** is a serious injury in which a portion of the skin and sometimes other soft tissue is partially or completely torn away (Figure 10-5). A partially avulsed piece of skin may remain attached but hangs like a flap. Bleeding is usually significant because avulsions often involve deeper soft tissue layers.

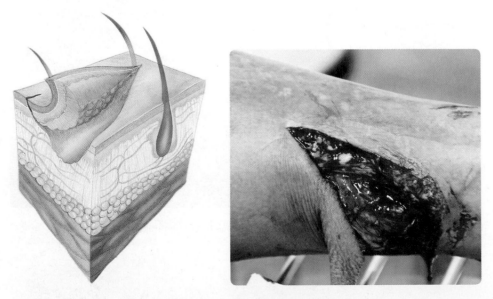

Figure 10-5. In an avulsion, part of the skin and other soft tissue is torn away.

Amputations

Sometimes a body part, such as a finger, may be severed (Figure 10-6). Such an injury is called an **amputation.** Although damage to the tissue is severe when a body part is severed, bleeding may not be as bad as you might expect. The blood vessels usually constrict and retract (pull in) at the point of injury, slowing bleeding and making it relatively easy to control with direct pressure. In the past, a completely severed body part could not be successfully reattached. With today's medical technology, reattachment is sometimes possible, making it important to carefully handle and send the severed body part to the hospital with the patient.

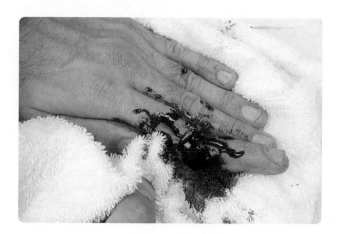

Figure 10-6. An amputation is a complete severing of a part of the body.

Punctures/Penetrations

A **puncture/penetration wound** results when the skin is pierced with a pointed object, such as a nail, a piece of glass, a splinter or a knife (Figure 10-7). A gunshot wound is also a puncture wound. Because the skin usually closes around the penetrating object, external bleeding is generally not severe. However, internal bleeding can be severe if the penetrating object damages major blood vessels or internal organs.

An object that remains in the open wound is called an **embedded object** (Figure 10-8). An object may also pass completely through a body part, creating two open wounds—one at the entry point and one at the exit point.

Although puncture wounds generally do not bleed profusely, they are more likely to become infected. Objects penetrating the soft tissues carry microorganisms that cause infections. Of particular danger is the microorganism that causes tetanus, a severe infection.

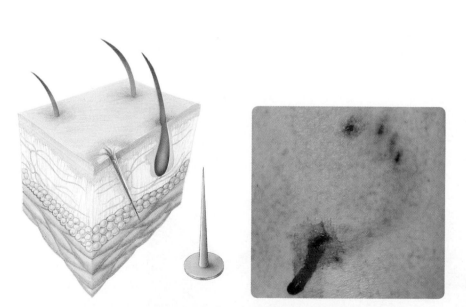

Figure 10-7. A puncture wound results when skin is pierced by a pointed object.

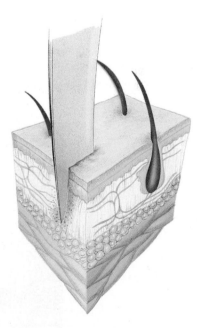

Figure 10-8. An object can become embedded in a wound.

Crush Injuries

A **crush injury** is the result of a body part, usually an extremity, being subjected to a high degree of pressure, in most cases after being compressed between two heavy objects (Figure 10-9). This type of injury may result in serious damage to underlying tissues and cause bleeding, bruising, fracture, laceration and **compartment syndrome,** which is swelling and an increase in pressure within a limited space that presses on and compromises blood vessels, nerves and tendons that run through that space. In a severe crush injury to the torso, internal organs may rupture. Crush injuries can be open or closed.

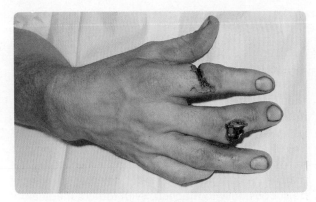

Figure 10-9. Crush injuries occur when a body part is subjected to a high degree of pressure.

Crush syndrome is also common in people who are trapped in collapsed structures due to, for example, an earthquake or act of terrorism. The injury does not happen at the time that the tissue is crushed, but once the crushed muscle is released from compression and the tissue is reperfused with blood. At that point, multiple adverse processes occur, as the products of muscle breakdown are released into the blood. The person may suffer major shock and renal failure, and death may occur.

General Care for Open Wounds

General care for open wounds includes controlling bleeding and preventing infection. Using dressings and bandages assists in both goals.

Using Dressings and Bandages

All open wounds need some type of covering to help control bleeding and prevent infection. These coverings are commonly referred to as dressings and bandages, and there are many types.

Dressings are pads placed directly on the wound to absorb blood and other fluids and to prevent infection. To minimize the chance of infection, dressings should be sterile. Standard dressings include varying sizes of cotton gauze, commonly ranging from 2 to 4 inches square. Much larger dressings are used to cover very large wounds and multiple wounds in one body area. Some dressings have nonstick surfaces to prevent the dressing from sticking to the wound (Figure 10-10).

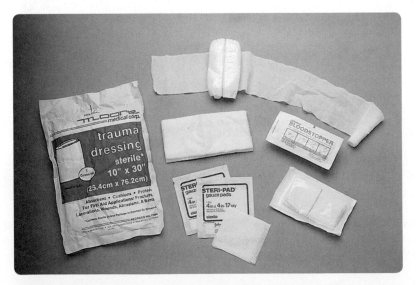

Figure 10-10. Dressings are pads placed directly on the wound. They come in various sizes. Some have surfaces that will not stick to a wound.

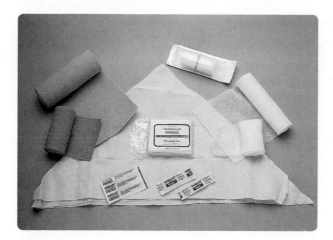

Figure 10-11. Different types of bandages are used to hold dressings in place, apply pressure to a wound, protect the wound from infection and provide support to an injured area.

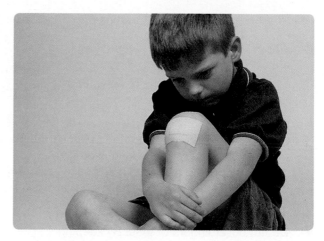

Figure 10-12. A common type of bandage is an adhesive compress.

An **occlusive dressing** is a dressing that closes a wound or damaged area of the body and prevents it from being exposed to the air or water. By preventing exposure to the air, occlusive dressings help to further prevent infection. Occlusive dressings help keep in medications that are applied to the affected area. They also help keep in heat, body fluids and moisture. Occlusive dressings can be manufactured or improvised. An example of an improvised occlusive dressing is plastic wrap secured with medical tape. This type of dressing is used for certain abdominal injuries that will be discussed in Chapter 14.

A bandage is any material that is used to wrap or cover any part of the body. Bandages are used to hold dressings in place, to apply pressure to control bleeding, to protect a wound from dirt and infection, and to provide support to an injured limb or body part. Any bandage applied snugly to create pressure on a wound or an injury is called a **pressure bandage.** Many different types of bandages are available commercially (Figure 10-11).

A common type of bandage is a commercially made **adhesive compress** or adhesive bandage (Figure 10-12). Available in assorted sizes, adhesive bandages consist of a small pad of nonstick gauze on a strip of adhesive tape that is applied directly to minor wounds.

A **bandage compress** is a thick gauze dressing attached to a bandage that is tied in place. Bandage compresses are specially designed to help control severe bleeding and usually come in sterile packages.

A **roller bandage** is usually made of gauze or gauze-like material. Roller bandages are available in assorted widths from ½ to 12 inches and lengths from 5 to 10 yards. A narrow bandage would be used to wrap a hand or wrist. A medium-width bandage would be used for an arm or ankle. A wide bandage would be used to wrap a leg. A roller bandage is generally wrapped around the body part. It can be tied or taped in place. A roller bandage may also be used to hold a dressing in place, secure a splint or control external bleeding (Figure 10-13).

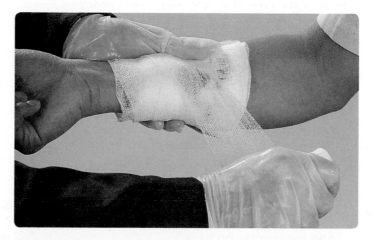

Figure 10-13. Roller bandages can be used to secure a dressing in place.

Follow these general guidelines when applying a roller bandage:

- Check for feeling, warmth and color of the area distal to (below) the injury site, especially fingers and toes, before and after applying the bandage.

- Secure the end of the bandage in place with a turn of the bandage. Wrap the bandage around the body part until the dressing is completely covered and the bandage extends several inches beyond the dressing. Tie or tape the bandage in place.

- Do not cover fingers or toes. By keeping these parts uncovered, you will be able to see if the bandage is too tight. If fingers or toes become cold or begin to turn pale, blue or ashen, the bandage is too tight and should be loosened slightly.

Elastic roller bandages, sometimes called elastic wraps, are designed to keep continuous pressure on a body part (Figure 10-14). Elastic bandages are available in 2-, 3-, 4- and 6-inch widths. As with roller bandages, the first step in using an elastic bandage is to select the correct size of bandage: a narrow (2- or 3-inch) bandage is used to wrap a hand or wrist; a medium-width (3- to 4-inch) bandage is used for an arm or ankle, and a wide (6-inch) bandage is used to wrap an upper leg or shoulder.

When properly applied, an elastic bandage can effectively control swelling or support an injured limb, as in the care for a venomous snakebite (see Chapter 17). An improperly applied elastic bandage can restrict blood flow, which is not only painful but can also cause tissue damage if not corrected. To apply an elastic roller bandage:

- Check for feeling, warmth and color of the area distal to (below) the injury site, especially the fingers and toes, before *and* after applying the bandage. By checking both before and after bandaging, you will be able to tell if any tingling or numbness is from the bandaging or the injury.

- Place the end of the bandage against the skin and use overlapping turns.

- If blood soaks through the bandage, apply more manual direct pressure over the wound and an additional dressing and another bandage as needed. Do not remove the original blood-soaked dressing that is on the wound. Disturbing the dressing may disrupt the formation of a clot and restart the bleeding. To control severe, life-threatening bleeding, consider alternative techniques such as tourniquets and hemostatic dressings.

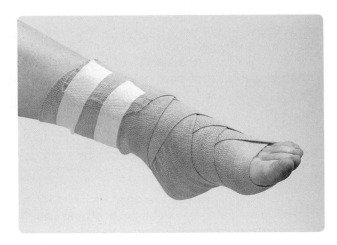

Figure 10-14. Elastic roller bandages can be applied to control swelling or support an injured limb.

- Gently stretch the bandage as you continue wrapping (Figure 10-15, A). The wrap should cover a long body section, such as an arm or a calf, beginning at the point farthest from the heart. For a joint like an ankle, knee or elbow, use figure-eight turns to support the joint.

- Secure the end of the bandage in place (Figure 10-15, B). Check the snugness of the bandaging—a finger should easily, but not loosely, pass under the bandage.

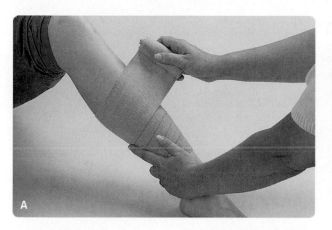
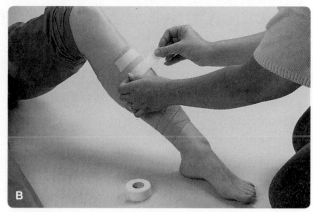

Figure 10-15, A–B. To apply an elastic bandage: Place the bandage against the skin and use overlapping turns. **A,** Gently stretch the bandage as you continue wrapping. The wrap should cover a long body section, such as an arm or calf, beginning at the point farthest from the heart. **B,** Secure the end of the bandage in place.

Specific Care for Minor Open Wounds

In minor open wounds, such as abrasions, damage is only superficial and bleeding is normally minimal. To care for a minor open wound, follow these general guidelines:

- Use a barrier between your hand and the wound. If readily available, put on disposable latex-free gloves and place a sterile dressing on the wound.

- Apply direct pressure for a few minutes to control any bleeding.

- Wash the wound thoroughly with soap and water and gently dry with clean gauze. If possible, irrigate an abrasion for 5 minutes with clean, warm, running tap water.

- Cover the wound with a clean dressing and a bandage (or with an adhesive bandage) to keep the wound moist and prevent drying. Apply an antibiotic ointment or wound gel to the dressing or bandage first if the person has no known allergies or sensitivities to the medication. Do not apply the ointment or gel directly to the wound as doing so may contaminate the tube.

- Wash your hands immediately after giving care, even if you wore gloves.

Placement of Stitches

Suturing a wound closed can speed the healing process, reduce the chance for infection and minimize scarring. Stitches should be placed within the first few hours after the injury. If you think that a wound needs stitches, it probably does, so have the wound evaluated by a healthcare provider as quickly as possible. In general, the following types of wounds often require stitches or another type of wound closure that is applied by a healthcare professional such as skin staples:

- Wounds that are deep or longer than ½ inch

- Wounds on parts of the body where scarring could impair appearance or function (for example, the face, hands or feet)

- Wounds caused by human or animal bites

- Wounds with jagged edges that gape open

- Wounds that are bleeding heavily and uncontrollably

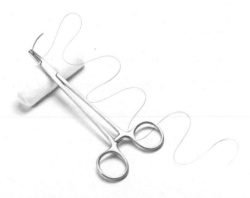

Specific Care for Major Open Wounds

A major open wound may have severe bleeding, deep or extensive destruction of tissue, or a deeply embedded or **impaled object.** To care for a major open wound, follow these general guidelines:

- Call 9-1-1 or the designated emergency number.

- Put on disposable latex-free gloves. If blood has the potential to splatter, you may need to wear eye and face protection.

- Control external bleeding using the general steps below:

  - Cover the wound with a dressing, and press firmly against the wound with a gloved hand until the bleeding stops.

  - Apply a pressure bandage over the dressing to maintain pressure on the wound and to hold the dressing in place.

  - If blood soaks through the bandage, this is a sign that bleeding is uncontrolled. Reapply manual direct pressure with greater force, and check that you are applying pressure in the proper location.

- If bleeding continues, consider alternative techniques for hemorrhage control, such as a tourniquet or hemostatic dressing combined with direct pressure (see Chapter 8). Continue to monitor the person's condition. Observe the person closely for signs that may indicate that the person is developing shock, such as faster or slower breathing, changes in skin color and restlessness.

- Take steps to minimize shock. A person with severe, life-threatening bleeding should not be standing or sitting—assist them to lie down flat on their back. Also, keep the person from getting chilled or overheated.

- Have the person rest comfortably and reassure them.

- Wash your hands immediately after giving care, even if you wore gloves.

There is *no* evidence to support using elevation to control external bleeding and there is evidence *against* using pressure points to control external bleeding.

> **What if...** *A person has a small- to medium-size superficial wound on his arm that is gaping open? I have heard that Super Glue® can be used to close the wound rather than seeking medical care. Is this true?*
>
> *While it is true that healthcare providers do sometimes use medical-grade glue to close a wound, "fast-acting" adhesives (cyanoacrylate) such as Super Glue® or Krazy Glue® are toxic and should not be used. There is also evidence that when these glues are placed in contact with cotton and other fabrics, they may cause a powerful, rapid heating reaction that creates the risk for thermal burns. When a healthcare provider uses glue to close a wound, they do so based on a set of established criteria, and the glue is medical-grade glue designed to be nontoxic and less irritating to skin tissue. The use of medical-grade glue is restricted to licensed healthcare providers.*

Special Considerations When Caring for Open Wounds

Amputations

If the person has an amputation in which a body part has been completely severed:

- Call 9-1-1 or the designated emergency number.

- Put on disposable latex-free gloves.

- First care for the wound as described above in Specific Care for Major Open Wounds.

- After controlling external bleeding, locate and care for the severed body part (or have another person on the scene follow these steps while you control the bleeding):

  ○ Wrap the severed body part in sterile gauze or any clean material, such as a washcloth. Moisten the cloth with sterile saline if available.

  ○ Place the wrapped part in a sealable plastic bag or container. Label it with the person's name and the time and date it was placed in the bag.

  ○ Keep the bag cool by placing it in a larger bag or container of an ice and water slurry (Figure 10-16)—*not* on ice alone and *not* on dry ice.

  ○ Make sure the bag or container is transported to the medical facility by emergency medical services (EMS) personnel with the injured person.

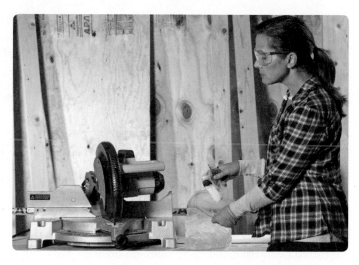

Figure 10-16. Wrap a severed body part in sterile gauze, place it in a sealable plastic bag, and put the bag in an ice and water slurry.

What if... *A person has an embedded object that has gone through both sides of the body? Do I stabilize the object on both sides?*

Yes, you will need to apply bulk-dressing support to both sides of the object to stabilize it. Stabilization of one side and not the other increases the risk for moving the object and causing further tissue damage.

Embedded/Impaled Objects

In some cases, an object that causes a wound may remain in the wound. If the embedded object is large (for example, a large piece of glass or metal), do not attempt to remove it. Any movement of the object can result in further tissue damage. Call 9-1-1 or the designated emergency number and put on disposable latex-free gloves. Place several dressings around the object to begin to control blood loss, and then pack bulk dressings or roller bandages around the embedded object to keep it from moving (Figure 10-17). Bandage the bulk dressings or roller bandages in place around the object. Remember to monitor the person for signs and symptoms of shock. Wash your hands immediately after giving care.

A small partially embedded object, such as a small splinter less than a ¼ inch in size, can usually be removed using first aid techniques; however, medical care should be sought if the splinter is deep, completely embedded in the skin, located under the nail or in the eye, or if there is severe pain upon trying to remove it. To remove a simple shallow splinter, grasp the end of the splinter with clean tweezers and pull it out.

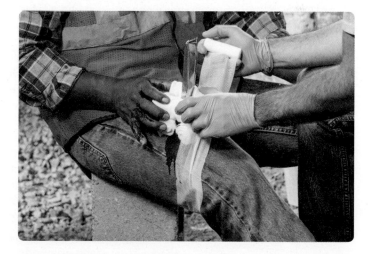

Figure 10-17. Use bulky dressings to support an embedded object, and then place bandages over the dressing and around the object to control bleeding.

After removing the splinter from the skin, wash the area with soap and water and rinse the area with tap water for about 5 minutes. After drying the area, cover it with a dressing and bandage to keep it clean. Apply antibiotic ointment or wound gel to the dressing first if there are no known allergies or sensitivities to the medication.

If the splinter is embedded in the eye, do not attempt to remove it. Call 9-1-1 or the designated emergency number.

Using Tourniquets and Hemostatic Dressings When Help Is Delayed

For a wound on an extremity that is bleeding severely, if direct pressure fails to control bleeding or is not possible, and professional medical help is not available or is delayed, application of a manufactured (commercial) tourniquet by a properly trained responder can be considered. Manufactured tourniquets are preferred over makeshift or homemade devices. For wounds not on an extremity, a hemostatic dressing with direct pressure may be considered, following the manufacturer's instructions. See Chapter 8 for details on applying a tourniquet and using a hemostatic dressing.

Infection

Any break in the skin can provide an entry point for microorganisms that can cause infection. Even a small, seemingly minor laceration, abrasion or burn has the potential to become infected. An infection can range from being merely unpleasant to being life threatening. Of particular danger is the microorganism that causes **tetanus** (Box 10-1).

Proper wound care helps to lower the risk for infection, but sometimes infections develop anyway. An untreated wound infection can cause complications, including delayed wound healing; infection of nearby skin (cellulitis) or bone (osteomyelitis); or infection throughout the body (sepsis, which can be fatal). See your

---

Box 10-1. **Tetanus Prophylaxis**

When a wound is deep or dirty, you should seek care from a healthcare provider, especially if you do not know or cannot remember when you last had a tetanus booster shot, or if it has been more than 5 years since your last tetanus booster shot. Tetanus is a severe bacterial infection that can result from a puncture wound or a deep laceration. The bacteria that cause tetanus are commonly found in soil and animal manure. Once introduced into the body via a deep or dirty wound, they produce a powerful toxin that can cause muscle paralysis and death. Signs and symptoms of tetanus infection include muscle spasms and stiffness. The spasms and stiffness begin in the jaw and neck, leading to difficulty swallowing (a classic sign of tetanus). As the infection progresses, the muscle spasms and weakness spread to the abdomen and then to the rest of the body.

Although the effects of the tetanus toxin can be managed through administration of an antitoxin, prevention through immunization is a better strategy. The initial tetanus vaccine series is usually given during childhood, and then immunity is maintained through a booster shot given at least every 10 years. Death rates from tetanus infection are highest among those who were never immunized against tetanus and those who fail to maintain adequate immunization through regular booster shots.

healthcare provider if you notice signs and symptoms of infection or if the wound does not seem to be healing. Signs and symptoms of an infected wound may include:

- Increased pain, swelling, redness or warmth in the area of the wound.

- Red streaks extending from the area of the wound.

- Pus (a thick yellow or green fluid) draining from the wound (Figure 10-18).

- Fever.

The healthcare provider may use advanced wound-care strategies, antibiotics or both to eliminate the infection and promote wound healing.

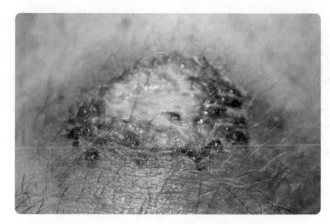

Figure 10-18. The area around an infected wound becomes swollen and red. There may be a pus discharge. *Photo: © Fedor Kondratenko, 2010. Used under license from Shutterstock.com.*

Care for Infection

If you see any signs of infection, keep the area clean, soak it in clean, warm water and apply an antibiotic ointment to the wound covering if the person has no known allergies or sensitivities to the medication. Coverings over the wound should be changed daily. If a fever or red streaks develop, the infection is worsening and a healthcare provider should be contacted to determine what additional care is necessary.

Burns

Burns are another kind of soft tissue injury caused by exposure to heat, chemicals, electricity or radiation. Burns caused by exposure to heat are the most common. Burns account for about 25 percent of all soft tissue injuries. Like other types of soft tissue injuries, burns can damage the top layer of skin or the skin and the layers of adipose, muscle and bone beneath.

More severe burns break the skin and thus can cause infection, fluid loss and loss of body temperature control. Burns can also damage the respiratory system and the eyes. The severity of a burn depends on:

- The temperature of the source of the burn.

- The length of exposure to the source.

- The location of the burn.

- The extent of the burn.

- The person's age and medical condition.

Because their skin is thinner and more delicate, older adults and young children are particularly susceptible to severe burns. People with chronic medical problems also tend to have more complications from severe burns, especially if they are not well nourished or have heart or kidney problems. People with nerve damage resulting from paralysis or other medical conditions may have no sensation. Therefore, they become burned more easily because they do not feel heat.

Types of Burns

Burns are classified by depth. The deeper the burn, the more severe it is. The three classifications of burns include **superficial burns** (formerly referred to as first degree), **partial-thickness burns** (formerly referred to as second degree) and **full-thickness burns** (formerly referred to as third degree). Burns are also classified by their source: heat (thermal), chemical, electrical or radiation (such as from the sun).

Signs and Symptoms of Burns

Signs and symptoms of burns depend on whether the burn is superficial, partial-thickness or full-thickness:

- Superficial burns:

  - Involve only the top layer of skin (Figure 10-19).

  - Cause skin to become red and dry, are usually painful, and the area may swell.

  - Usually heal within a week without permanent scarring.

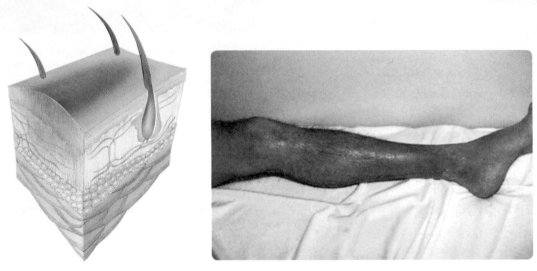

Figure 10-19. A superficial burn involves only the top layer of skin. *Photo: courtesy of Alan Dimick, M.D., Professor of Surgery, Former Director of UAB Burn Center*

- Partial-thickness burns:

  - Involve the top layers of skin (epidermis and dermis) (Figure 10-20).

  - Cause skin to become red; are usually painful; have blisters that may open and weep clear fluid, making the skin appear wet; may appear mottled; and often swell.

  - Usually heal in 3 to 4 weeks and may scar.

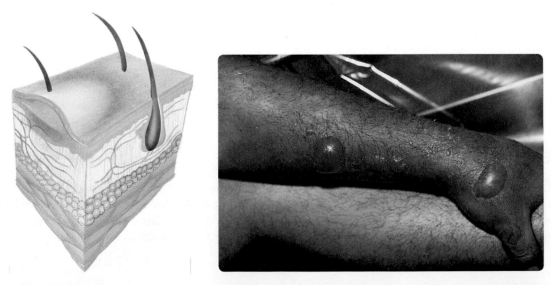

Figure 10-20. A partial-thickness burn involves the epidermis and dermis. *Photo: courtesy of Alan Dimick, M.D., Professor of Surgery, Former Director of UAB Burn Center*

- Full-thickness burns:

  ○ May destroy all layers of skin and some or all of the underlying structures—fat, muscles, bones and nerves.

  ○ The skin may be brown or black (charred), with the tissue underneath sometimes appearing white, and can either be extremely painful or relatively painless (if the burn destroys nerve endings) (Figure 10-21).

  ○ Healing requires medical assistance; scarring is likely.

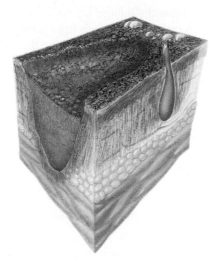 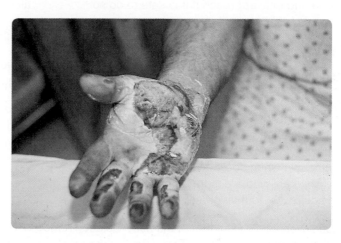

Figure 10-21. A full-thickness burn destroys both layers of skin in addition to any or all of the underlying structures, including fat, muscles, bones and nerves. *Photo: courtesy of Alan Dimick, M.D., Professor of Surgery, Former Director of UAB Burn Center*

Identifying Critical Burns

A ***critical burn*** requires immediate medical attention. Critical burns are potentially life threatening, disfiguring and disabling. Knowing whether you should call 9-1-1 or the designated emergency number for a burn is often difficult. It is not always easy or possible to assess the severity of a burn immediately after injury. Even superficial burns to large areas of the body or to certain body parts can be critical. You cannot judge severity of a burn by the pain the person feels because nerve endings may be destroyed.

Call 9-1-1 or the designated emergency number immediately if the person:

- Has trouble breathing.

- Has burns covering more than one body part (e.g., upper leg or chest) or a large surface area.

- Has burns encircling an extremity (**circumferential burns**).

- Has suspected burns to the airway. Burns to the mouth and nose may be a sign of this (Figure 10-22).

- Has burns to the head, face, neck, hands, feet or genitals.

- Has a partial- or full-thickness burn and is younger than age 5 or older than age 60.

- Has a burn resulting from chemicals, explosions, lightning or electricity.

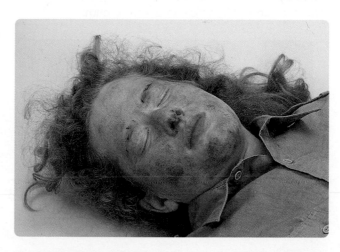

Figure 10-22. Burns around the mouth and nose may indicate that the airway is burned.

Care for Heat (Thermal) Burns

Myth-Information. *Myth: Soothe a burn with butter.* Not a good idea! Putting butter, mayonnaise, petroleum jelly or any other greasy substance on a burn is not effective for relieving pain or promoting healing. In fact, applying a greasy substance to the burn can seal in the heat and make the burn worse.

Follow these basic steps when caring for a heat burn:

- Check the scene for safety by performing a scene size-up and only approach if it is safe to do so.

- Stop the burning process by removing the person from the source of the burn.

- Check for life-threatening conditions.

- As soon as possible, cool the burn with large amounts of cold running water for at least 10 minutes or until pain is relieved (Figure 10-23, A). Be careful to not cause hypothermia when cooling large burns or burns on small children, who are more prone to hypothermia than adults due to their greater skin surface area.

- If possible, have the injured person remove all rings, bracelets or watches from a burned extremity. Once the extremity swells, this will be much more difficult to do.

- Cover the burn loosely with a dry, sterile dressing (Figure 10-23, B).

- Take steps to minimize shock. Have the person lie down flat on their back and prevent them from getting chilled or overheated.

- Comfort and reassure the person.

Remember, even after the source of the burn has been removed, soft tissue will continue to burn for minutes afterward, causing more damage. Therefore, it is essential to cool any burned areas immediately with large amounts of cold water. Do *not* use ice or ice water. Ice or ice water causes the body to lose critical heat and further damages delicate tissues, making the burn deeper. Use whatever resources are available to flush the area—a tub, shower or garden hose. You can apply clean soaked towels, sheets or other wet cloths to a burned face or other area that cannot be immersed. Be sure to keep these compresses cool and moist by adding more water. Otherwise, the compresses will quickly absorb the heat from the skin's surface, dry out and stick to the skin.

Allow several minutes for the burned area to cool. If pain continues when the area is removed from the water, continue cooling. When the burn is cool, remove all rings, bracelets, watches and clothing from the area by carefully removing or cutting material away. Do *not* try to remove any clothing that is stuck to the skin. Remove jewelry only if doing so will not further injure the person, as swelling may occur.

Burns often expose sensitive nerve endings. Cover the burned area to keep out air and help reduce pain. Use dry, sterile dressings if possible and loosely bandage them in place. Do *not* touch a burn with anything except a clean covering. The bandage should not put pressure on the burn surface. If the burn covers a large area of the body, cover the burned area with clean, dry sheets or other cloth. Covering the burn also helps to prevent infection. Do *not* try to clean a severe burn.

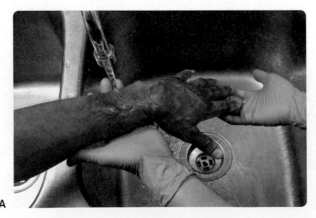 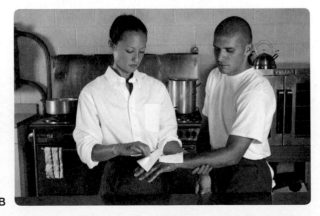

A B

Figure 10-23, A–B. A, Cool a heat (thermal) burn with large amounts of cold running water until the pain is relieved. **B,** Cover the burned area loosely with a dry, sterile dressing.

Do not put ointments, butter, oil or other commercial or home remedies on blisters, deep burns or burns that may require medical attention. Oils and ointments seal in heat, do not relieve pain and will have to be removed by medical personnel. Other home remedies can contaminate open skin areas, causing infection. Do not break blisters. Intact skin helps prevent infection.

For small superficial burns that are not sufficiently severe or extensive enough to require medical attention, care for the burned area as an open wound. Wash the area with soap and water, and keep the area clean. Cover the burn with a dressing and bandage. Apply antibiotic ointment or wound gel to the dressing first if the person has no known allergies or sensitivities to the medication. Tell the person to watch for signs of infection.

Large partial-thickness and full-thickness burns can cause shock as a result of pain and loss of body fluids. In addition, when a person suffers a burn, they are less able to regulate body temperature. As a result, a person who has been burned has a tendency to become chilled. To help maintain normal body temperature and prevent hypothermia, keep the person warm and away from drafts. Have the person lie down unless they are having trouble breathing. Also remember that cooling a burn over a large area of the body can bring on hypothermia. Be aware of this risk and look for signs and symptoms of hypothermia (see Chapter 19).

Care for Chemical Burns

Chemical burns are common in industrial settings but also occur in the home. Typically, burns result from chemicals that are strong acids or alkalis. Cleaning solutions, such as household bleach, drain cleaners, toilet bowl cleaners, paint strippers, and lawn or garden chemicals, are common sources of chemicals that can eat away or destroy tissues. These substances can quickly injure the skin. Signs and symptoms of a chemical burn include:

- Pain.
- Burning.
- Numbness.
- Change in level of consciousness.

- Respiratory distress.
- Oral discomfort or swelling.
- Eye discomfort.
- Change in vision.

As with heat burns, the stronger the chemical and the longer the contact, the more severe the burn. The chemical will continue to burn as long as it is on the skin. You must remove the chemical from the body as quickly and safely as possible and call 9-1-1 or the designated emergency number. To care for a chemical burn:

- It the chemical is dry or in a powdered form, brush the chemical from the skin with a gloved hand or a towel and remove any contaminated clothing or jewelry. Be careful not to get the chemical on yourself or on a different area of the person's skin.

- Flush the burn with large amounts of cool running tap water (under pressure). Continue flushing the burn for at least 20 minutes or until EMS personnel arrive. Do not use a forceful flow of water from a hose; the force may further damage burned skin.

- Take steps to minimize shock. Keep the person from getting chilled or overheated.

- If an eye is burned by a chemical, flush the affected eye with water for at least 20 minutes or until EMS personnel arrive. Tilt the head so that the affected eye is lower than the unaffected eye as you flush (Figure 10-24). This position helps prevent the chemical from getting into the unharmed eye. Flush from the nose outward. If both eyes are affected, direct the flow to the bridge of the nose and flush both eyes from the inner corner outward.

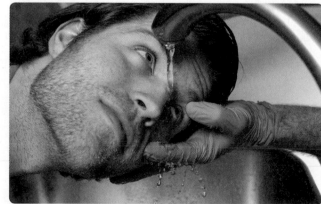

Figure 10-24. If an eye is burned by a chemical, flush the affected eye with cool water until EMS personnel take over.

- Be aware that chemicals can be inhaled, potentially damaging the airway or lungs. Call 9-1-1, the national Poison Help line at 1-800-222-1222 or the designated emergency number if you believe chemicals have been inhaled and give that information to the call taker.

> **What if...** *A person has a chemical burn and the water reacts with the burn while flushing it, making the situation worse?*
>
> *While there are some substances that dissolve readily in water to form a corrosive solution (e.g., ammonia and hydrogen chloride), flushing the area with large amounts of water for at least 20 minutes should adequately dilute the solution to avoid additional damage. If the solution penetrates clothing, ask the person to remove the contaminated clothing while continuing to flush the skin with water. Be careful not to contaminate yourself while giving care.*

Care for Electrical Burns

The human body is a good conductor of electricity. When someone comes in contact with an electric source, such as a power line, a malfunctioning household appliance or lightning, electricity is conducted through the body. Electrical resistance of body parts produces heat, which can cause burn injuries (Figure 10-25). The severity of an electrical burn depends on the type and amount of contact, the current's path through the body and how long the contact lasted. Electrical burns are often deep. The person may have an entrance wound and an exit wound where the current entered and exited the body. Although these wounds may look superficial, the tissues below may be severely damaged.

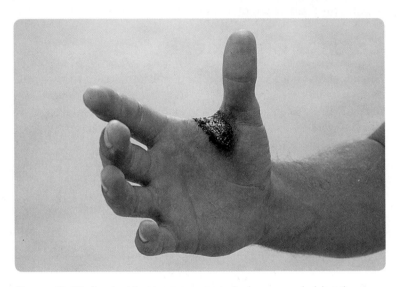

Figure 10-25. An electrical burn may severely damage underlying tissues.

Electrical injuries also cause problems in addition to burns. Electricity running through the body can make the heart beat erratically. As a result, the person's heart or breathing may stop. The person may also have fractured bones caused by strong muscle spasms. The signs and symptoms of electrical injury include:

- Unresponsiveness.
- Dazed, confused behavior.
- Obvious burns on the skin's surface.
- Trouble breathing or no breathing.
- Burns both where the current entered and where it exited the body, often on the hand or foot.

Suspect a possible electrical injury if you hear a sudden loud pop or bang or see an unexpected flash. If you encounter a person with an electrical burn:

- Scene safety is of the utmost importance—never go near the person until you have confirmed that they are *not* still in contact with the power source.
- If possible, turn off the power at its source and care for any life-threatening emergencies. (If you cannot safely turn the power off at its source, call 9-1-1 or the designated emergency number and wait for help to arrive.)

- Call 9-1-1 or the designated emergency number. Any person who has suffered an electric shock needs to be evaluated by a medical professional to determine the extent of the injury.

- Remember that electrocution can cause cardiac and breathing emergencies. Be prepared to perform CPR and use an automated external defibrillator (AED).

- Care for shock and thermal burns.

- Look for entry and exit wounds and give appropriate care.

- Check for additional injuries, such as fractures, which may result from severe muscle contractions that occur in resistance to the electric current.

Care for Radiation Burns

Radiation burns may occur from exposure to nuclear radiation, X-rays or as a side effect of radiation therapy. They can also be caused by tanning beds or solar radiation from the sun. Solar burns are similar to heat burns. Usually solar burns are mild but can be painful (Figure 10-26). They may blister, involving more than one layer of skin. Care for sunburns as you would any other heat burn. Cool the burn and protect the burned area from further damage by keeping it away from the sun. Do not break blisters. Intact skin helps prevent infection.

People are rarely exposed to other types of radiation unless working in special settings, such as certain types of medical, industrial or research facilities. If you work in such settings, you should be informed of the risks and will be required to take precautions to prevent overexposure.

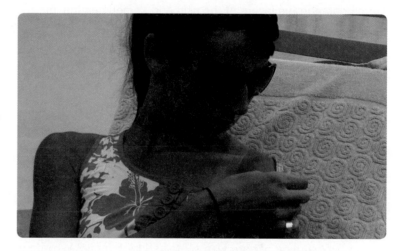

Figure 10-26. Radiation burns, such as sunburn, are usually mild, but they can be painful and blister when involving more than one layer of skin.

SMART MOVES > PREVENTING BURNS

- Heat burns can be prevented by following safety practices that prevent fire and by being careful around sources of heat.

- Chemical burns can be prevented by following safety practices around all chemicals and by following manufacturers' guidelines when handling chemicals.

- Electrical burns can be prevented by following safety practices around electrical lines and equipment and by leaving outdoor areas when lightning could strike.

- Sunburn (radiation burn) can be prevented by wearing appropriate clothing (i.e., clothing made of dark-colored, tightly woven materials containing sun protection factor [SPF]) and using sunscreen. Use a broad-spectrum sunscreen with an SPF of at least 30, and reapply it regularly.

Summary

Caring for soft tissue injuries involves a few simple steps. With closed wounds, minor injuries require no special medical care, although applying cold can help minimize pain and swelling. If you suspect the possibility of a serious internal injury, always call 9-1-1 or the designated emergency number. With open wounds, you need to control bleeding and minimize the risk for infection. Remember that with minor wounds, your primary concern is to cleanse the wound to prevent infection. With major wounds, you should control the bleeding quickly and seek medical attention. Wear disposable latex-free gloves or use a barrier, such as plastic wrap, dressings or a clean folded cloth, to avoid contact with blood. Dressings and bandages, when correctly applied, help control bleeding and minimize the danger of infection.

Burns damage the layers of the skin and sometimes the internal structures as well. Heat, chemicals, electricity and radiation all cause burns. When caring for a person with burns, always first ensure your personal safety. When the scene is safe, approach the person and check for life-threatening conditions, followed by non-life-threatening conditions, if necessary. Follow the steps for burn care. In addition, always check for inhalation injury if the person has a heat or chemical burn. With electrical burns and victims of a lightning strike, check carefully for additional conditions, such as trouble breathing, cardiac arrest and fractures.

READY TO RESPOND? >

Think back to Jeremy's burn injury in the opening scenario, and use what you have learned to respond to these questions:

1. What type of burn was sustained by Jeremy? Why do you think so?

2. Will the burn require medical attention? Why or why not?

3. What steps would you take to care for Jeremy's burns?

Study Questions

1. **Match each term with the correct definition.**

   a. Soft tissue   c. Critical burn   e. Closed wound

   b. Open wound   d. Bandages   f. Full-thickness burn

   ____ Any burn that is potentially life threatening, disabling or disfiguring

   ____ A burn that destroys skin and underlying tissues

   ____ The layers of the skin, adipose and muscles

   ____ Wrappings that hold dressings in place

   ____ Injury resulting in tissue damage beneath the skin's surface, while the skin remains intact

   ____ Injury resulting in a break in the skin's surface

2. **Match each type of injury to its example.**

   a. Abrasion   b. Puncture   c. Avulsion   d. Contusion

   ____ Torn earlobe

   ____ Black eye

   ____ Scraped knee

   ____ Gunshot wound

3. **Match each type of wound with the appropriate care.**

   a. A major open   b. A minor open   c. A major open   d. A severed
   wound   wound   wound with an   body part
                                                           impaled object

   ____ Cover with dressing and pressure bandage.

   ____ Wash the wound thoroughly with soap and water.

   ____ Wrap the part and place it in a plastic bag, and then in an ice and water slurry.

   ____ Use bulky dressings to stabilize.

4. **List five signs and symptoms of infection.**

5. **List two of the purposes of bandaging.**

(*Continued*)

Study Questions continued

6. List and briefly describe six types of open wounds.

7. List four sources of burns.

8. Describe the following types of burns:

   a. Superficial burn   b. Partial-thickness burn   c. Full-thickness burn

In questions 9 through 22, circle the letter of the correct answer.

9. To prevent infection of a minor open wound, you should—

   a. Wash the area with soap and water.
   b. Apply a pressure bandage.
   c. Remove all jewelry.
   d. Wrap the affected area with moist sterile dressings.

10. A sign of an infected open wound is—

   a. Red streaks extending from the wound.
   b. Swelling and redness around the wound.
   c. The affected area is cool to the touch.
   d. a and b

11. Which should you do to care for an infected wound?

   a. Keep the area clean.
   b. Apply an antibiotic ointment.
   c. Change coverings daily.
   d. All of the above

12. Which statement applies to all open wounds?

   a. They always bleed heavily.
   b. They are at risk for infection.
   c. They must always be cleaned immediately before bleeding is controlled.
   d. They are life threatening.

13. Which should you do in caring for a major open wound?

   a. Apply direct pressure with a dressing to control bleeding.
   b. Wash the wound.
   c. Apply an occlusive dressing.
   d. Apply an antibiotic ointment.

(Continued)

Study Questions continued

14. Which should you do when caring for an injury in which the body part has been completely severed?

a. Place the part directly on ice.

b. Seek medical assistance and make sure the part is transported with the person.

c. Wash the body part thoroughly with soap and water.

d. Secure the part back in place using sterile roller bandages.

15. A 6-year-old girl falls on a sharp object. The object is sticking out of her leg. What should you do?

a. Allow the area to bleed freely.

b. Remove the object and control bleeding.

c. Wash the wound with soap and water.

d. Control bleeding and stabilize the object in the position in which you find it.

16. Which is the step you should take to control external bleeding (minor)?

a. Elevate the injured area.

b. Apply direct pressure.

c. Apply a pressure point.

d. Apply a tourniquet.

17. Which could swelling and discoloration indicate?

a. A closed wound

b. Damage to underlying structures

c. Internal bleeding

d. All of the above

18. Which action would you take when caring for a minor closed wound?

a. Apply a warm compress over the wound.

b. Apply cold for 20 minutes using a barrier between the skin and cold pack.

c. Keep the injured area below the level of the heart.

d. Call 9-1-1 or the designated emergency number.

19. What is the first step you should take when caring for an electrical burn?

a. Check for life-threatening conditions.

b. Make sure the scene is safe (the power source is turned off).

c. Look for an entry and exit wound.

d. Check for non-life-threatening conditions.

(Continued)

Study Questions continued

20. **Which burns require professional medical attention?**

    a. Burns that cover more than one body part

    b. Burns that cause the person to have trouble breathing

    c. Burns resulting from electricity, explosions or chemicals

    d. All of the above

21. **The student at the lab table near you spills a liquid corrosive chemical on his arm. Which would you do first?**

    a. Remove the chemical with a clean cloth.

    b. Put a sterile dressing over the burn site.

    c. Flush the arm with water.

    d. Have the person immediately remove contaminated clothes.

22. **Luke's grandmother was burned on one leg and foot when a pan of boiling water tipped off the stove. Which should Luke have done first to care for her?**

    a. Put ice cubes on the burned area.

    b. Immediately put a dry, sterile dressing on the burned area.

    c. Help her put her foot and leg in the bathtub and flood it with cold water.

    d. Wash the area and then apply a burn ointment.

Answers are listed in the Appendix.

11

MUSCULOSKELETAL INJURIES

You are running soccer practice for the team you coach when one of the players, Kelly, stumbles on a rough spot in the field while running and dribbling the ball. She grabs her ankle and grimaces. With the big tournament ahead, you wonder if she has sprained her foot badly, or if it is just a simple muscle strain that could heal quickly.

Learn and Respond ▶

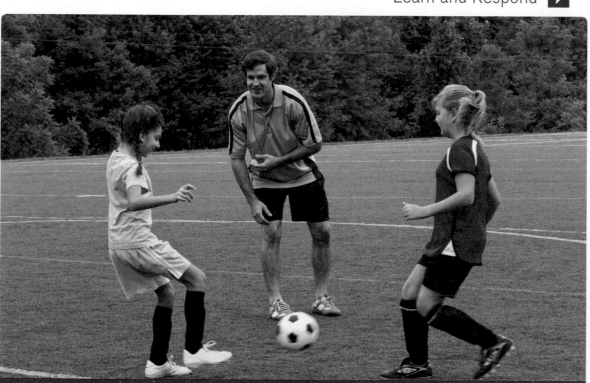

Introduction

Injuries to the musculoskeletal system are common. Millions of people at home, at work or at play injure their muscles, bones or joints. No age group is exempt. A person may fall and bruise their hip. A person who braces a hand against a dashboard in a car crash may injure the bones at the shoulder, disabling the arm. A person who falls while skiing may twist a leg, tearing the supportive tissues of a knee and making it impossible to stand or move.

Although musculoskeletal injuries are almost always painful, they are rarely life threatening when cared for properly. However, when not recognized and cared for properly, musculoskeletal injuries can have serious consequences and even result in permanent disability or death. In this chapter, you will learn how to recognize and care for musculoskeletal injuries. Developing a better understanding of the structure and function of the body's framework will help you assess musculoskeletal injuries and give appropriate care.

The Musculoskeletal System

The musculoskeletal system is made up of muscles and bones that form the skeleton, as well as connective tissues, tendons and ligaments. Together, these structures give the body shape, form and stability. Bones and muscles connect to form various body segments. They work together to provide body movement.

Muscles

Muscles are soft tissues that are able to contract and relax. The body has over 600 muscles (Figure 11-1). Most are *skeletal muscles,* which attach to the bones. Skeletal muscles account for most of your lean body weight (body weight without excess fat). Skeletal muscles protect the bones, nerves and blood vessels. All body movements result from the brain directing skeletal muscles to contract and relax via a pathway of nerves. Skeletal muscle actions are under our conscious control. Because you move them voluntarily, skeletal muscles are also called voluntary muscles.

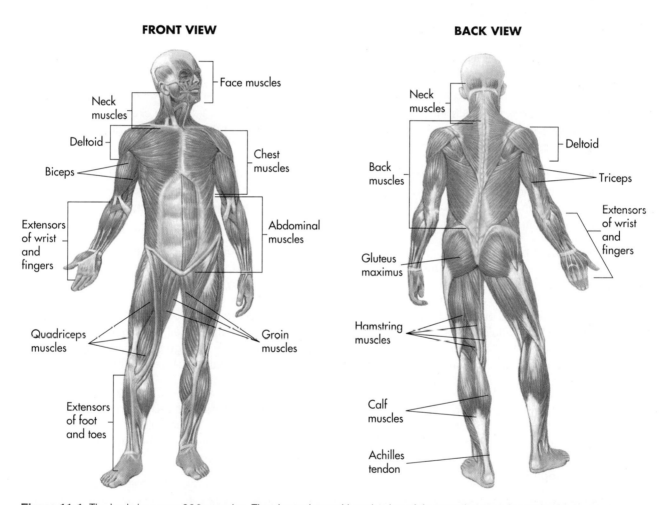

FRONT VIEW

- Face muscles
- Neck muscles
- Deltoid
- Biceps
- Chest muscles
- Extensors of wrist and fingers
- Abdominal muscles
- Quadriceps muscles
- Groin muscles
- Extensors of foot and toes

BACK VIEW

- Neck muscles
- Back muscles
- Deltoid
- Triceps
- Extensors of wrist and fingers
- Gluteus maximus
- Hamstring muscles
- Calf muscles
- Achilles tendon

Figure 11-1. The body has over 600 muscles. The shortening and lengthening of the muscles are what make the body move.

Most skeletal muscles are anchored to bone at each end by strong, cordlike, fibrous tissues called *tendons* (Figure 11-2). Muscles and their adjoining tendons extend across joints. When the brain sends a command to move, nerve impulses travel through the spinal cord and nerve pathways to the individual muscles and stimulate the muscle fibers to contract. When the muscle fibers contract, pulling the ends of the muscle closer together, the muscles pull the bones, causing motion at the joint.

Muscles in a group often pull at the same time. For instance, the hamstring muscles are a group of muscles at the back of the thigh. When the hamstrings contract, the leg bends at the knee joint. The biceps are a group of muscles at the front of the upper arm. When the biceps contract, the arm bends at the elbow joint. Generally, when one group of muscles contracts, another group of muscles on the opposite side of the body part relaxes. Even simple tasks, such as bending to pick up an object from the floor, involve a complex series of movements in which different muscle groups contract and relax.

Injuries to the brain, spinal cord or nerves can affect muscle control. A loss of muscle movement is called **paralysis.** Less serious or isolated muscle injuries may affect only strength because adjacent muscles can often do double duty and take over for the injured muscle.

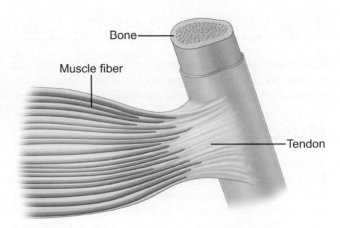

Figure 11-2. Most of the body's muscles are attached to bones by tendons.

Bones

The skeleton is formed from 206 bones of various sizes and shapes (Figure 11-3). The skeleton protects vital organs and other soft tissues. The skull protects the brain. The ribs protect the heart and lungs. The bones that form a canal called the spinal column protect the **spinal cord.**

Bones are hard, dense **tissues.** The strong, rigid structure of bones helps them to withstand stresses that cause injuries. The shape of bones depends on what the bones do and the stresses placed on them. For instance, although similar to the bones of the arms, the bones of the legs are much larger and stronger because they carry the body's weight.

Bones are classified as long, short, flat or irregular (Figure 11-4). Long bones are longer than they are wide and include the bones of the upper arm (humerus), the forearm (radius and ulna), the thigh (femur) and the lower leg (tibia and fibula). Short bones are about as wide as they are long and include the small bones of the hand (carpals) and feet (tarsals). Flat bones have a relatively thin, flat shape. Flat bones include the breastbone (sternum), the ribs and the shoulder blade (scapula). Bones that do not fit into the other categories are called irregular bones. Examples include the vertebrae and the bones that make up the skull, including the bones of the face. Bones are weakest at the points where they change shape, so they usually fracture at these points. In children, the bones are weakest at the growth plates, located at the ends of long bones.

Bones have a rich supply of blood and nerves. Some bones store and manufacture red blood cells within the sponge-like inner marrow and supply them to the circulating blood. Bone injuries can bleed and are usually painful. The bleeding can become life threatening if not properly cared for. Bones heal by developing new bone cells within a fibrous network of tissue that forms between the broken bone ends. Bone is the only body tissue that can regenerate in this way.

The bones of young children are softer and more porous than the bones of adults, so they bend and break more easily. Therefore, children are less likely to sprain a joint and more likely to break a bone. At puberty, a child's bones become as hard as an adult's. As people age, their bones lose mass and density and are more likely to give way to everyday stresses, which can cause significant injuries. For instance, an older person with significant bone loss can easily break the strongest bone in the body, the femur (thighbone), just by pivoting their weight on one leg. The gradual, progressive weakening of bone is called **osteoporosis.**

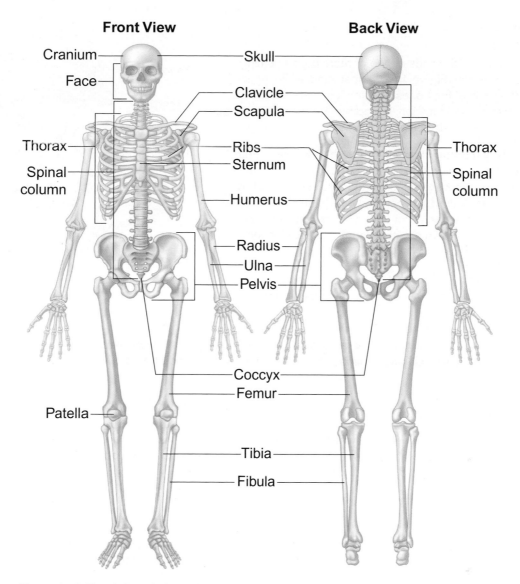

Front View   Back View

Cranium

Face

Skull

Clavicle

Scapula

Thorax

Ribs

Sternum

Spinal column

Humerus

Thorax

Spinal column

Radius

Ulna

Pelvis

Coccyx

Femur

Patella

Tibia

Fibula

Figure 11-3. The skeleton is formed from 206 bones in various sizes and shapes. The skeleton protects many of the organs inside the body.

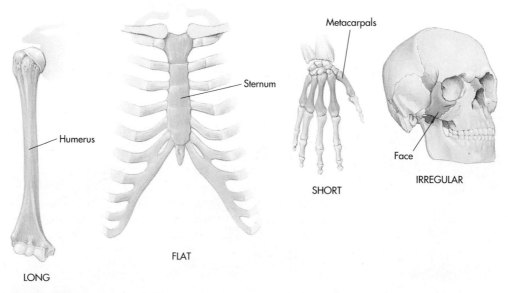

Metacarpals

Sternum

Humerus

Face

IRREGULAR

SHORT

LONG

FLAT

Figure 11-4. Bones vary in shape and size. Bones are weakest at the points where they change shape and usually fracture at these points.

Joints

A *joint* is formed by the ends of two or more bones coming together at one place (Figure 11-5). Most joints allow motion. However, the ends of the bones at some joints are fused together, which restricts motion. Fused bones, such as the bones of the skull, form solid structures that protect their contents.

Joints that allow movement are held together by tough, fibrous connective tissues called *ligaments.* Because ligaments actually resist joint movement, joints that are surrounded by ligaments have restricted movement, while joints that have few ligaments move more freely. For instance, the shoulder joint, with few ligaments, allows greater motion than the hip joint, although their structures are similar.

Joints that move more freely, such as the ankle and shoulder, have less natural support, which makes them more prone to injury. However, all joints have a normal range of movement. When a joint is forced beyond its normal range, ligaments stretch and tear, making the joint unstable. Unstable joints can be disabling, particularly when they are weight bearing, such as the knee or ankle. Unstable joints are also prone to re-injury and often develop arthritis in later years.

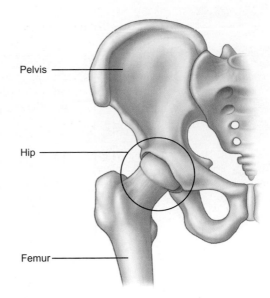

Figure 11-5. The ends of two or more bones coming together at one place form a joint.

Injuries to the Musculoskeletal System

Muscles, bones and joints are injured when a force is applied to them. Knowing the cause of injury can give you important clues about which parts of the body may be injured, what other hidden injuries might exist along with the more obvious ones and how serious the injuries may be.

There are three basic causes of musculoskeletal injury:

- Direct force causes injury at the point of impact and can either be blunt or penetrating (Figure 11-6, A). For example, a person might be hit by a loose pitch during a baseball game, fracturing the bone in the ankle. Or, penetrating objects, such as bullets and knives, can injure structures beneath the skin at the point where they penetrate.

- Indirect force transmits energy through the body and causes injury to a body part away from the point of impact (Figure 11-6, B). For example, a fall on an outstretched hand may result in an injury to the shoulder or collarbone.

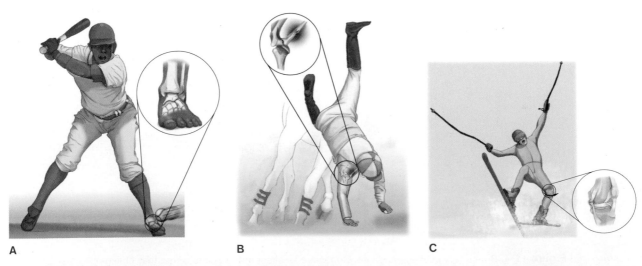

A   B   C

Figure 11-6, A–C. The three basic causes of musculoskeletal injury are **A,** direct force, **B,** indirect force and **C,** twisting force.

- Twisting force, or rotating force, causes injury when one part of the body remains still while the rest of the body is twisted or turned away from it (Figure 11-6, C). For example, if a ski and its binding keep the lower leg in one position while the body falls in another, the knee may be forced beyond its normal range of motion, causing injury. Twisting injuries are not always this complex. Twisting injuries more often occur from simply stepping off a curb (ankle) or turning to reach for an out-of-the-way object (back).

Types of Musculoskeletal Injuries

The four basic types of musculoskeletal injuries are fractures, dislocations, sprains and strains.

Fractures

A **fracture** is a break or disruption in bone tissue. Fractures include bones that are chipped or cracked, as well as bones that are broken all the way through (Figure 11-7). Direct and indirect forces, such as from a fall or a blow, commonly cause fractures. However, if strong enough, twisting forces can also cause a fracture. Some fractures are obvious, but others may not be easy to detect without further assessment. While most isolated fractures are not considered critical or life threatening, if the femur or pelvis is fractured, the person is at serious risk for excessive blood loss, shock and death. Fractures to the spine can also result in damage to the spinal cord.

Fractures are classified as either open or closed. **Closed fractures** leave the skin unbroken and are more common than open fractures (Figure 11-8, A). **Open fractures** occur when the skin over the fracture site is broken (Figure 11-8, B). An example of an open fracture is when a limb is severely angulated or bent, causing bone ends to tear the skin and surrounding soft tissues. Another example is when an object penetrates the skin and breaks the bone. Bone ends do not have to be visible in an open fracture. Open fractures are more serious than closed fractures because of the risks for severe blood loss and infection. Although fractures are rarely an immediate threat to life, any fracture involving a large bone, such as the femur or pelvis, can cause severe shock because bones and soft tissue may bleed heavily. Fractures can also be life threatening if they cover an artery or affect breathing.

Fractures are not always obvious unless a telltale sign, such as an open wound with protruding bone ends or a severely deformed body part, is present. The way in which the injury occurred, however, is often enough to suggest a possible fracture. A fall from a significant height or a motor vehicle crash could suggest a possible fracture.

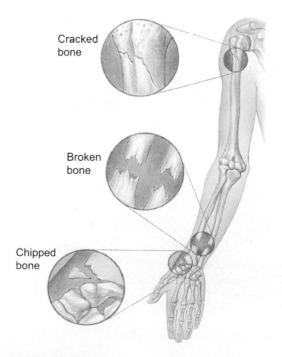

Figure 11-7. A fracture is a crack, complete break or chip in a bone.

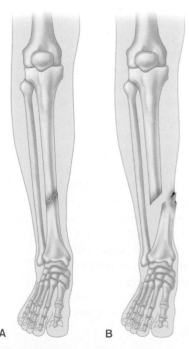

A   B

Figure 11-8, A–B. A, Closed fracture. **B,** Open fracture.

Dislocations

Dislocations are usually more obvious than fractures. A ***dislocation*** is a displacement or separation of a bone from its normal position at a joint (Figure 11-9). This movement is usually caused by a violent force tearing the ligaments that hold the bones in place. However, if a joint has been dislocated once and the ligaments holding the bones in place were damaged, subsequent dislocations are then more likely to occur. In some cases, dislocation can become chronic so that relatively minor movements can cause joint instability. When a bone is moved out of place, the joint no longer functions. The displaced end of the bone often forms a bump, a ridge or a hollow that does not normally exist.

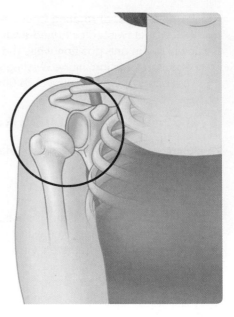

Figure 11-9. A dislocation is a separation of a bone from its normal position at a joint.

> **What if...** *A person has a dislocated finger? Is it OK to "pop" it back into place? I know people who have done this before without any problems.*
>
> *As a trained lay responder, you should never attempt to "pop" (or technically speaking, reduce) a dislocated joint, not even a finger. This can cause additional damage to the normal articulation of the bone as well as associated tendon, ligament, vascular and neurological damage. Only a licensed medical professional should perform reduction or realignment of a joint dislocation if deemed appropriate.*

Some joints, such as the shoulder or finger, dislocate easily because they are relatively exposed and not as well protected by ligaments. Other joints, such as joints of the elbow or spine, are well protected because of the shape of the bones and the way they fit together; therefore, they dislocate less easily.

A force strong enough to cause an initial dislocation can also cause a fractured bone, bleeding and nerve damage. It is important to check for those injuries as well. A dislocation can be extremely painful.

Sprains

A ***sprain*** is the partial or complete tearing or stretching of ligaments and other tissues at a joint (Figure 11-10). A sprain usually results when the bones that form a joint are forced beyond their normal or usual range of motion. The more ligaments are stretched or torn, the more severe the injury. The sudden, violent forcing of a joint beyond its range of motion can completely rupture ligaments and even dislocate the bones. Severe sprains may also involve a fracture of the bones that form the joint. Ligaments may pull bone away from their point of attachment. Young children are more likely to have a fracture than a sprain because their ligaments are stronger than their bones.

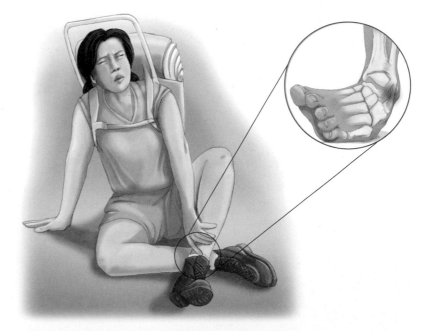

Figure 11-10. A sprain is the tearing of ligaments at a joint.

Mild sprains, which stretch ligament fibers, generally heal quickly. The person may have only a brief period of pain or discomfort and quickly return to activity with little or no soreness. For this reason, people often neglect sprains and the joint is often re-injured. Severe sprains or sprains that involve a fracture usually cause pain when the joint is moved or used. The weight-bearing joints of the ankle and knee and the joints of the fingers and wrist are those most commonly sprained.

Surprisingly, a sprain can be more disabling than a fracture. When fractures heal, they usually leave the bone as strong as it was before, or stronger, decreasing the likelihood that a second break will occur at the same spot. On the other hand, ligaments cannot regenerate. If a torn ligament(s) is not repaired, it can render the joint less stable and may impede motion. The injured area may also be more susceptible to re-injury.

Strains

A **strain** is the excessive stretching and tearing of muscle fibers or tendons (Figure 11-11). A strain is sometimes called a muscle pull or tear. Because tendons are tougher and stronger than muscles, tears usually occur in the muscle itself or where the muscle attaches to the tendon. Strains often result from overexertion, such as lifting something too heavy or working a muscle too long. They can also result from sudden or uncoordinated movement. Strains commonly involve the muscles in the neck or back, the front or back of the thigh, or the back of the lower leg. Strains of the neck and lower back can be particularly painful and therefore disabling.

Like sprains, strains are often neglected, which commonly leads to re-injury. Strains sometimes recur

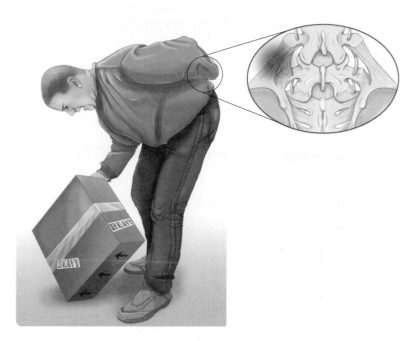

Figure 11-11. A strain is the stretching and tearing of muscles or tendons.

chronically, especially to the muscles of the neck, lower back and the back of the thigh. Neck and back problems are two of the leading causes of absenteeism from work, accounting annually for billions of dollars in workers' compensation claims and lost productivity.

Checking for Musculoskeletal Injuries

You will identify and care for injuries to the musculoskeletal system during the head-to-toe check for non-life-threatening conditions. Because musculoskeletal injuries look alike, you may have difficulty determining exactly what type of injury has occurred. Usually only a trained medical professional can tell the difference between a sprain, strain, fracture or dislocation, often with the use of an X-ray, computed tomography (CT) scan or magnetic resonance imaging (MRI). However, you do not need to know what kind of injury a person has in order to give the appropriate care. The primary goal of care is to prevent further injury and get medical attention for the person.

As you check the person, think about how the body normally looks and feels. Ask how the injury happened and if there are any areas that are painful. Visually inspect the entire body, beginning with the head. Compare the two sides of the body. Then, carefully visually check each body part. Do not ask the person to move any areas in which they have pain or discomfort or if you suspect injury to the head, neck or spine. Start with the neck, followed by the shoulders, the chest and so on. Check each extremity separately so you can determine where any pain originated. As you conduct the check, look for clues that may indicate a musculoskeletal injury.

Keep in mind that if there was sufficient force to fracture a bone or dislocate a joint, that force may also cause internal injuries leading to internal bleeding and the possibility of shock. Fractures and dislocations can cause severe pain, and the person may be so focused on the pain that they will not mention other problems, such as abdominal pain, which may actually indicate more serious injuries.

Signs and Symptoms of Musculoskeletal Injuries

Always suspect a serious musculoskeletal injury when any of the following signs or symptoms are present:

- There was a snapping sound. If a bone has fractured, the person may report hearing or feeling the bone snap or break.

- There is pain. One of the most common symptoms in any muscle, bone or joint injury is pain. The injured area may be very painful to touch or move.

- There is significant bruising and swelling. The area may be swollen and red or bruised.

- There is significant deformity. The area may be twisted or strangely bent compared with the uninjured side (Figure 11-12).

- The injured area has visible abnormal lumps, ridges and hollows (i.e., deformities).

- The person is unable to use the affected part normally. This may be due to pain or a dislocated joint.

- There are bone fragments sticking out of a wound.

- The person feels bones grating. Crepitus, or a grating sound or feeling, occurs when two pieces of bone rub together.

- The injured area is cold, numb and tingly.

- The cause of the injury suggests that it may be severe.

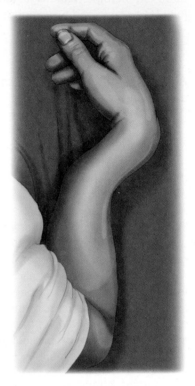

Figure 11-12. Areas of serious bone or joint injury may appear deformed.

Obvious deformities, such as abnormal lumps, ridges, depressions or unusual angles in body parts, are often a sign of a fracture or dislocation. Dislocations are generally more obvious than other musculoskeletal injuries because the joint appears deformed. Comparing the injured part with an uninjured part may help you detect a deformity.

Pain, swelling and discoloration of the skin commonly occur with any significant musculoskeletal injury. The injured area may be painful to touch and to move. Swelling and discoloration of the skin surrounding the injury may be evident; these are due to bleeding from damaged blood vessels and tissues in the injured area. Swelling may appear rapidly at the site of injury, develop gradually or not appear at all. At first, the skin may only look red. As blood seeps to the skin's surface, the area begins to look bruised.

A person's inability to move or use an injured part may also indicate a significant injury. The person may tell you they are unable to move the part or that moving the injured part is simply too painful. For injuries to a leg, a person may not be able to put weight onto their foot for walking. Often, the muscles of an affected area contract in an attempt to hold the injured part in place. This muscle contraction helps to reduce pain and prevent further injury. Similarly, a person often supports the injured part in the most comfortable position. To manage musculoskeletal injuries, avoid any movement of an injured body part that causes pain.

A lack of sensation in the affected part can indicate serious injury or injury in another area. Fingers or toes, for example, can lose sensation if the arm or leg is injured. Also, check the person's skin below the injured site (toward the fingers or toes) for feeling, warmth and color. Skin that is cold to the touch or bluish in color indicates a lack of or reduced circulation below the site of the injury.

Care for Musculoskeletal Injuries

A gentle, reassuring approach is important in caring for a person with muscle, bone and joint injury. The person is likely to be experiencing severe pain and may be frightened. Avoid moving the injured part of the person's body; keep the injured area stable in the position found until more advanced medical personnel take over.

Call 9-1-1 or the designated emergency number for a musculoskeletal injury if:

- There is obvious deformity.

- There is moderate or severe swelling and discoloration.

- Bones sound or feel like they are rubbing together.

- A snap or pop was heard or felt at the time of the injury.

- There is a fracture with an open wound at, or bone piercing through, the injury site.

- The injured person cannot move or use the affected part normally.

- The injured area is cold and numb.

- The injury involves the head, neck or spine.

- The injured person has trouble breathing.

- The cause of the injury suggests that the injury may be severe.

- It is not possible to safely or comfortably move the person to a vehicle for transport to a hospital.

The general care for musculoskeletal injuries includes following the mnemonic RICE: rest, immobilize, cold and elevate.

> **What if...** *A person has an angulated fracture of the tibia or radius? On television they always seem to realign these fractures to prevent further injury. Should I do this too?*
>
> *You should* never *attempt to realign an angulated fracture. Instead, follow the care steps outlined in this chapter, and call 9-1-1 or the designated emergency number immediately so that the person can receive advanced medical care as quickly as possible.*

Rest

Avoid any movements or activities that cause pain. Do not move or straighten the injured area; do not try to straighten angulated fractures. Help the person find the most comfortable position to rest in until help arrives.

If you suspect injuries to the head, neck or spine, remind the person to remain still, and avoid moving their head or neck until EMS arrives. Do *not* hold the person's head or try to forcibly restrict their movement as this may only lead to further complications. If you are alone and have to leave to get help, place the person in the recovery position (see Chapter 5).

Immobilize

If you suspect a serious musculoskeletal injury, you must ***immobilize*** the injured part (keep it from moving) before giving the additional care described below. The purposes of immobilizing an injury are to:

- Lessen pain.

- Prevent further damage to soft tissues.

- Reduce the risk for severe bleeding.

- Reduce the possibility of loss of circulation to the injured part.

- Prevent closed fractures from becoming open fractures.

An injured area should be stabilized in the position found. Often, this is as simple as using the ground to provide support to an injured leg, ankle or foot; or letting the person cradle an injured elbow or arm in a position of comfort.

Splint the injured part only if the injured person must be moved or transported by non-professional emergency personnel to a medical facility for treatment. When using a splint, follow these four basic principles:

- Splint *only* if you have to move the injured person and can do so without causing more pain and discomfort to the person.

- Splint an injury in the position in which you find it. Do not move, straighten or bend angulated bones or joints.

- Splint the injured area and the joints or bones above and below the injury site.

- Check for proper circulation (feeling, warmth and color) before and after splinting. If circulation has changed with splinting, loosen the splint slightly and reassess circulation.

Chapter 12 discusses splinting in detail.

Do not use a pressure immobilization bandage as there is no evidence to support its effectiveness in the care of an injured extremity.

Cold

Cold helps reduce swelling and eases pain and discomfort. You can make a cold pack by filling a plastic bag with ice and water or by using a large bag of frozen vegetables, such as peas. You can also use a commercial cold pack if other options are not available. Always place a layer of gauze or cloth between the source of cold and the skin to prevent damage to the skin.

Leave a cold pack on the injured part for no longer than 20 minutes. If continued cold is needed, remove the cold pack for 20 minutes, then reapply a new cold pack for an additional 20 minutes. If 20 minutes cannot be tolerated, apply a cold pack for periods of 10 minutes.

Do not apply a cold pack to an open fracture. This could put pressure on the open fracture site, which could cause discomfort to the person and possibly make the injury worse. Instead, place the cold packs around the site. Do not apply heat to any acute musculoskeletal injury as there is no evidence that applying heat helps.

Myth-Information. *Myth: Apply heat to a muscle, bone or joint injury to speed healing.* Although applying heat is commonly used to relieve pain associated with chronic muscle, bone and joint conditions such as arthritis, it is not the best treatment for an acute muscle, bone or joint injury. Applying heat causes the blood vessels in the area to dilate (widen), bringing more blood to the area and increasing swelling. Cold, on the other hand, causes blood vessels to constrict (narrow), reducing blood flow to the area, helping to reduce swelling. In addition, applying cold slows nerve impulses, helping to reduce pain.

What if… *A friend or family member has a sprained ankle for which emergency medical care is not needed? How long should a cold pack be used on the injury?*

Soft tissue injuries such as joint sprains and strains respond well to the application of a cold pack. Specifically, the application of cold assists in decreasing hemorrhaging and swelling by causing a narrowing of the blood vessels (vasoconstriction). The reduction in swelling also assists in reducing the effects of inflammation and may ease a person's pain and discomfort. That said, the length of application of a cold pack is dependent on the severity of the injury and the presence of the signs and symptoms of inflammation (e.g., heat, redness, swelling, pain and loss of function) rather than a predetermined time frame. Use cold packs as long as needed to help the person see a reduction in pain and swelling.

Elevate

Elevating the injured area above the level of the heart helps slow the flow of blood, reducing swelling. Elevation is particularly effective in controlling swelling in extremity injuries. However, you should only elevate the injured part if it does not cause more pain. In addition, do not attempt to elevate a seriously injured area of a limb unless it has been immobilized.

Considerations for Transporting a Person

Some injuries, such as a suspected broken finger, may not require you to call 9-1-1 or the designated emergency number, yet they still need medical attention. When transporting the person to a medical facility, bring someone along or have someone else drive. This way you can keep an eye on the person and give care if needed. Injuries to the pelvis, hip or thigh can be life threatening. A person with such an injury should not be moved unnecessarily. Minimizing movement until emergency medical services (EMS) personnel take over can help to prevent the injury from becoming worse.

Summary

Sometimes it is difficult to tell whether an injury is a fracture, dislocation, sprain or strain. Because you cannot be sure which type of injury a person might have, always care for the injury as if it were serious. If EMS personnel are on the way, do not move the person. Control any bleeding. Take steps to minimize shock, monitor the person's airway and breathing, and reassure and comfort the person. If you need to transport the person to a medical facility yourself, be sure to immobilize the injury before moving the person.

READY TO RESPOND? >

Think back to Kelly in the opening scenario, and use what you have learned to respond to these questions:

1. What types of musculoskeletal injuries could Kelly have as a result of her fall?

2. What would indicate that Kelly's injury is severe?

3. What can you do to make Kelly more comfortable?

Study Questions

1. **Match each item with the correct definition.**

   a. Bone   d. Joint   g. Skeletal muscles   j. Strain

   b. Dislocation   e. Ligaments   h. Splint   k. Tendon

   c. Fracture   f. Muscle   i. Sprain

   ____ Device used to keep body parts from moving

   ____ Displacement of a bone from its normal position at a joint

   ____ Tissue that contracts and relaxes to create movement

   ____ Broken bone

   ____ Dense, hard tissue that forms the skeleton

   ____ Injury that stretches and tears ligaments and other soft tissues at joints

   ____ Fibrous band attaching muscle to bone

   ____ Structure formed where two or more bones meet

   ____ Injury that stretches and tears muscles and tendons

   ____ Muscles that attach to bones

   ____ Fibrous bands holding bones together at joints

2. **List the reasons to call 9-1-1 or the designated emergency number for a musculoskeletal injury.**

3. **List four principles of splinting.**

In questions 4 through 8, circle the letter of the correct answer.

4. **Which should you do when caring for an injured joint?**

   a. Have the person immediately move the injured area.

   b. Straighten the injured area before splinting.

   c. Apply cold to the injured area.

   d. Keep the injured area below the level of the heart.

(Continued)

Study Questions continued

5. Signs of a serious musculoskeletal injury include—

a. Feeling, warmth and color below the site of the injury.

b. Deformity or bone fragments protruding from a wound.

c. The person was hit in the thigh by a softball.

d. Ability to move the injured area.

6. You find a person lying quietly on the ground. Their right leg is twisted at an unusual angle and you can see protruding bones and blood. The scene is safe and there is *no* severe, life-threatening bleeding. Which do you do first?

a. Straighten the leg.

b. Check for life-threatening conditions.

c. Use direct pressure to stop the bleeding.

d. Look for material to use to immobilize the injured area.

7. Why should you immobilize a musculoskeletal injury?

a. To prevent further injury to soft tissues

b. To eliminate all discomfort or pain

c. To control severe bleeding

d. To help the person to heal

8. Which step would you take before and after splinting an injury?

a. Tell the person to move the injured area.

b. Check for feeling, warmth and color.

c. Slide the splint down to extend below the injured area.

d. Elevate the legs 8 inches.

Answers are listed in the Appendix.

12

INJURIES TO THE EXTREMITIES

You decide to run a few miles to the park to meet your friend Sue and do some additional exercise with her. As you prepare to set off again together, Sue suddenly loses her balance and falls backwards. Luckily, she does not hit her head, but she does cut her leg near her ankle. Her leg is bleeding and she cannot move her ankle without serious pain.

Learn and Respond ▶

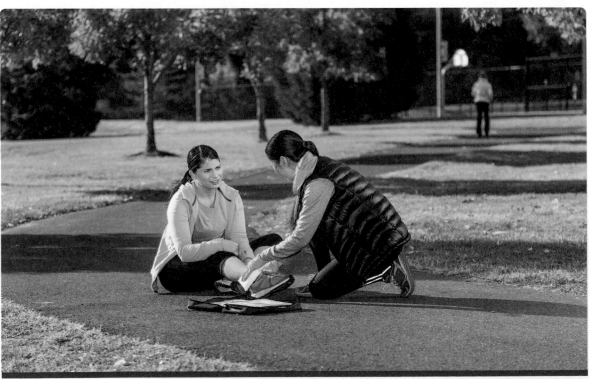

After reading this chapter, you should be able to:

- Describe the reasons for immobilizing an injury to an extremity.

- Describe the general guidelines for splinting.

- Describe how to care for injuries to the shoulder, upper arm and elbow.

- Describe how to care for injuries to the forearm, wrist and hand.

- List three specific signs and symptoms of a fractured femur.

- Describe how to care for injuries to the femur, knee and lower leg.

- Describe how to care for injuries to the ankle and foot.

After reading this chapter and completing the class activities, you should be able to:

- Demonstrate how to effectively immobilize an injured extremity using an anatomic, soft or rigid splint.

- Demonstrate how to effectively immobilize an upper extremity injury using a sling and a binder.

```
┌  KEY TERMS  ┐
```

Binder: A cloth wrapped around a person to securely hold the arm against the person's chest to add stability; also called a *swathe*.

Extremity: A limb of the body; *upper extremity* is the arm; *lower extremity* is the leg.

Forearm: The part of the upper extremity from the elbow to the wrist.

Lower extremity: The parts of the body from the hip to the toes.

Lower leg: The part of the lower extremity from the knee to the ankle.

Thigh: The part of the lower extremity from the pelvis to the knee.

Upper arm: The part of the upper extremity from the shoulder to the elbow.

Upper extremity: The parts of the body from the shoulder to the fingers.

Introduction

Injuries to an ***extremity***—an arm or leg—are quite common. They can range from a simple contusion to a severe, painful, life-threatening injury, such as a fracture of the femur (thighbone). The prompt care you give can help prevent further pain, damage and a lifelong disability.

The extremities consist of bones, soft tissues, blood vessels and nerves. They are subject to various kinds of injury. Injury can affect the soft tissues, resulting in open or closed wounds. Injury can also affect the musculoskeletal system, resulting in sprains, strains, fractures or dislocations. You learned about giving care for soft tissue and musculoskeletal injuries in Chapters 10 and 11. This chapter will provide more specific information on how to care for these types of injuries when they involve the extremities.

Immobilizing Serious Extremity Injuries

As you learned in Chapter 11, if you suspect a serious musculoskeletal injury, you must immobilize the injured part before moving the injured person or giving additional care, such as applying cold or elevating the injured extremity. Always suspect a serious extremity injury when any of the following signs or symptoms are present:

- Pain or tenderness
- Swelling
- Discoloration
- Deformity of the limb
- Inability to move or use the limb

- Inability to bear weight on an injured leg
- Severe external and/or internal bleeding
- Loss of sensation or feeling, or tingling
- A limb that is cold to the touch

Immobilizing an injury serves to:

- Lessen pain.
- Prevent further damage to soft tissues.
- Reduce the risk for severe bleeding.

- Reduce the possibility of loss of circulation to the injured part.
- Prevent closed fractures from becoming open fractures.

Generally, immobilizing an injury simply requires stabilizing it in the position found. For example, an injured leg stretched out on the ground is supported by the ground. However, if a person must be moved or transported in order to seek additional medical attention, and it does not cause more pain, you will use a splint to immobilize the extremity before moving the person.

A tool or device used to immobilize an injured extremity is called a splint. There are many commercially manufactured types of splints, but if necessary one can be improvised from items available at the scene.

Types of Splints

Splints are commercially made or can be improvised from materials on hand. As a trained lay responder, there are three types of splints you are likely to use—soft, rigid and anatomic:

- Soft splints, as the name suggests, include soft materials such as folded blankets, towels, pillows or a folded triangular bandage (cravat) (Figure 12-1). A sling is a specific kind of soft splint that uses a triangular bandage to provide stability and support when the shoulder, elbow or upper arm has been injured. A sling may be used in conjunction with a **binder** (also referred to as a *swathe*) to immobilize the injury and support the weight of the arm.

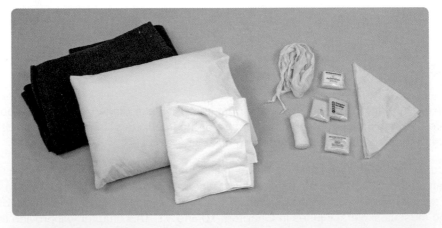

Figure 12-1. Folded blankets, towels, pillows or a triangular bandage tied as a sling can be used as soft splints.

- Rigid splints include padded boards, folded magazines or newspapers, and padded metal strips that do not have any sharp edges (Figure 12-2).

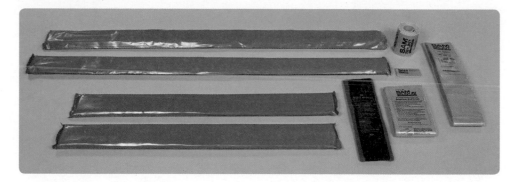

Figure 12-2. Commercially made rigid splints are available (shown), but many items, such as padded boards or folded newspapers, can be used.

- Anatomic splints use the person's own body as a splint (Figure 12-3). For example, an arm can be splinted to the chest; an injured leg can be splinted to the uninjured leg.

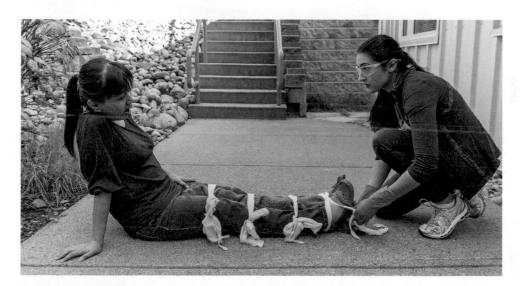

Figure 12-3. An anatomic splint uses a part of the body as the splint. *Photo: courtesy of the Canadian Red Cross*

Applying a Splint

No matter where the splint will be applied, or what the injury is, there are some general rules for splinting (see Skill Sheets 12-1 to 12-4). To splint an injured body part:

- Support the injured part in the position in which you find it. If possible, have the person or a bystander help you.

- Check the body part that is on the other side of the injury for circulation (feeling, warmth and color) before and after splinting to make sure the splint is not too tight.

- Apply the splint to immobilize the bones or joints both above and below an injured area (Figure 12-4). For example, if a bone in the lower leg is broken, use the splint to immobilize the knee and ankle.

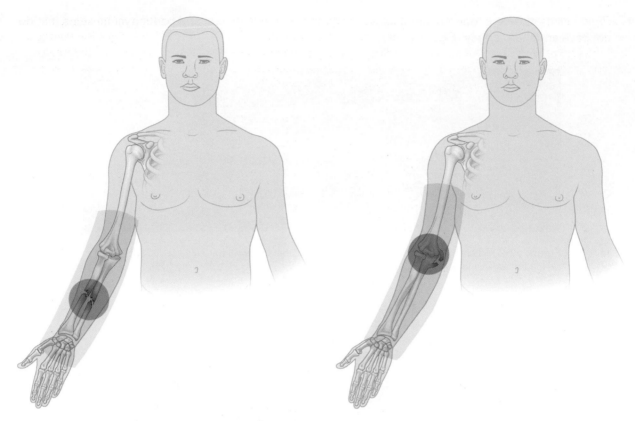

Figure 12-4. For fractures, splint the joints both above and below the site of the injury.

■ Cut off or remove any clothing around the injury site. If the person is wearing a watch or jewelry near the injury, these should be removed as swelling may occur beyond the actual injury site. For example, if an elbow is injured, any bracelets, watches or rings should be removed and given to the injured person for storage.

■ Cover any bleeding or open wounds, including open fractures, with sterile dressings and carefully bandage with minimal pressure before splinting.

■ Do *not* try to push protruding bones back below the skin.

■ Do *not* attempt to straighten any angulated fracture; always splint the limb in the position found.

■ Do *not* allow the person to bear weight on an injured lower extremity.

■ Pad the splints you are using so that they will be more comfortable and conform to the shape of the injured body part.

■ Secure the splint in place with cravats, roller bandages or other wide strips of cloth. Avoid securing the splint directly over an open wound or the injury.

■ Elevate the splinted part if doing so does not cause the person discomfort.

After the injured extremity has been immobilized, apply cold to the injured area to help minimize pain and swelling. Be sure to place a thin barrier between the source of cold and the skin. Help the person rest in the most comfortable position, and comfort and reassure them. Do *not* apply ice or a cold pack directly over an open fracture, because doing so would require you to put pressure on the open fracture site and could cause discomfort to the person. Instead, place cold packs around the site. Do *not* apply heat to an acute musculoskeletal injury.

Take steps to minimize shock, including placing the person in a lying or supine position and preventing the person from becoming chilled or overheated. As you determine what additional care might be needed, continue to watch for signs of shock, including monitoring the person's level of consciousness, breathing, skin color and temperature. Be alert for any signs such as changes in breathing rate, skin color or level of consciousness that may indicate the person's condition is worsening.

Upper Extremity Injuries

The term **upper extremity,** or arm, describes the parts of the body from the shoulders to the fingers. The bones of the upper extremities include the collarbone **(clavicle),** shoulder blade **(scapula),** bone from the shoulder to the elbow **(humerus),** forearm **(radius** and **ulna),** wrist **(carpals),** hand **(metacarpals)** and fingers **(phalanges).** The upper extremities also include several major blood vessels and nerves. Figure 12-5 shows the major structures of the upper extremities.

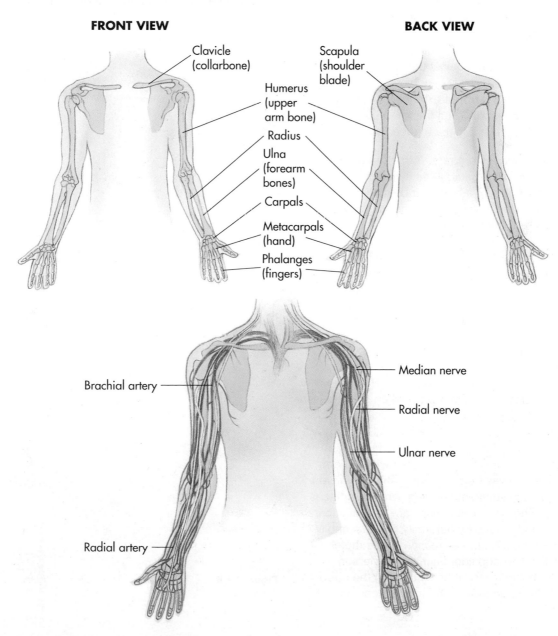

Figure 12-5. Major structures of the upper extremities.

The upper extremities are among the most commonly injured areas of the body. The most frequent cause of injury is falling on the hand of an outstretched arm. Because a falling person instinctively tries to break their fall by extending the arms and hands, these areas receive the force of the body's weight, which can cause a serious injury.

Shoulder Injuries

The shoulder consists of three bones that meet to form the shoulder joint. These bones are the clavicle, scapula and humerus. The most common shoulder injuries are sprains. However, injuries to the shoulder may also involve a fracture or dislocation of one or more of these bones.

The most frequently injured bone of the shoulder is the clavicle. Clavicle injuries are more common in children than adults. Typically, the clavicle is fractured or separates from its normal position at either end of the bone as a result of a fall onto the shoulder (Figure 12-6). An injury commonly occurs when the impact from a fall forces the outer end of the clavicle to separate from the joint where it touches the scapula. The person usually feels pain in the shoulder area, which may radiate down the upper extremity. A person with a clavicle injury usually attempts to ease the pain by holding the arm against the chest. Because the clavicle lies directly over major blood vessels and nerves to the upper extremity, it is especially important to immobilize a fractured clavicle promptly to prevent injury to these structures.

Scapula fractures are rare. A fracture of the scapula typically results from a violent force, such as a fall from a height or being hit by a car. Because it takes great force to fracture the scapula, you should look for additional injuries to the head, neck, spine or chest. The most significant signs and symptoms of a fractured scapula are extreme pain in the upper back over the shoulder blade and the inability to move the shoulder. If the chest cavity is injured, the person may have trouble breathing.

A dislocation of the shoulder joint is another common type of shoulder injury. Like fractures, dislocations often result from falls. They also often result from a direct blow when the arm is in the throwing position. Such dislocations happen frequently in sports, such as football and rugby, when a player attempts to break a fall with an outstretched arm or gets tackled with the arm positioned away from the body. This movement can result in ligaments tearing, which displaces bones. Shoulder dislocations are painful and can often be identified by deformity and the inability to bring the affected extremity across the chest. As with other shoulder injuries, the person often tries to minimize the pain by holding the upper extremity in the most comfortable position.

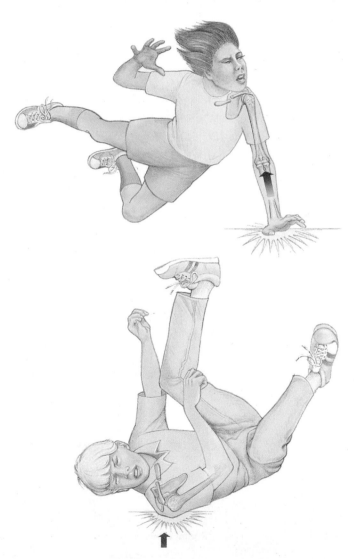

Figure 12-6. A clavicle fracture is usually caused by a fall onto the shoulder.

Care for Shoulder Injuries

To care for shoulder injuries:

- Do not move or straighten the injured area. Stabilize the injury in the position found. If an injured person is holding the forearm securely against the chest, do not change the position. Holding the arm against the chest is an effective method of immobilization. Allow the person to continue to support the upper extremity in the position in which they are holding it, usually the most comfortable position.

- Control any external bleeding with direct pressure, unless the bleeding is located directly over a suspected fracture. With a fracture, apply pressure around the area. Always wear disposable latex-free gloves or use another protective barrier.

- If the person is holding the upper extremity away from the body, use a pillow, rolled blanket or similar object to fill the gap between the upper extremity and chest to provide support for the injured area.

- If you must transport or move the person, and it does not cause more pain, splint the upper extremity in place using the guidelines described earlier in the chapter. Place the upper extremity in a sling and, if possible and tolerable for the person, bind it to the chest with cravats (sling and binder) to further stabilize the injury (Figure 12-7). For a suspected shoulder dislocation, you may need to use pillows under the arm between the chest and shoulder to support the area.

- Apply a cold pack.

- Take steps to minimize shock.

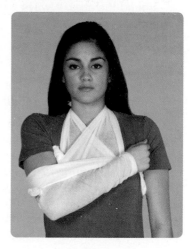

Figure 12-7. Splint for a shoulder injury.

Upper Arm Injuries

The **upper arm** is the area that extends from the shoulder to the elbow. The bone of the upper arm is the humerus. The humerus is the largest bone in the arm.

The humerus can be fractured at any point, although it is usually fractured at the upper end near the shoulder or in the middle of the bone. The upper end of the humerus often fractures in older adults and in young children as a result of a fall onto the shoulder and upper arm. Breaks in the middle of the bone mostly occur in young adults. When the humerus is fractured, the blood vessels and nerves supplying the entire upper extremity may be damaged. Most humerus fractures are very painful and the person will most likely not be able to use the injured arm. Do not permit the person to use the arm. A humerus fracture can also cause considerable deformity.

> **What if...** *I need to transport someone with a shoulder injury and I do not have a splint or triangular bandages in my kit to immobilize the injury?*
>
> *In a majority of cases, a responsive person with an injury to the shoulder (i.e., scapula or clavicle) will attempt to ease the pain by holding the arm against the chest. However, if you need to transport the person and splinting material is not readily available, an improvised sling and binder, or at least a sling, can be produced easier than you may think. Two simple methods are using a belt as a sling and/ or placing the involved extremity inside a jacket or button-down shirt as a binder. Even better, when designing a first aid kit for home or recreational use, consider adding at least four 40 × 40 × 56-inch triangular bandages. While many preassembled kits come with one such bandage, a minimum of four would be necessary to immobilize a forearm injury or lower leg injury, while two or three are needed for a sling and binder, depending on a person's torso size. A small pillow makes an excellent improvised soft splint for shoulder dislocations. Gently wedge the pillow between the arm and chest or abdomen and secure it around the chest with two end-to-end cravats.*

Care for Upper Arm Injuries

In general, care for upper arm injuries in the same way as for shoulder injuries.

■ Do not move or straighten the injured area. Stabilize the injury in the position found.

■ Control any external bleeding with direct pressure, unless the bleeding is located directly over a suspected fracture. With a fracture, apply pressure around the area. Always wear disposable latex-free gloves or use another protective barrier.

■ If you must transport or move the person, and it does not cause more pain, splint an upper arm injury using a padded rigid splint on the outside of the arm.

○ If the elbow can be comfortably bent, place the upper extremity in a sling and binder to further stabilize the injury.

○ If the elbow cannot be comfortably bent, or if the rigid splint you are using is longer than the upper arm, keep the arm straight at the person's side and wrap bandages or binders around the arm and chest (Figure 12-8).

■ Apply a cold pack.

■ Take steps to minimize shock. Most people with an injured shoulder or upper arm will prefer to be in a seated or semi-recumbent position and will have difficulty lying down.

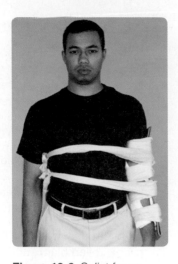

Figure 12-8. Splint for an upper arm injury.

Elbow Injuries

The elbow is a joint formed by the humerus and the two bones of the forearm, the radius and the ulna. Injuries to the elbow can cause permanent disability, because all the nerves and blood vessels to the forearm and hand go through the elbow. Therefore, treat elbow injuries seriously.

Like other joints, the elbow can be sprained, fractured or dislocated. Injuries to a joint such as the elbow can be made worse by movement because movement can easily damage the nerves and blood vessels located in the elbow. An injured elbow may be in a bent or straight position.

Care for Elbow Injuries

To give care for elbow injuries:

■ Do not move or straighten the injured area. Stabilize the injury in the position found.

■ Control any external bleeding with direct pressure, unless the bleeding is located directly over a suspected fracture. With a fracture, apply pressure around the area. Always wear disposable latex-free gloves or use another protective barrier.

■ If you must transport or move the person, and it does not cause more pain, splint the arm from the shoulder to the wrist in the best way possible in the position you find it.

○ If the elbow is bent, even if it is deformed, splint with a sling and consider the use of a binder if necessary and tolerable for the person (Figure 12-9).

○ If the elbow is straight, immobilize the elbow with rigid splints along the length of both sides of the arm, from fingertips to the underarm.

■ Apply a cold pack.

■ Shock is unlikely with isolated upper extremity injuries. If shock is suspected, assess the person for other injuries and have the person lie down flat on their back if possible.

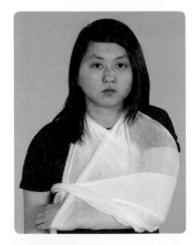

Figure 12-9. Splint for an elbow injury.

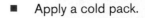

Forearm, Wrist and Hand Injuries

The **forearm** is the area between the elbow and the wrist. The wrist is a joint formed by the hand and forearm. Injuries to the wrist may involve one or both of the two forearm bones, the radius and ulna. The hand consists of many small bones—the carpals, metacarpals and phalanges. Serious injuries to the wrists and hands can significantly impact a person's daily activities.

If a person falls on an outstretched upper extremity, both forearm bones may break. When both forearm bones fracture, the arm may look S-shaped (Figure 12-10). Because the radial artery and nerve are close to these bones, a fracture may cause severe bleeding or loss of movement in the wrist and hand. The wrist is a common location for sprains and fractures. It is often difficult to tell the extent of the injury.

Because the hands are used in so many daily activities, they are susceptible to injury. Most injuries to the hands and fingers involve minor soft tissue damage. However, a serious injury may damage nerves, blood vessels and bones. Home, recreational and industrial mishaps often produce lacerations, avulsions, burns and fractures of the hands.

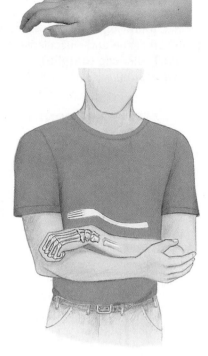

Figure 12-10. Fractures of both forearm bones often have a characteristic S-shaped deformity.

Care for Forearm, Wrist and Hand Injuries

To give care for forearm, wrist or hand injuries:

- Do not move or straighten the injured area. Stabilize the injury in the position found.

- Control any external bleeding with direct pressure, unless the bleeding is located directly over a suspected fracture. With a fracture, apply pressure around the area. Always wear disposable latex-free gloves or use another protective barrier.

- If you must transport or move the person, and it does not cause more pain:

  ○ Support an injured forearm or wrist by placing a rigid splint underneath the forearm, from the elbow to the fingertips. A sling and binder can then be applied to support the arm against the chest.

  ○ If a single finger is injured, you may be able to create an anatomic splint by taping the injured finger to the one beside it. You can also improvise a rigid splint by taping the injured area to a small object, such as a popsicle stick or tongue depressor (Figure 12-11).

  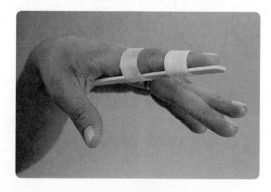

  Figure 12-11. A popsicle stick or tongue depressor can be used to splint a finger injury.

  ○ For several broken fingers or when the back of the hand is involved in the injury, place a rolled up bandage or a small ball in the palm of the person's hand with the fingers curled naturally around it, then wrap the entire hand and splint the lower arm and wrist with a rigid splint. A sling can be added to help support the arm.

- Apply a cold pack.

- Take steps to minimize shock. If shock is suspected, assess the person for other injuries and have the person lie down flat on their back if possible.

Lower Extremity Injuries

Injuries to the leg, or ***lower extremity***—the part of the body from the hip (pelvis) to the toes—can involve both soft tissue and musculoskeletal damage. The lower extremity includes the pelvic bones, thighbone **(femur),** kneecap **(patella),** two bones in the lower leg **(tibia** and **fibula),** bones of the ankle **(tarsals),** foot **(metatarsals)** and toes **(phalanges).** Figure 12-12 shows the major structures of the lower extremities.

FRONT VIEW

BACK VIEW

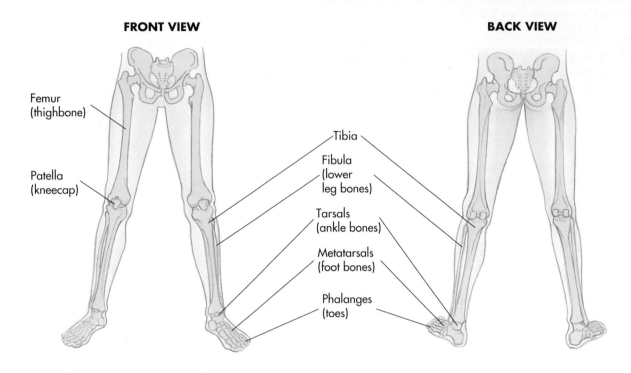

Femur (thighbone)

Patella (kneecap)

Tibia

Fibula (lower leg bones)

Tarsals (ankle bones)

Metatarsals (foot bones)

Phalanges (toes)

Figure 12-12. Major structures of the lower extremities.

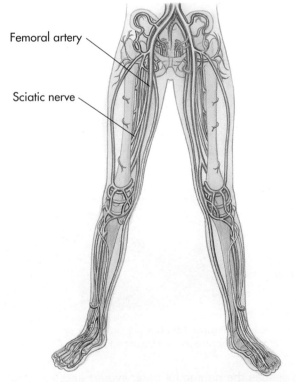

Femoral artery

Sciatic nerve

Thigh Injuries

The femur is the largest bone in the body. It is located in the *thigh,* which is located between the pelvis and the knee. The **femoral arteries** are the major supplier of blood to the lower extremities. Because of the size and strength of the femur, a significant amount of force is required to cause a fracture. When the femur is fractured, the adjacent blood vessels and nerves may be damaged. If a femoral artery is damaged, the blood loss can be life threatening.

Thigh injuries range from bruises and torn muscles to severe injuries, such as fractures or hip or knee dislocations. Most femur fractures involve the upper end of the bone where the femur meets the pelvis at the hip joint (Figure 12-13). Although the hip joint is not involved, such injuries are often called hip fractures.

A fracture of the femur usually produces a characteristic deformity. Because the thigh muscles are so strong, they pull the ends of the broken bone together, causing them to overlap. This pulling may cause the injured leg to be noticeably shorter than the other leg. The injured leg may also be turned outward (Figure 12-14). Other signs or symptoms of a fractured femur include severe pain and inability to move the lower extremity. Do not attempt to splint a suspected femur fracture (this requires special training and equipment). A fractured femur is a serious life-threatening injury that requires immediate medical attention.

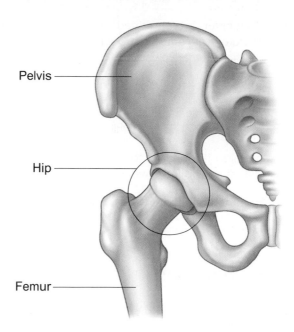

Figure 12-13. Most femur fractures involve the upper end of the bone where the femur meets the pelvis at the hip joint.

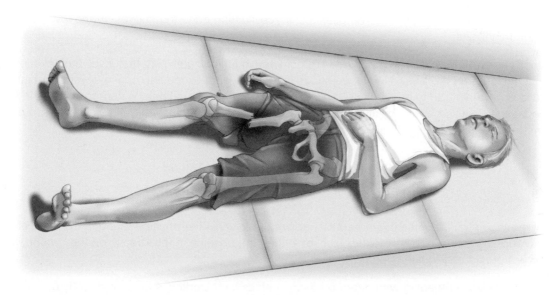

Figure 12-14. A fractured femur often produces a characteristic deformity. The injured leg is shorter than the uninjured leg and may be turned outward.

Care for Femur Injuries

Initial care for a serious injury to the thigh includes the following:

■ Do not move or straighten the injured area.

■ Control any external bleeding with direct pressure, unless the bleeding is located directly over a suspected fracture. With a fracture, apply pressure around the area. Always wear disposable latex-free gloves or use another protective barrier.

■ Call 9-1-1 or the designated emergency number immediately.

Emergency medical services (EMS) personnel are much better prepared to care for and transport a person with a serious thigh injury. While waiting for EMS personnel to arrive:

■ Stabilize the injury in the position found. If the person's leg is supported by the ground, do not move it. Rather, use rolled towels or blankets to support the leg in the position in which you found it.

■ Help the person rest in the most comfortable position.

■ Apply a cold pack.

■ Take steps to minimize shock, remembering that a fractured femur can result in serious internal bleeding and the likelihood of shock is considerable:

    ○ Keep the person lying down and try to keep them calm.

    ○ Keep the person from becoming chilled or overheated and make sure to call 9-1-1 or the designated emergency number.

    ○ Monitor the person's breathing and their general condition.

    ○ Watch for changes in the person's level of consciousness.

Knee Injuries

The knee joint is highly vulnerable to injury. The knee comprises the upper ends of the tibia and fibula, the lower end of the femur and the patella. The patella is a free-floating bone that moves on the lower front surface of the thighbone.

Sprains, fractures and dislocations of the knee are common in athletic activities that involve quick movements or exert unusual force on the knee. Deep lacerations in the area of the knee can cause severe joint infections. The patella is very vulnerable to bruises and lacerations, as well as dislocations. Violent forces to the front of the knee, such as those caused by hitting the dashboard of a motor vehicle or falling and landing on bent knees, can fracture the kneecap or cause a dislocation of the knee or hip.

Care for Knee Injuries

To care for an injured knee:

■ Do not move or straighten the injured area. Stabilize the injury in the position found. If the knee is bent, you can support it on a pillow or folded blanket in the bent position. If the knee is on the ground, the ground will provide adequate support.

■ Control any external bleeding with direct pressure, unless the bleeding is located directly over a suspected fracture. With a fracture, apply pressure around the area. Always wear disposable latex-free gloves or use another protective barrier.

■ Call 9-1-1 or the designated emergency number.

- If you must transport or move the person, and it does not cause more pain:

  ○ Use padded rigid splints running around either side of the knee to immobilize the knee. If the knee is straight, use two padded rigid splints on either side of the affected leg. The inside splint should start at the groin and extend past the bottom of the foot. The outside splint should start at the hip and also extend past the foot. Cravats will help keep the splint in place.

  ○ If the knee is straight, you might also splint by securing the injured knee to the uninjured leg, as you would do for a lower leg injury.

- Apply a cold pack.

- Take steps to minimize shock.

Lower Leg Injuries

The **lower leg** is the area between the knee and the ankle. The tibia and fibula are the two bones in the lower leg. A fracture in the lower leg may involve the tibia, the fibula or both bones. Sometimes both are fractured simultaneously. However, a blow to the outside of the lower leg can cause an isolated fracture of the smaller bone (fibula). Since the fibula is not a major weight-bearing bone, these fractures can be harder to detect.

Because these two bones lie just beneath the skin, open fractures are common. Lower leg fractures may cause a severe deformity in which the lower leg is angulated, as well as pain and inability to move the leg. Lower leg fractures can cause significant swelling that can affect circulation, resulting in severe leg pain, tingling, pallor or weakness. These signs and symptoms may indicate a decrease in blood flow below the injury site, which requires immediate advanced medical care.

Care for Lower Leg Injuries

To care for a lower leg injury:

- Do not move or straighten the injured area. Stabilize the injury in the position found. Do not forget that the ground acts as an adequate splint. If the person's lower extremity is supported by the ground, do not move it. Rather, use rolled towels or blankets to support the leg in the position in which you found it.

- Control any external bleeding with direct pressure, unless the bleeding is located directly over a suspected fracture. With a fracture, apply pressure around the area. Always wear disposable latex-free gloves or use another protective barrier.

- Call 9-1-1 or the designated emergency number immediately.

- If you must transport or move the person, and it does not cause more pain, you can create an anatomic splint by securing the injured lower extremity to the uninjured lower extremity with several wide cravats placed above and below the site of the injury:

  ○ If one is available, place a pillow or rolled blanket between the lower extremities and bind them together above and below the site of the injury (Figure 12-15).

- Apply a cold pack.

- Take steps to minimize shock.

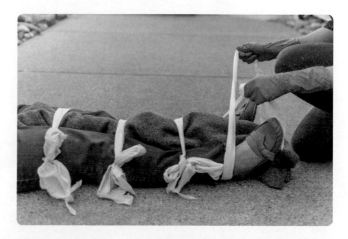

Figure 12-15. Place padding between the lower extremities and bind them together with cravats, above and below the injury site. *Photo: courtesy of the Canadian Red Cross*

Ankle and Foot Injuries

The foot consists of many small bones—the tarsals, metatarsals and phalanges. The ankle is a joint formed by the foot and the lower leg. Ankle and foot injuries are commonly caused by twisting forces. Injuries range from minor sprains with little swelling or pain to fractures and dislocations.

Many common ankle and foot injuries are caused by severe twisting forces that occur when the foot turns in or out at the ankle as a person steps down from a height, such as a curb or step. Fractures of the feet and ankles can also occur from forcefully landing on the heel. The force of the impact may be transmitted up the lower extremities. This transmitted force can result in an injury elsewhere in the body, such as the lower back. Always suspect that a person who has fallen or jumped from a height may also have additional injuries to the thigh, pelvis, head, neck or spine. Foot injuries may involve the toes. Although toe injuries are painful, they are rarely serious. Anatomic splinting of the toes with tape ("buddy taping") is an effective splint for toe injuries.

> **What if...** *A person has a musculoskeletal injury to the ankle? Should I remove their shoe?*
>
> *The decision for or against removing a shoe is not based on specific scientific evidence. There are just as many reasons to remove the shoe as there are for leaving it in place. If the footwear is supporting the injury, leave it in place and allow it to act as splint. If a person has a suspected broken bone, consider calling EMS and allowing them to decide (in conjunction with the responsive person's requests) whether to remove the footwear or not.*

Care for Ankle and Foot Injuries

To care for an ankle or foot injury:

- Do not move or straighten the injured area. Stabilize the injury in the position found.

- Control any external bleeding with direct pressure, unless the bleeding is located directly over a suspected fracture. With a fracture, apply pressure around the area. Always wear disposable latex-free gloves or use another protective barrier.

- If you must transport or move the person, and it does not cause more pain, immobilize the entire foot and ankle by using a soft splint, such as a pillow or rolled blanket (Figure 12-16). Wrap the injured area with the soft splint, and secure it with two or three cravats.

- Apply a cold pack.

- Take steps to minimize shock.

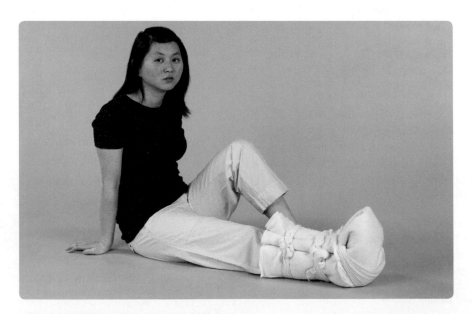

Figure 12-16. Splint for an ankle or foot injury.

Summary

You can care for musculoskeletal and soft tissue injuries to the extremities by giving care that focuses on minimizing pain, further damage to the injured area and shock. Remember: it is not always possible to distinguish between minor and severe injuries. Injuries to the pelvis and femur are potentially critical because of the major blood vessels running through these parts of the body. In addition, a force strong enough to cause injury to an extremity may also have been strong enough to cause other injuries.

With any injury to an extremity, first care for any life-threatening conditions and call 9-1-1 or the designated emergency number if necessary. Be sure to control any severe external bleeding. Then immobilize the injured area, apply a cold pack and take steps to minimize shock. Only use a splint if you must move or transport the person, and can do so without causing more pain. If you do apply a splint, be sure to follow the guidelines contained in this chapter, including splinting injuries in the position found, splinting the bones or joints both above and below an injury, using padding for comfort and support, and checking for adequate circulation before and after splinting.

READY TO RESPOND? ❭

Think back to Sue in the opening scenario, and use what you have learned to respond to these questions:

1. Could Sue have sustained a serious injury? Why or why not?

2. What steps should you take to help Sue?

Study Questions

1. Match each term with the correct definition.

   a. Upper arm   b. Forearm   c. Femur   d. Lower leg

____ The part of the lower extremity from the pelvis to the knee

____ The part of the upper extremity from the elbow to the wrist

____ The part of the lower extremity from the knee to the ankle

____ The part of the upper extremity from the shoulder to the elbow

2. Identify the most frequent cause of upper extremity injuries.

Base your answers for questions 3 through 5 on the scenario below.

A person attempting to leap a 4-foot gate catches one foot on the gate and falls hard on the other side. They appear to be unable to get up. The person says their left leg and arm both hurt. When you check, you find that they are unable to move their leg, which is beginning to swell. Their left arm looks deformed at the shoulder, and there is no sensation in the fingers of that arm. The arm is beginning to look bruised and is painful. The person says they feel a little nauseated and dizzy, and there is also a scrape on their hand.

3. What type of injury does the person likely have?

4. Identify the signs and symptoms that support your answer.

5. Describe the steps you would take to help the person.

6. List two specific signs and symptoms of a fractured femur.

7. List three types of splints used to immobilize an extremity.

(Continued)

Study Questions continued

In questions 8 and 9, circle the letter of the correct answer.

8. A man who has fallen down a steep flight of stairs is clutching his right arm to his chest. He says his shoulder hurts, and he cannot move his arm. How should you care for him?

   a. Give him some ice and tell him to go home.

   b. Immobilize the arm in the position you found it.

   c. Tell him to move the arm back to its normal position.

   d. Check the stairs to see what caused him to trip.

9. A child has fallen from a bicycle onto the pavement and landed on her elbow. The elbow is bent, and the girl says she cannot move it. What do you do after calling 9-1-1 or the designated emergency number?

   a. Straighten the elbow and splint it.

   b. Drive her to the hospital.

   c. Immobilize the elbow in the bent position.

   d. Ask her to continue to try to move the elbow.

10. You just finish mountain biking on a little-used local nature path when your friend unexpectedly hits a loose patch of dirt and slams down hard on the ground. Your friend is lying on the ground, awake and breathing. Their lower leg is bleeding profusely from a gash and seems to be bent at an odd angle. With no one around, and no mobile phone, you think you might need to transport your friend to the hospital yourself. List the guidelines you should follow in applying a splint to immobilize the injury.

Answers are listed in the Appendix.

Applying a Sling and Binder

AFTER CHECKING THE SCENE AND THE INJURED PERSON

---

1. Get consent.

---

2. Support the injured part.

   ■ Support both above and below the site of the injury.

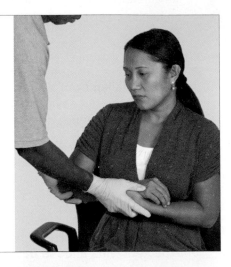

---

3. Check for circulation.

   ■ Check for feeling, warmth and color beyond the injury.

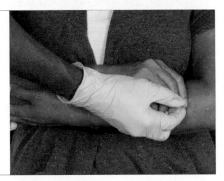

---

4. Position the sling.

   ■ Place a triangular bandage under the injured arm and over the uninjured shoulder to form a sling.

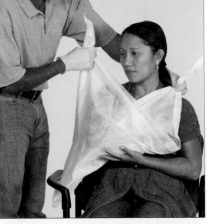

(Continued)

Applying a Sling and Binder *Continued*

5. Secure the sling.

   ■ Tie the ends of the sling at the side of the neck.

   TIP: *Pad the knots at the neck and side of the binder for comfort.*

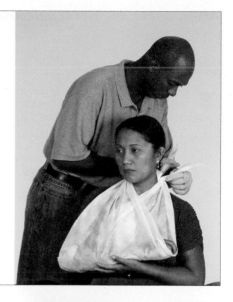

6. Bind with the bandage.

   ■ Bind the injured body part to the chest with a folded triangular bandage.

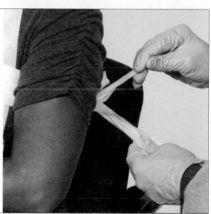

7. Recheck for circulation.

   ■ Recheck for feeling, warmth and color.

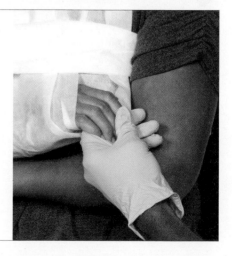

Applying a Rigid Splint

AFTER CHECKING THE SCENE AND THE INJURED PERSON

1. Get consent.

2. Support the injured part.

   ■ Support both above and below the site of the injury.

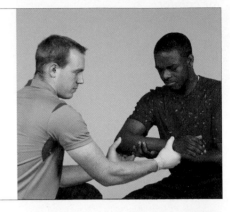

3. Check for circulation.

   ■ Check for feeling, warmth and color beyond the injury.

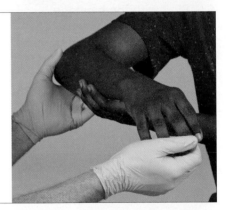

4. Place the splint.

   ■ Place an appropriately sized rigid splint (e.g., padded board) under the injured body part.

   TIP: *Place padding such as roller gauze under the palm of the hand to keep it in a natural position.*

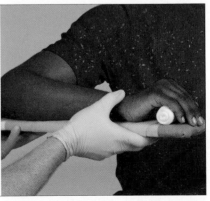

(Continued)

Applying a Rigid Splint *Continued*

5. Secure the bandages.

   ■ Tie several folded triangular bandages above and
   below the injured body part.

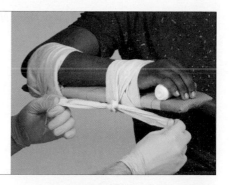

6. Recheck for circulation.

   ■ Recheck for feeling, warmth and color.

TIP: *If a rigid splint is used on an injured forearm,
immobilize the wrist and elbow. Bind the arm to the chest
using folded triangular bandages or apply a sling. If
splinting an injured joint, immobilize the bones on either
side of the joint.*

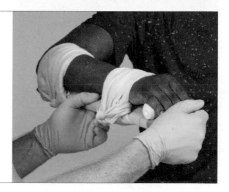

Applying an Anatomic Splint

AFTER CHECKING THE SCENE AND THE INJURED PERSON

1. Get consent.

2. Support the injured part.
   - Support both above and below the site of the injury.

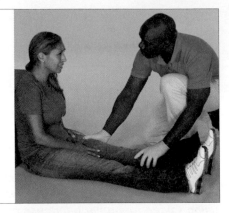

3. Check for circulation.
   - Check for feeling, warmth and color beyond the injury.

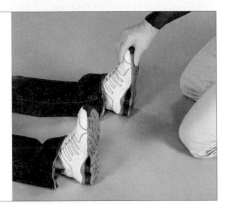

4. Position the bandages.
   - Place several folded triangular bandages above and below the injured body part.

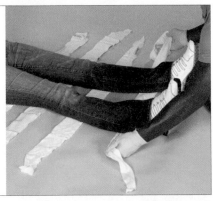

(Continued)

Applying an Anatomic Splint *Continued*

5. Align body parts.

   ■ Place the uninjured body part next to the injured body part.

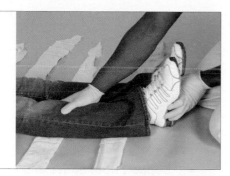

6. Place padding between the body parts and fill any voids. Tie the bandages securely around both legs.

   Photo: courtesy of the Canadian Red Cross

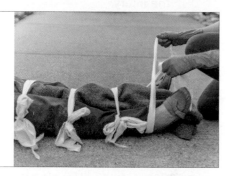

7. Recheck for circulation.

   ■ Recheck for feeling, warmth and color.

   TIP: *If you are not able to check warmth and color because a sock or shoe is in place, check for feeling.*

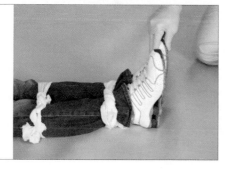

Skill Sheet 12-4

Applying a Soft Splint

AFTER CHECKING THE SCENE AND THE INJURED PERSON

1. Get consent.

2. Support the injured part.

   ■ Support both above and below the site of the injury.

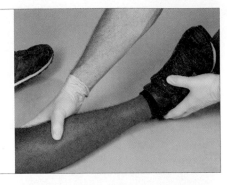

3. Check for circulation.

   ■ Check for feeling, warmth and color beyond the injury.

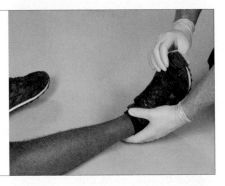

4. Position the bandages.

   ■ Place several folded triangular bandages above and below the injured body part.

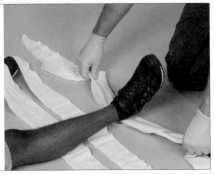

(Continued)

Applying a Soft Splint *Continued*

5. Wrap with a soft object.

 ▪ Gently wrap a soft object (e.g., a folded blanket or pillow) around the injured body part.

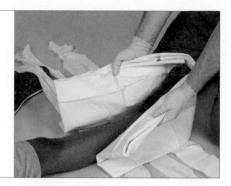

6. Tie the bandages securely.

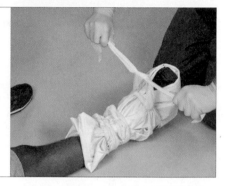

7. Recheck for circulation.

 ▪ Recheck for feeling, warmth and color.

TIP: *If you are not able to check warmth and color because a sock or shoe is in place, check for feeling.*

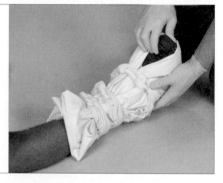

13

INJURIES TO THE HEAD, NECK OR SPINE

You and your friends are having a great time playing a game of touch football in the park. The score is tied when your quarterback throws a long pass. As the intended receiver jumps to grab the pass, the guy on defense gets overzealous, grabbing onto the receiver's back and sending them both crashing headfirst into the ground. One player stands up quickly and offers a hand to the other. You are all alarmed when the player on the ground says he cannot move his arms.

Learn and Respond ❯

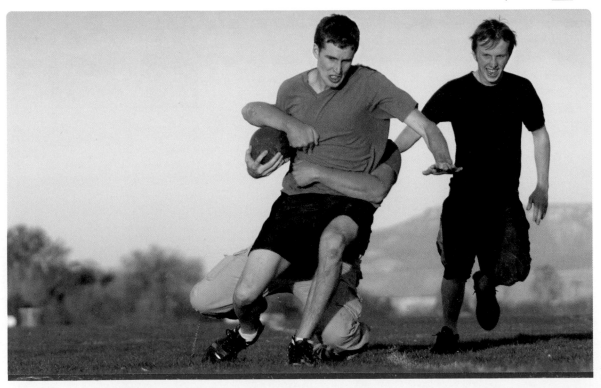

```
OBJECTIVES
```

After reading this chapter, you should be able to:

- Identify the most common causes of head, neck and spinal injuries.

- List 10 situations that might indicate serious head, neck and spinal injuries.

- List the signs and symptoms of head, neck and spinal injuries.

- Describe how to care for specific injuries to the head, face, neck and lower back.

- Know how to prevent head, neck and spinal injuries.

```
KEY TERMS
```

Concussion: A temporary loss of brain function caused by a blow to the head.

Spine: The series of vertebrae extending from the base of the skull to the tip of the tailbone (coccyx); also referred to as the spinal column or the vertebral column.

Traumatic brain injury (TBI): An injury to the brain resulting from an external force such as a blow to the head or a penetrating injury to the brain. TBIs are associated with temporary and/or permanent impairment to brain function, including physical, emotional and cognitive functioning. A concussion is a common type of TBI.

Vertebrae: The 33 bones of the spine.

Introduction

Although injuries to the head, neck or spine account for only a small percentage of all injuries, they cause more than half of the fatalities. Each year, nearly 2 million Americans suffer a head, neck or spinal injury serious enough to require medical care. Most of those injured are males between the ages of 15 and 30. Motor-vehicle collisions account for about half of all head, neck and spinal injuries (Figure 13-1). Other causes include falls, sports-related mishaps, incidents related to recreational activities and violent acts such as assault.

Causes of Head, Neck and Spinal Injuries

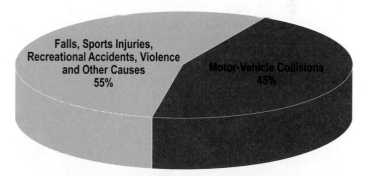

Figure 13-1. Motor-vehicle crashes account for nearly half of all head, neck and spinal injuries.

Besides those who die each year in the United States from head, neck and spinal injury, nearly 80,000 people become permanently disabled. These survivors have a wide range of physical and mental impairments, including **traumatic brain injury (TBI),** paralysis, speech and memory problems, and behavioral disorders.

Fortunately, prompt, appropriate care can help minimize the damage from most head, neck and spinal injuries. In this chapter, you will learn how to recognize a serious head, neck or spinal injury. You will also learn how to give appropriate care to minimize these injuries.

Recognizing Serious Head, Neck and Spinal Injuries

Injuries to the head, neck or spine often damage both bone and soft tissue, including brain tissue and the spinal cord. It is usually difficult to determine the extent of damage in head, neck and spinal injuries, so treat all such injuries as serious.

The Head

The head contains the brain, special sense organs, the mouth and nose and related structures (Figure 13-2). It is easily injured because it lacks the padding of muscle and adipose that are found in other areas of the body. The head is formed by the skull and the face. The broad, flat bones of the skull are fused together to form a hollow shell. This hollow shell, the cranial cavity, contains the brain. The face is on the front of the skull. The bones of the face include the bones of the cheek, forehead, nose and jaw.

The Brain

Injuries to the head can affect the brain. The brain can be bruised or lacerated when extreme force causes it to move in the skull, stretching and tearing tissue or bumping against the skull. Extreme force, or trauma, can fracture the thick bones of the skull. The major concern with skull fractures is damage to the brain.

Swelling and bleeding from a ruptured vessel in the brain can accumulate within the skull (Figure 13-3). Because the skull contains very little free space, bleeding can build pressure that can further damage brain tissue. Bleeding within the skull can occur rapidly or slowly over a period of days. This bleeding will affect the brain, resulting in changes in the level of consciousness. Unresponsiveness, or drifting in and out of responsiveness, is often the first and most important sign of a serious head injury.

The Face

The face contains both bones and soft tissues. Although some injuries to the face are minor, many can be life threatening. With a facial injury, consider whether the force that caused the injury may have been sufficiently strong to fracture facial bones and damage the brain or the spine. Facial injuries can also affect the airway and the person's ability to breathe.

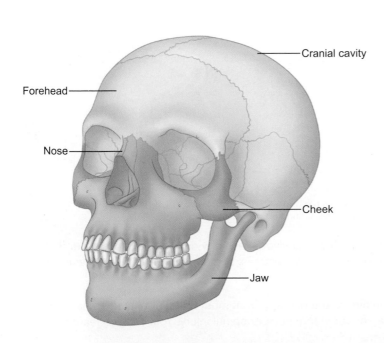

Figure 13-2. The head.

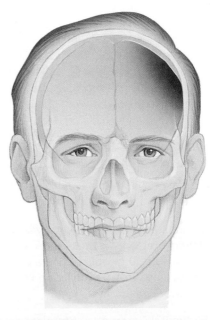

Figure 13-3. Injuries to the head can rupture blood vessels in the brain. Pressure builds within the skull as blood accumulates, causing brain injury.

The Neck

The neck contains the esophagus, larynx and part of the trachea. It also contains major blood vessels, muscles and tendons, and the cervical bones of the spine. Any injury to the neck must be considered serious. Crushing, rotating, tension or penetrating forces that cause the neck to stretch or bend too far can injure the neck. Sharp-edged objects can lacerate the neck's soft tissues and blood vessels.

The Spine

The *spine,* which is also called the **spinal column** or **vertebral column,** is a strong, flexible column of small bones called ***vertebrae,*** extending from the base of the skull to the tip of the tailbone. The spine supports the head and the trunk and protects the spinal cord. The vertebrae are separated from each other by cushions of cartilage called disks (Figure 13-4, A). This cartilage acts as a shock absorber when a person walks, runs or jumps. The **spinal cord,** which is a bundle of nerves that originate in the brain, runs through circular openings in the vertebrae. Nerve branches extend to various parts of the body through openings on the sides of the vertebrae.

The spine is divided into five regions: the cervical (neck) region, the thoracic (upper and middle back) region, the lumbar (lower back) region, the sacrum (triangular bone at the lower end of the spinal column) and the coccyx (tailbone), which is the small final segment of the spinal column (Figure 13-4, B).

Injuries to the spine can fracture the vertebrae and sprain or tear the ligaments. These injuries usually heal without problems. With severe injuries, however, the vertebrae may shift and compress or sever the spinal cord, causing temporary or permanent paralysis, or even death. The parts of the body that are paralyzed depend on which area of the spinal cord is damaged (Figure 13-4, C).

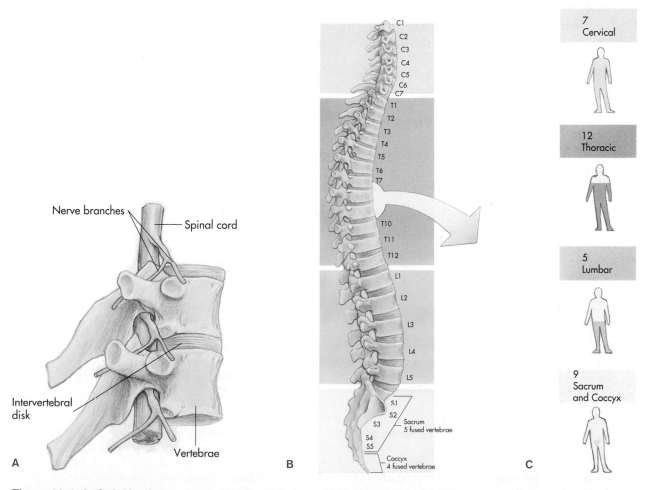

Figure 13-4, A–C. A, Vertebrae are separated by cushions of cartilage called disks. **B,** The spine is divided into five regions. **C,** Traumatic injury to a region of the spine can paralyze specific body areas.

Checking the Scene and the Person

When you encounter an injured person, you will evaluate the scene during the scene size-up for clues as to whether a head, neck or spinal injury may have occurred. As you evaluate the scene and gather an initial impression, think about the forces involved in the injury. Strong forces are likely to cause severe injury to the head, neck or spine. For example, a driver whose head hits and breaks a car windshield in a crash may receive a potentially serious head, neck or spinal injury. Similarly, a swimmer who dives into shallow water and strikes their head on the bottom may sustain a serious injury.

In general, you should consider the possibility of a serious head, neck or spinal injury if the injured person:

- Is unresponsive.

- Was involved in a motor-vehicle crash or subjected to another significant force.

- Was injured as a result of a fall from greater than the person's standing height.

- Is wearing a safety helmet that is broken.

- Complains of neck or back pain.

- Has tingling or weakness in the extremities.

- Is not fully alert.

- Appears to be intoxicated.

- Appears to be frail.

- Is older than 65 years.

- Is a child younger than 3 years with evidence of a head or neck injury.

Approach the person from the front so they can see you without turning their head, and tell the person to respond verbally to your questions. Ask the responsive person the following questions to further assess the situation:

- Does your head, neck or back hurt?

- What happened?

- Where specifically does it hurt?

- Can you move your hands and feet?

Signs and Symptoms of Serious Head, Neck or Spinal Injuries

When you are checking a person with a suspected head, neck or spinal injury, look for any swollen or bruised areas, but do not put direct pressure on any area that is swollen, depressed or soft. You may also find certain signs and symptoms that indicate a serious injury. These signs and symptoms include:

- Changes in the level of consciousness.

- Severe pain or pressure in the head, neck or spine.

- Tingling or loss of sensation in the extremities.

- Partial or complete loss of movement of any body part.

- Observable, unusual bumps or depressions on the head or neck.

- Sudden loss of memory.

- Blood or other fluids in the ears or nose.

- Profuse external bleeding of the head, neck or back.

- Seizures in a person who does not have a seizure disorder.

- Impaired breathing or impaired vision as a result of injury.

- Nausea or vomiting.

- Persistent headache.

- Loss of balance.

- Bruising of the head, especially around the eyes or behind the ears (Figure 13-5, A–B).

These signs and symptoms may be immediately obvious or develop later. Alone, these signs and symptoms do not always suggest a serious head, neck or spinal injury, but they may when combined with the cause

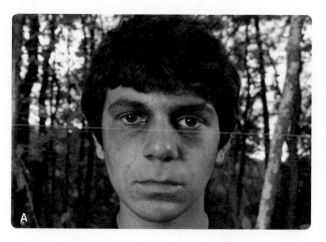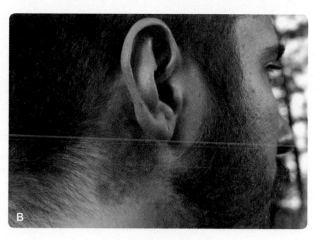

Figure 13-5, A–B. A, Bruising around the eyes or **B,** bruising behind the ears indicates a serious head injury.

of the injury. Regardless of the situation, always call 9-1-1 or the designated emergency number when you suspect a serious head, neck or spinal injury.

Care for Serious Head, Neck or Spinal Injuries

Head, neck and spinal injuries can become life-threatening emergencies. A serious injury to the head or neck can cause a person to stop breathing. When such an injury is suspected, always call 9-1-1 or the designated emergency number. Give the following care while waiting for emergency medical services (EMS) personnel to arrive:

- Minimize movement of the head, neck or spine by asking the person to remain still. Do *not* hold their head or restrict the person's movement as this may make the situation worse. Because excessive movement of the head, neck or spine can damage the spinal cord irreversibly, remind the person to remain as still as possible and provide comfort and reassurance to them until EMS personnel arrive and take over.

- If the person is wearing a helmet, do *not* remove it unless you are *specifically* trained to do so *and* it is necessary to assess the person's airway.

- Check for life-threatening conditions.

- Monitor responsiveness and breathing.

- Control any external bleeding with direct pressure unless the bleeding is located directly over a suspected fracture. Do *not* apply direct pressure if there are any signs of an obvious skull fracture.

- Do *not* attempt to remove a penetrating object; rather, stabilize it with a bulky dressing.

- Wear disposable latex-free gloves or use another barrier.

- Take steps to minimize shock. Keep the person from becoming chilled or overheated.

- If you need to leave the person, such as to call 9-1-1 or get an AED, carefully place them in the recovery position to protect their airway if they begin to vomit. However, do *not* place a person with a head, neck or spinal injury in the recovery position if you are able to remain with the person and monitor their condition.

What if... *A person has a suspected spinal injury and I have access to a cervical collar? Should I use it? I have seen EMS personnel apply them before.*

The short answer is no. Immobilization devices, such as cervical collars, should not be used by trained lay responders. The reason for this is twofold. As a trained lay responder, your training does not include the appropriate use of such devices, and you should not give care for which you are not trained. The second reason is that the benefit of using immobilization devices has not been proven and, in fact, using such devices may be harmful even when used appropriately by trained professional responders.

What if... *I suspect an injury to the spine and the person is not breathing? Which is more important— keeping the spine from moving or giving CPR?*

While the general rule is to always leave a person's head, neck or spine in the position found without any movement or alignment with the body, if the person is unresponsive and not breathing, giving CPR must take precedence over not moving the head and neck. If you must move the person to open the airway during CPR, slowly and cautiously extend the head and neck until the airway is opened, and then continue with CPR as necessary.

Check for Life-Threatening Conditions

You do not always have to put a person onto their back to check breathing. A cry of pain, chest movement as a result of inhaling and exhaling, or the sound of breathing tells you the person is breathing, so you do not need to move them to check. If the person is breathing normally, support the person in the position in which they were found. If the person is not breathing or you cannot tell, roll the person gently onto their back, but avoid twisting the spine. Carefully tilt the head and lift the chin just enough to open the airway to give rescue breaths if needed during CPR.

If the person begins to vomit, carefully roll them into the recovery position as described in Chapter 5.

Monitor Responsiveness and Breathing

Observe the person's level of consciousness and breathing. A serious head injury can result in changes in responsiveness. The person may give inappropriate responses to name, time, place or when describing what happened. They may speak incoherently (in a way that cannot be understood). The person may be drowsy, appear to lapse into sleep and then suddenly awaken, or completely become unresponsive. Breathing may become rapid or irregular. Because injuries to the head or neck can paralyze chest nerves and muscles, breathing can stop. If breathing stops, give CPR immediately.

Control External Bleeding

Some head and neck injuries involve soft tissue damage. Because many blood vessels are located in the head and two major arteries (the carotid arteries) and the jugular veins are located in the neck, the person can lose a significant amount of blood quickly. If the person is bleeding externally, control it promptly with dressings, direct pressure and bandages. Do *not* apply pressure to both carotid arteries simultaneously, and do *not* put a bandage around the neck. Doing so could cut off or seriously diminish the oxygen supply to the brain. If there is severe, life-threatening bleeding, consider the use of a hemostatic dressing with pressure if direct pressure fails to stop the bleeding.

Take Steps to Minimize Shock

A serious injury to the head or spine can disrupt the body's normal heating or cooling mechanism. When this disruption occurs, the person is more susceptible to shock. For example, a person suffering a serious head, neck or spinal injury while outside on a cold day will be more likely to develop hypothermia because the normal shivering response to rewarm the body may not work. For this reason, it is important to take steps to minimize shock by having the person lie flat on their back, covering them with a blanket, and keeping them from becoming chilled or overheated.

Specific Injuries

The head is easily injured because it lacks the padding of muscle and fat found in other areas of the body. You can feel bone just beneath the surface of the skin over most of the head, including the chin, cheekbones and scalp. When you are checking a person with a suspected head injury, look for any swollen or bruised areas, but do not put direct pressure on any area that is swollen, depressed or soft.

Concussions

A **concussion** is a common type of traumatic brain injury that involves a temporary loss of brain function. Concussions are particularly common sports-related injuries, but they can occur whenever a person experiences a bump, blow or jolt to the head or body that results in rapid movement of the head. A person who has had one concussion is at increased risk for subsequent concussions.

A concussion can result from even a seemingly minor bump, blow or jolt and may be tricky to recognize. Many people who experience a concussion do not lose consciousness, or they may only lose consciousness very briefly. Your best clues that a person may have a concussion are often changes in the person's behavior noted after the person has experienced a bump, blow or jolt. For example, the person may seem confused, dazed or stunned; lose the ability to remember or follow simple instructions; or ask repeatedly what happened. The person may complain of a headache, feel nauseated or vomit, have blurred or double vision, complain of dizziness, or be especially sensitive to light or noise. Many people who have experienced a concussion say that the concussion caused them to feel "sluggish," "groggy" or just "not right." Signs and symptoms of a concussion (Table 13-1) usually are apparent soon after the injury, although some can appear hours or days later. For example, the person may sleep more or less than usual. Children may show changes in playing or eating habits. The effects of the concussion can last for several days, weeks or longer.

If you think that a person has sustained a concussion, advise the person to stop the activity they were engaged in when the incident occurred. The person should follow up with a healthcare provider for a full evaluation. A healthcare provider is best able to evaluate the severity of the injury and make recommendations about when the person can return to normal activities. And, while rare, permanent brain injury and death are potential consequences of failing to identify and respond to a concussion in a timely manner.

Table 13-1. **Signs and Symptoms of a Concussion**

Thinking and Remembering	Physical	Emotional	Behavioral
■ Difficulty thinking clearly ■ Difficulty remembering events that occurred just prior to the incident and just after the incident ■ Difficulty remembering new information ■ Difficulty concentrating ■ Feeling mentally "foggy" ■ Difficulty processing information	■ Headache ■ Blurry vision ■ Nausea or vomiting ■ Dizziness ■ Sensitivity to noise or light ■ Balance problems ■ Feeling sluggish (lack of energy)	■ Irritability ■ Sadness ■ Heightened emotions ■ Nervousness or anxiety	■ Changes in sleeping habits (sleeping more or less than usual, difficulty falling asleep) ■ Changes in playing and eating habits (in children)

> **Myth-Information.** *Myth: A person with a concussion who falls asleep could die.* It is generally considered safe for a person with a concussion to go to sleep. However, the person's healthcare provider may recommend that you wake the person periodically to make sure that their condition has not worsened.

Care for Concussions

Every suspected concussion should be treated seriously. **The person should always follow up with a healthcare provider for a full evaluation.** If you are unsure of the seriousness of the concussion, call 9-1-1 or the designated emergency number. While waiting for help to arrive, monitor the person for any changes in their condition and try to comfort and reassure the person. Encourage the person to talk with you to help keep the person calm.

Scalp Injuries

Scalp bleeding can be minor or severe. However, minor lacerations can appear to bleed heavily because the scalp contains many blood vessels.

Care for Scalp Injuries

If the person has an open wound to the scalp, control the bleeding with direct pressure:

- Apply several dressings and hold them in place with your gloved hand. If gloves are not available, use a protective barrier.

- Be sure to press gently at first because the skull may be fractured. If you feel a depression, spongy area or bone fragments, do *not* put direct pressure on the wound. Attempt to control bleeding with pressure on the area *around* the wound (Figure 13-6).

- Secure the dressings with a roller bandage or triangular bandage.

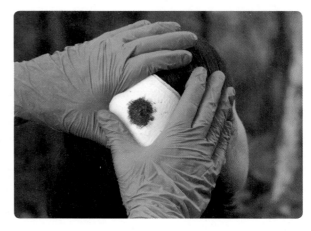

Figure 13-6. To avoid putting pressure on a deep scalp wound, apply pressure around the wound.

Examine the injured area carefully because the person's hair may hide part of the wound. Call 9-1-1 or the designated emergency number if you are unsure about the extent of the injury. EMS personnel will be better able to evaluate the injury. Severe bleeding from the scalp can cause shock in young children and infants.

Nose and Mouth Injuries

Facial trauma can range from minor injuries (cuts and abrasions, bruises, bloody noses and knocked-out teeth) to more severe injuries, such as a fracture of one or more of the facial bones. A person with a facial injury may also have a head, neck or spinal injury, such as a concussion.

> Although open wounds on the face and scalp can seem to bleed profusely, the bleeding is usually easily controlled with direct pressure and time.

Nose Injuries

Falling or getting hit in the nose can result in a nosebleed. Other, nontraumatic causes of nosebleeds include breathing dry air and changes in altitude. Certain medical conditions (such as hypertension, or high blood pressure) and the use of certain medications (such as blood thinners) can make a person more susceptible to nosebleeds.

In most cases, you can stop a nosebleed by having the person pinch their nostrils together while sitting with the head slightly forward (Figure 13-7). (Sitting with the head slightly forward helps to keep blood from pooling in the back of the throat, which can lead to choking or, if the blood is swallowed, vomiting.) Keep the nostrils pinched shut for at least 5 minutes before checking to see if the bleeding has stopped. If the bleeding has not stopped after 5 minutes, keep pinching the nostrils shut for another 5 minutes. If the bleeding is severe or gushing, call 9-1-1 or the designated emergency number.

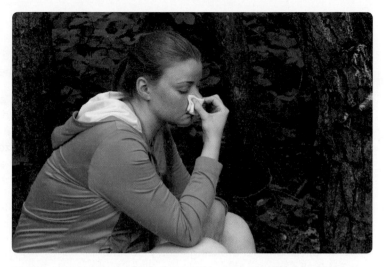

Figure 13-7. To control a nosebleed, have the person lean forward and pinch the nostrils together until bleeding stops (about 10 minutes).

Mouth Injuries

Injuries to the mouth may cause breathing problems if blood or loose teeth block the airway, so make sure the person is able to breathe. If the person is bleeding from the mouth and you do not suspect a serious head, neck or spinal injury, place the person in a seated position leaning slightly forward. This will allow any blood to drain from the mouth. If this position is not possible, place the person on their side in the recovery position. Have the person hold a gauze pad at the site of the bleeding and apply direct pressure to stop the bleeding. (If the person is responsive, having the person apply direct pressure to a wound inside their own mouth is easier and safer than doing it for the person.)

Lip and Tongue Injuries

For injuries that penetrate the lip, place a rolled gauze pad between the lip and the gum. You can place another gauze pad on the outer surface of the lip. If the tongue is bleeding, apply a gauze pad and direct pressure. Applying a cold pack wrapped in a dry towel to the lips or tongue can help to reduce swelling and ease pain.

Dental Injuries

If a tooth is knocked out, control the bleeding by placing a rolled gauze pad into the space left by the missing tooth and have the person gently bite down to maintain pressure (Figure 13-8). Try to locate and save the tooth, because a dentist or other healthcare provider may be able to reimplant it. Place the tooth in Hanks' Balanced Salt solution (e.g., Save-A-Tooth®), if available. If you do not have Hanks' Balanced Salt solution, place the tooth in egg white, coconut water or whole milk. If these are not available, place the tooth in the injured person's saliva. Be careful to pick up the tooth only by the crown (the part of the tooth that is normally visible above the gum line) rather than by the root. The person should seek dental or emergency care as soon as possible after the injury. The sooner the tooth is reimplanted, the better the chance that it will survive. Ideally, reimplantation should take place within 30 minutes.

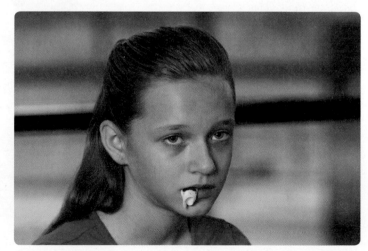

Figure 13-8. If a tooth is knocked out, place a sterile dressing directly in the space left by the tooth. Tell the person to bite down.

Cheek Injuries

Injury to the cheek usually involves only soft tissue. You may have to control bleeding on either the outside, inside or both sides of the cheek depending on the severity of the injury.

If an object passes completely through the cheek and becomes embedded, and you cannot control bleeding with the object in place, the object should be removed so that you can control bleeding and keep the airway clear. *This circumstance is the only exception to the general rule not to remove embedded objects from the body.* An embedded object in the cheek cannot be easily stabilized, makes control of bleeding more difficult, and may become dislodged and obstruct the airway. To care for a person with an embedded object in the cheek that is not embedded in another location in the mouth:

- Remove the object by pulling it out in the same direction it entered.

- Fold or roll several dressings and place them inside the mouth. Also, apply dressings to the outside of the cheek. Be sure not to obstruct the airway.

- If there are no suspected head, neck or spinal injuries, place the person in a seated position, leaning slightly forward, so that blood will not drain into the throat.

- As with any severe bleeding or embedded object, call 9-1-1 or the designated emergency number.

Eye Injuries

Injuries to the eye can involve the bone and soft tissue surrounding the eye or the eyeball. Blunt objects, such as a fist or a baseball, may injure the eye area, or a smaller object may penetrate the eyeball. Injuries that penetrate the eyeball are very serious and can cause blindness. Foreign bodies, such as dirt, sand, or slivers of wood or metal that get in the eye are irritating and can cause significant damage. The eye immediately produces tears in an attempt to flush out such objects. Pain from the irritation is often severe. The person may have difficulty opening the eye because light further irritates it.

Care for Eye Injuries

Care for open or closed wounds around the eyeball as you would for any other soft tissue injury. Never put direct pressure on the eyeball.

To care for a foreign body in the eye:

- Try to remove the foreign body by telling the person to blink several times, then try gently flushing the eye with water.

- If the object remains, the person should receive more advanced medical care. The eye should be flushed continuously until EMS personnel arrive.

- Flushing the eye with water is also appropriate if the person has any chemical in the eye (Figure 13-9). Flush the eye continuously until advanced medical personnel arrive. If only one eye is affected, make sure you do *not* let the water run into the unaffected eye.

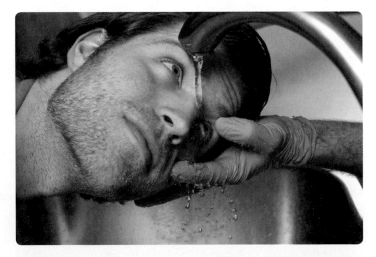

Figure 13-9. Gently flush an eye that has been exposed to chemicals by placing the affected eye on the bottom.

Follow these guidelines when giving care for an eye with an embedded object:

- Place the person in a face-up position and enlist someone to help stabilize the person's head.

- Do *not* attempt to remove any object embedded in the eye.

- Stabilize the object by encircling the eye with a gauze dressing or soft sterile cloth, being careful *not* to apply any pressure to the area.

- Position bulky dressings, such as roller gauze, around the impaled object and then cover it with a shield such as a paper cup. Do *not* use Styrofoam®-type materials, as small particles can break off and get into the eye.

- The shield should *not* touch the object. Bandage the shield and dressing in place with a self-adhering bandage and roller bandage covering the person's injured eye, as well as the uninjured eye, to keep the object stable and minimize movement.

- Comfort and reassure the person. Do *not* leave the person unattended.

What if... *A person has a relatively large object embedded in the eye and I do not have a paper cup to stabilize it with?*

As with all embedded objects, your goal is to attempt to stabilize the object as best you can. If no paper cup is readily available, consider the use of bulky dressings to secure the object. As discussed in this chapter, be careful to avoid placing direct pressure on the eye itself. Bandage the dressings loosely and seek immediate medical attention.

Ear Injuries

External injuries to the ear are common. Open wounds, such as lacerations or abrasions, can result from recreational injuries, such as being struck by a racquetball or falling off a bike. An avulsion of the ear may occur when a pierced earring catches on something and tears away from the ear.

The ear can also be injured internally. A foreign object, such as dirt, an insect or cotton, can easily become lodged in the ear canal. A direct blow to the head may rupture the eardrum. Sudden pressure changes, such as those caused by an explosion or a deep-water dive, can also injure the ear internally. The person may lose hearing or balance or experience inner ear pain. These injuries require more advanced medical care.

Care for Ear Injuries

You can control bleeding from the soft tissues of the ear by applying direct pressure to the affected area with a gloved hand or other barrier.

For a foreign object in the ear:

- If you can easily see and grasp the object, remove it.

- Do not try to remove any object by using a pin, toothpick or a similar sharp item. You could force the object farther back or puncture the eardrum.

- If you cannot easily remove the object, the person should seek more advanced medical care.

If the person has a serious head injury, blood or other fluid may be in the ear canal or may be draining from the ear. Do *not* attempt to stop this drainage with direct pressure. Instead, loosely cover the ear with a sterile dressing. Call 9-1-1 or the designated emergency number.

Lower Back Injuries

Certain injuries to the neck and back are not life threatening but can be extremely painful and temporarily disabling and may occur without warning. These injuries usually occur from forcing the back beyond its limits in strength or flexibility. Using improper lifting techniques when lifting or moving heavy objects is one way to injure the back. Working in a cramped space in a bent-over or awkward position may cause back pain, as can sitting or standing in one position for a long period of time. Often acute back pain that develops suddenly is a result of one of the following causes:

- Ligament pulls and muscle strains: violent movement or unaccustomed effort stretches or tears muscles in the back or neck, or the ligaments that bind together or surround each section of the spine.

- Vertebrae displacement: twisting movement causes two vertebrae to slip out of place, and facets (bony projections) lock in a position that puts pressure on a nerve or irritates the joint, often causing muscles to go into spasm.

- Slipped (prolapsed) disk: pressure and wear and tear on one of the cartilage disks that separate the vertebrae cause the soft center of the disk to protrude through the disk's outer layer. This center part presses on a nerve, often causing muscles to spasm.

Signs and Symptoms of Lower Back Injuries

Signs and symptoms of a lower back injury include:

- Shooting pain in the lower back.

- Sharp pain in one leg.

- Sharp pain and tightness across the lower back.

- A sudden, sharp pain in the back and a feeling that something snapped.

- Inability to bend over without pain.

Regardless of the possible cause of back pain, call 9-1-1 or the designated emergency number immediately if the person has any of the following accompanying signs or symptoms:

- Numbness or tingling in any extremity

- Difficulty moving

- Loss of bladder or bowel control

These signs and symptoms indicate possible damage to the spinal cord. Wait for EMS personnel to arrive and keep the person warm and quiet.

A person with pain on one side of the small of the back who also has a fever or feels ill should call a physician. The person may have a kidney infection. Older adults with back pain may have a life-threatening emergency called an aortic **aneurysm.** For older adults with severe back pain, call 9-1-1 or the designated emergency number.

Care for Lower Back Injuries

Because the care for lower back injuries varies depending on the nature of the injury, the person should consult a physician. As indicated above, there are also instances where you should always call 9-1-1 or the designated emergency number, including:

- Signs or symptoms of possible spinal cord damage

- An older adult with severe back pain

Cold treatment is usually recommended for musculoskeletal injuries initially. Bed rest and pain-relieving medications, such as acetaminophen or ibuprofen, generally provide relief for strains and muscle spasms. Exercises are frequently recommended to strengthen the back and abdominal muscles after the pain has gone and should only be done at the direction of a physician or rehabilitation specialist.

While some injuries are unavoidable, many others are preventable by being aware of potential dangers in the environment and taking appropriate safety measures. These measures include:

- Correctly wear safety belts (including lap and shoulder restraints), and place children in car safety seats.

- Correctly wear approved helmets, eyewear, faceguards and mouthguards for activities for which they are recommended.

- Take steps to prevent falls such as ensuring that hallways and stairways in your home are well lit, and stairways have handrails and nonslip treads. Rugs should be secured with double-sided tape or appropriate mats.

- Use non-slip mats in the bathtub or use handrails.

- Always use a step stool or step ladder to reach objects that are up high. Do not attempt to pull down heavy objects that are out of reach over your head.

- Use proper lifting techniques when lifting and carrying heavy objects.

- Obey rules in sports and recreational activities.

- Avoid inappropriate use of alcohol and other drugs.

- Inspect work and recreational equipment periodically.

- Do not dive into a body of water if you are unsure of the depth.

- Think and talk about safety and use good common sense.

Summary

In this chapter, you have learned how to recognize and care for serious head, neck and spinal injuries; specific injuries to the head and neck; and lower back problems. Like injuries elsewhere on the body, injuries to the head, neck or spine often involve both soft tissue and bone. Often the cause of the injury is the best indicator of whether or not it is serious. If you have any doubts about the seriousness of a head, neck or spinal injury, call 9-1-1 or your designated emergency number.

READY TO RESPOND? >

Think back to the touch football game in the opening scenario, and use what you have learned to respond to these questions:

1. Is it safe to assume that the football player who stands up right away does not have a head, neck or spinal injury? Why or why not?

2. While one of the other players runs off to alert a police officer he sees patrolling the park, you head over to the person who is lying there, awake and alert. What should your priority be?

Study Questions

1. **Match each term with the correct definition.**

   a. Concussion   b. Traumatic brain   c. Spine   d. Vertebrae
                                 injury

   ____ The 33 bones of the spine

   ____ An injury associated with temporary and/or permanent impairment to brain function, including physical, emotional and cognitive functioning

   ____ A temporary loss of brain function caused by a blow to the head

   ____ Series of vertebrae extending from the base of the skull to the tip of the tailbone

2. **List five situations that might indicate the possibility of a serious head, neck or spinal injury.**

3. **List six signs and symptoms of head, neck or spinal injuries.**

4. **List the steps of care for an eye injury in which the eyeball has been penetrated.**

In questions 5 through 11, circle the letter of the correct answer.

5. **Which are among the most common causes of serious head, neck and spinal injury?**

   a. Motor-vehicle   b. Sports-related   c. Falls   d. All of the above
       collisions   injuries

6. **Serious injuries to the head, neck or spine can damage—**

   a. Soft tissues.   b. Nerve tissues.   c. Bones.   d. All of the above

7. **Which of the following situations would cause you to suspect a serious head, neck or spinal injury?**

   a. A man complains   b. Two people   c. A high school   d. A child trips and
       of lower back pain   bump their heads   football player is   falls onto her
       after working out in   together while   holding his neck   hands and knees.
       the gym.   reaching for a   after making a
                   piece of paper   tackle headfirst.
                   on the floor.

(Continued)

Study Questions continued

8. **Which should you do when caring for a person with a suspected head, neck or spinal injury?**

   a. Help support the injured area by walking the person to the nearest wall.

   b. Call the person's physician for additional care.

   c. Remind the person to remain still while checking for life-threatening conditions.

   d. Have the person lie flat and elevate the legs 8 to 12 inches.

9. **At the scene of a car crash, a person has blood seeping from their ears. Which should you do?**

   a. Loosely cover the ears with a sterile dressing.

   b. Do nothing; this is a normal finding in a head injury.

   c. Collect the fluid in a sterile container for analysis.

   d. Pack the ears with sterile dressings to prevent further fluid loss.

10. **Which is your primary concern when caring for an injury to the mouth or neck?**

    a. Infection

    b. Airway obstruction

    c. Swelling

    d. Scarring

11. **Which is a sign or symptom of an injured ear?**

    a. Hearing loss

    b. Loss of balance

    c. Inner ear pain

    d. All of the above

12. **As you begin to apply direct pressure to control bleeding for a scalp injury, you notice a depression of the skull in the area of the bleeding. What should you do next?**

Answers are listed in the Appendix.

14

INJURIES TO THE CHEST, ABDOMEN AND PELVIS

Y ou are traveling home when you witness a crash. As debris falls off of a speeding truck, a bicyclist quickly swerves to avoid it but falls in the road from the sudden movement. The car traveling behind does get hit by the debris, but the driver manages to brake before hitting the man in the road. It looks like everyone is okay from a distance, but as you approach to help, you can see that the bicyclist is holding his chest and his breathing sounds shallow as if it is painful to breathe. Another bystander has called 9-1-1 and is setting up hazard signals to alert traffic. You are the only person trained in first aid, so you begin to check the bicyclist after getting his consent.

Learn and Respond ▶

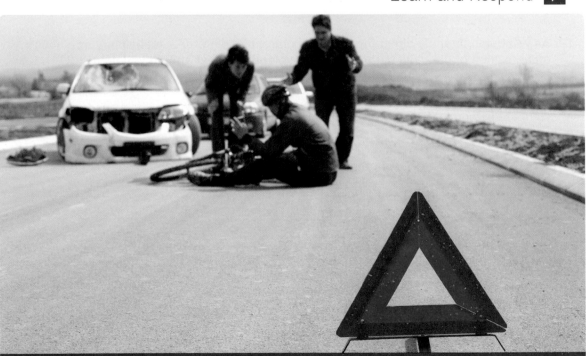

After reading this chapter, you should be able to:

- Explain why injuries to the chest, abdomen and pelvis can be life threatening.

- List the signs and symptoms of a chest injury.

- Describe how to care for rib fractures.

- Describe how to care for an open chest wound.

- List the signs and symptoms of abdominal and pelvic injuries.

- Describe the care for open and closed abdominal and pelvic injuries.

- Describe how to care for injuries to the genitals.

KEY TERMS

Abdomen: The middle part of the trunk, containing the stomach, liver, intestines and spleen.

Chest: The upper part of the trunk, containing the heart, major blood vessels and lungs.

Genitals: The external reproductive organs.

Pelvis: The lower part of the trunk, containing the intestines, bladder and internal reproductive organs.

Rib cage: The cage of bones formed by the 12 pairs of ribs, the sternum and the spine.

Sternum: The long, flat bone in the middle of the front of the rib cage; also called the breastbone.

Introduction

Many injuries to the chest, abdomen and pelvis involve only soft tissues. Often these injuries, like those that occur elsewhere on the body, are only minor cuts, scrapes, burns and bruises. Occasionally, a violent force or mechanism known as trauma results in more severe injuries. These include fractures and injuries to organs that cause severe bleeding or impair breathing. Fractures and lacerations often occur in motor-vehicle collisions to occupants not wearing seat belts. Falls, sports mishaps and other forms of trauma may also cause such injuries.

Because the chest, abdomen and pelvis contain many organs important to life, injury to any of these areas can be life threatening. You may recall from Chapter 13 that a force capable of causing severe injury in these areas may also cause injury to the spine.

This chapter describes the signs and symptoms of different injuries to the chest, abdomen and pelvis and the care you would give for them. In all cases, follow the emergency action steps as well as these basic guidelines:

- Call 9-1-1 or the designated emergency number.
- Control bleeding.

- Limit movement.
- Take steps to minimize shock.

- Monitor breathing and signs of life.

Chest Injuries

The **chest** is the upper part of the trunk. The chest is shaped by 12 pairs of ribs. Ten of the pairs attach to the **sternum** (breastbone) in front and to the spine in back. Two pairs, the floating ribs, attach only to the spine. The **rib cage,** formed by the ribs, the sternum and the spine, protects vital organs, such as the heart, major blood vessels and the lungs (Figure 14-1). Also in the chest are the esophagus, the trachea and the muscles of respiration.

Chest injuries are the second leading cause of trauma deaths each year in the United States. Injuries to the chest may result from a wide variety of causes, such as motor-vehicle collisions, falls, sports mishaps and crushing or penetrating forces (Figure 14-2, A–C). About 35 percent of deaths from motor-vehicle collisions involve chest injuries. Chest injuries may involve the bones that form the chest cavity or they may involve the organs or other structures in the cavity itself.

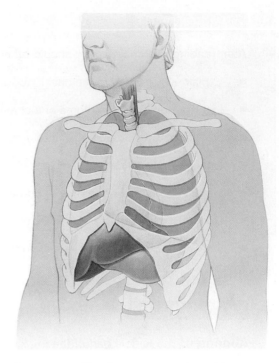

Figure 14-1. The rib cage surrounds and protects several vital organs.

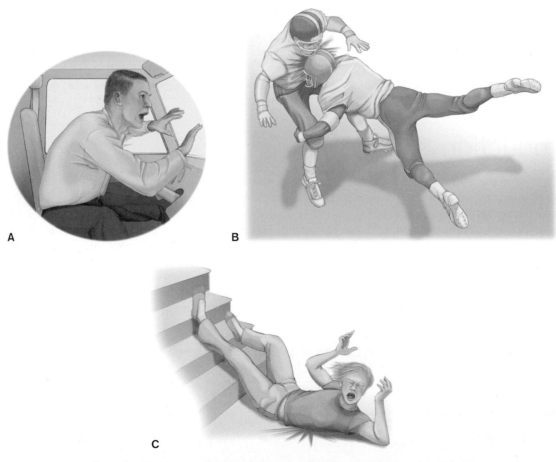

Figure 14-2, A–C. A, Crushing forces; **B,** direct blows; and **C,** falls can all lead to chest injuries.

Care for Abdominal Injuries

Call 9-1-1 or the designated emergency number for any signs or symptoms of an abdominal injury. With a severe open injury, abdominal organs sometimes protrude through the wound (Figure 14-8, A).

To care for an open wound to the abdomen, follow these steps:

- Put on disposable latex-free gloves or use another barrier.

- Do not apply direct pressure.

- Do not push any protruding organs back into the open wound.

- Remove clothing from around the wound (Figure 14-8, B).

- Apply a moist (clean, warm tap water can be used), sterile or clean dressing loosely over the wound (Figure 14-8, C).

- Cover the dressing loosely with plastic wrap, if available, making an occlusive dressing.

- Cover the dressing lightly with a folded towel to maintain warmth (Figure 14-8, D).

- Keep the person from getting chilled or overheated.

To care for a closed abdominal injury:

- Carefully position the person on their back with the knees bent, if that position does not cause pain. Bending the knees allows the muscles of the abdomen to relax.

- Avoid putting direct pressure on the area.

- Place rolled-up blankets or pillows under the person's knees if available.

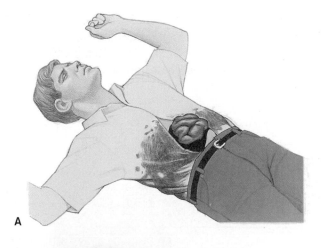
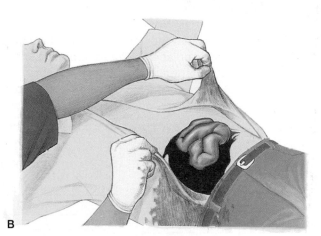
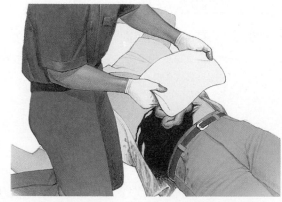
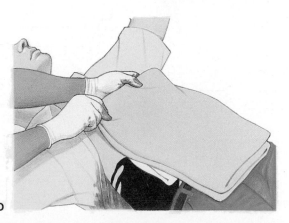

Figure 14-8, A–D. A, Severe injuries to the abdominal cavity can result in protruding organs. **B,** Carefully remove clothing from around the wound. **C,** Apply a large, moist, sterile dressing over the wound and cover it with plastic wrap. **D,** Place a folded towel over the dressing to maintain warmth.

Shock is likely to occur with any serious abdominal injury. Call 9-1-1 or the designated emergency number immediately, and take steps to minimize shock by having the person lie on their back. Keep the person from becoming chilled or overheated, and monitor breathing and how the skin looks and feels until emergency medical services (EMS) personnel arrive.

To care for an impaled object in the abdomen:

- Do *not* remove the object.

- Dress the wound around the object to control bleeding.

- Stabilize the object with bulky dressings to prevent movement.

What if... *I am giving care to someone with an open abdominal injury in which the organs are protruding, but I have only a small dressing available with which to cover the area?*

In the event of protruding abdominal organs, your small sterile dressings are most likely not going to adequately cover the open wound. In this situation, if you have access to plastic wrap, use this first. Then consider the use of clean sheets or blankets if they are available. Another option is using the lining of a jacket to cover the open wound and maintain warmth.

Pelvic Injuries

The **pelvis** is the lower part of the trunk. It contains the bladder, reproductive organs and part of the large intestine, including the rectum. Major arteries (the femoral arteries) and nerves pass through the pelvis. It includes a group of large bones that form a protective girdle around the organs inside of a person's sides and back, but not in front (Figure 14-9). A great force is required to cause serious injury to the pelvic bones.

Injuries to the pelvis may include fractures to the pelvic bone and damage to structures within. Fractured bones may puncture or lacerate these structures, or they can be injured when struck a forceful blow by blunt or penetrating objects. An injury to the pelvis sometimes involves the **genitals,** the external reproductive organs. Genital injuries are either closed wounds such as a bruise, or open wounds such as an avulsion or laceration. Any injury to the genitals is extremely painful.

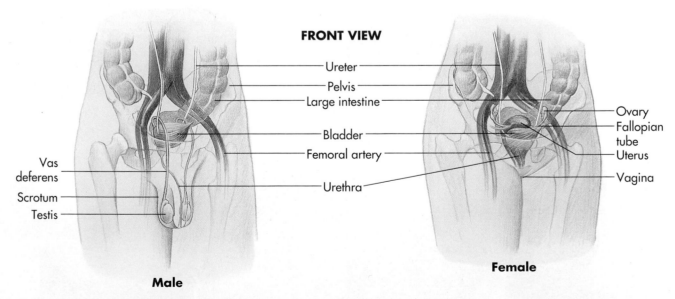

FRONT VIEW

Ureter · Pelvis · Large intestine · Bladder · Femoral artery · Urethra

Vas deferens · Scrotum · Testis

Male

Ovary · Fallopian tube · Uterus · Vagina

Female

Figure 14-9. The internal structures of the pelvis are well protected on the sides and back, but not in front.

Signs and Symptoms of Pelvic or Genital Injuries

Signs and symptoms of pelvic injury are the same as those for an abdominal injury. These signs and symptoms include:

- Severe pain.

- Bruising.

- External bleeding.

- Nausea and vomiting (sometimes containing blood).

- Weakness.

- Thirst.

- Pain, tenderness or a tight feeling in the area.

- Organs protruding from the area.

- Rigid abdominal muscles.

- Other signs and symptoms of shock.

Care for Pelvic or Genital Injuries

Always call 9-1-1 or the designated emergency number if you suspect a pelvic injury. Because an injury to the pelvis also can involve injury to the lower spine, it is best not to move the person. If possible, try to keep the person lying flat. Watch for signs of internal bleeding and take steps to minimize shock until EMS personnel take over.

Any injury to the genitals is extremely painful. Care for a closed wound to the genitals as you would for any closed wound, but with respect for the person's privacy. For injuries to the penis, wrap the injury in a soft, sterile dressing moistened with saline solution, and apply a cold compress to reduce pain and swelling. As with any injury, never remove an impaled object. Stabilize the object, and bandage it in place.

If the injury is an open wound, apply a sterile dressing and direct pressure with your gloved hand or the patient's hand, or use a protective barrier to avoid contact. If the penis is partially or completely amputated, apply a sterile pressure dressing to help stop bleeding, which may be significant. Aggressive direct pressure may also be needed if bleeding is excessive. If any parts are avulsed or completely amputated, wrap them in sterile gauze, moistened in sterile saline if available. Then place them in a plastic bag, labeled with the person's name and the time and date they were placed in the bag. Keep the bag cool by placing it in a larger bag or container of ice and water slurry, *not* on ice alone and *not* on dry ice. Give the bag to the EMS personnel when they arrive.

It is also possible for injuries to affect the scrotum and testicles. A blow to this area can rupture the scrotum and can cause pooling of blood, which is extremely painful. A ruptured testicle requires surgery. Apply a cold pack to the area to reduce swelling and pain and, if the scrotal skin has become avulsed, try to find it. Wrap the skin in sterile dressing and transport it with the person. The scrotum should be dressed with gauze sterilized and moistened with saline. Apply pressure to control bleeding.

To give care for an injury to the female genitals, control bleeding with pressure using compresses moistened with saline. Use a diaper-like dressing or feminine pad(s) for the wound and stabilize any impaled objects with a bandage. Straddle-type injuries may cause a closed wound with significant swelling, pain or inability to urinate. A feminine pad works well as a cushion dressing for these injuries, too. Use cold packs over the dressing to reduce swelling and ease pain. *Never* place anything in the vagina, including a dressing. Treat the person for shock as required.

Take care to provide the person with privacy by clearing the area of onlookers and draping a sheet or blanket over the person. Do *not* directly touch the genitals if possible while applying a dressing or cold pack. Always ask permission to give care. Ask if the person has suffered any other injuries, such as to the head. Be aware that if you are caring for a genital injury, sexual assault may be involved and you may be at a crime scene. If bleeding is life threatening, this will take priority over maintaining the integrity of a crime scene.

What if... *I am in a situation where a person has an open wound to the genitals, but the person is a minor?*

This can be a difficult situation, not because the care given is any different from the care given to an open wound to the forearm, but simply because of the age of the person and the location of the injury. To manage this situation after gaining consent, first, take time to slowly and clearly explain to the minor what care needs to occur. If the minor does not want you to help, and can follow your directions, walk them through the care steps. When assisting minors, always consider seeking additional assistance from a bystander who will be witness to your actions. Of course, if the minor's parents are available, in addition to obtaining consent, you should also solicit their assistance in giving care. Finally, while this can be an embarrassing situation for both the person and the first aid provider, remember to always act confidently.

Summary

Injuries to the chest, abdomen and pelvis can be serious. They can damage soft tissues, bones and internal organs. Although many injuries are immediately obvious, some may be detected only as the person's condition worsens over time. Watch for the signs and symptoms of serious injuries that require medical attention.

Care for any life-threatening conditions, and then give any additional care needed for specific injuries. Always call 9-1-1 or the designated emergency number as soon as possible. Have the person remain as still as possible. For open wounds to the chest, abdomen and pelvis, control bleeding. If you suspect a fracture, immobilize the injured part. Use occlusive dressings for open abdominal wounds when these materials are available. Your actions can make the difference in the person's chance of survival.

READY TO RESPOND? ❯

Think back to the bicyclist in the opening scenario, and use what you have learned to respond to these questions:

1. What signs and symptoms of injury does the bicyclist have, and what type of injury do they likely point to?

2. What steps should you take to help the person until EMS personnel arrive?

Study Questions

1. **Match each term with the correct definition.**

   a. Abdomen   b. Chest   c. Genitals   d. Pelvis   e. Sternum

   _____ External reproductive organs

   _____ The middle part of the trunk, containing the stomach, liver and spleen

   _____ The upper part of the trunk, containing the heart, major blood vessels and lungs

   _____ Long, flat bone in the middle of the front of the rib cage, also called the breastbone

   _____ The lower part of the trunk, containing the intestines, bladder and reproductive organs

2. **List five general guidelines for care for injuries to the chest, abdomen and pelvis.**

3. **List seven signs and symptoms of a chest injury.**

4. **List six signs and symptoms of an abdominal or pelvic injury.**

In question 5, circle the letter of the correct answer.

5. **Care for injuries to the chest, abdomen and pelvis includes—**

   a. Watching for changes in a person's breathing.   b. Controlling internal bleeding.   c. Giving the person fluids.   d. Minimizing bystander activity.

Base your answers for questions 6 through 8 on the scenario below.

You arrive at the local convenience store late Saturday night to satisfy your frozen yogurt craving. As you enter, you notice drops of blood on the floor. A robbery has just occurred—the store clerk appears to have been beaten and stabbed. The clerk is awake but in considerable pain and is having trouble breathing. You hear a sucking sound coming from the chest when the person breathes.

6. **What type of injury does the person have?**

7. **Identify the signs and symptoms that support your answer to question 6.**

8. **Describe the steps you would take to help this person.**

Answers are listed in the Appendix.

PART FIVE

Medical Emergencies

15 SUDDEN ILLNESSES

You've been asked to meet with Paul, a recruiter from a company you are interested in joining. When you arrive right on time at 1 p.m., the receptionist leads you to an open door, where you are both surprised to find Paul lying on the floor. He does not respond when the receptionist calls his name. With a look of panic on her face, she says something about diabetes and the fact that Paul ran out of time for lunch after going to the gym for a vigorous workout during his lunch break.

Learn and Respond ▶

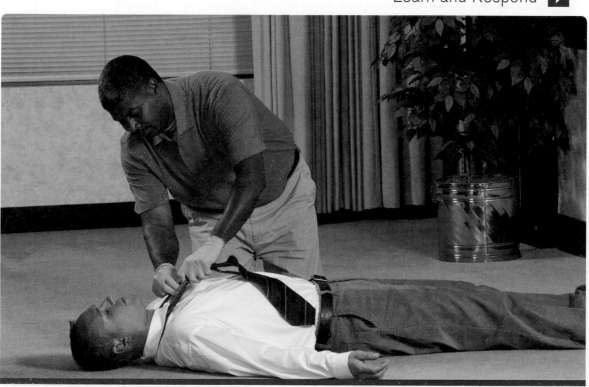

After reading this chapter, you should be able to:

- Recognize the signs and symptoms of a sudden illness.

- List the general guidelines for giving care to a person with a sudden illness.

- Describe how to care for a person who faints.

- Describe how to care for a person having a diabetic emergency.

- Describe how to care for a person having a seizure.

- Describe how to care for a person having a stroke.

- Identify ways to reduce the risk of a stroke or transient ischemic attack (TIA).

KEY TERMS

Absence seizure: A type of generalized seizure in which there are minimal or no movements; the person may appear to have a blank stare; also known as a petit mal or nonconvulsive seizure.

Aura phase: The first stage of a generalized seizure, during which the person experiences perceptual disturbances, often visual or olfactory in nature.

Clonic phase: The third phase of a generalized seizure, during which the person experiences the seizure itself.

Complex partial seizure: A type of partial seizure in which the person may experience an altered mental status or be unresponsive.

Diabetes: A disease in which there are high levels of blood glucose due to defects in insulin production, insulin action or both.

Diabetic emergency: A situation in which a person becomes ill because of an imbalance of insulin and sugar (glucose) in the bloodstream.

Epilepsy: A brain disorder characterized by recurrent seizures.

Fainting: Temporary loss of consciousness; usually related to temporary insufficient blood flow to the brain; also known as syncope, "blacking out" or "passing out."

Febrile seizure: Seizure activity brought on by a rapid increase or spike in body temperature in a young child or an infant.

Generalized tonic-clonic seizure: A seizure that affects most or all of the brain.

Glucose: A simple sugar that is the primary source of energy for the body's tissues.

Grand mal seizure: A type of generalized seizure that involves whole-body contractions with loss of consciousness.

Hyperglycemia: A condition in which too much sugar (glucose) is in the bloodstream, resulting in higher than normal blood glucose levels; also known as high blood glucose.

(Continued)

Hypoglycemia: A condition in which too little sugar (glucose) is in the bloodstream, resulting in lower than normal blood glucose levels; also known as low blood glucose.

Insulin: A hormone produced by the pancreas to help glucose move into cells; in persons with diabetes, it may not be produced at all or may not be produced in sufficient amounts.

Partial seizure: A seizure that affects only part of the brain; may be simple or complex.

Post-ictal phase: The fourth and final phase of a generalized seizure, during which the person becomes extremely fatigued.

Simple partial seizure: A seizure in which a specific body part experiences muscle contractions; does not affect memory or awareness.

Stroke: A disruption of blood flow to part of the brain that may cause permanent damage to brain tissue. The disruption can be caused by an obstruction (a clot) or by bleeding in the brain.

Tonic phase: The second phase of a generalized seizure, during which a person becomes unresponsive and muscles become rigid.

Transient ischemic attack (TIA): A condition that produces stroke-like symptoms but causes no permanent damage; may be a precursor to a stroke; sometimes called a mini-stroke.

Introduction

While some illnesses develop over time, others can strike without a moment's notice. If a person suddenly becomes ill, it is important to respond quickly and effectively. However, when illness happens suddenly, it can be hard to determine what is wrong and what you should do to help.

In this chapter, you will learn about the signs and symptoms of some common sudden illnesses, such as fainting, diabetic emergencies, seizures and strokes. You will also learn how to use the emergency action steps **CHECK—CALL—CARE** to help someone who becomes suddenly ill—whether or not you know the exact cause.

Sudden Illnesses

It usually is obvious when someone is injured and needs care. The person may be able to tell you what happened and what hurts. Checking the person also gives you clues about what might be wrong. However, when someone becomes suddenly ill, it is not as easy to tell what is physically wrong.

Sudden illness may result from a condition that has a rapid and severe onset **(acute),** or it may result from a persistent condition that continues or develops over a long period of time **(chronic).** Sometimes, there are no signs or symptoms to give clues about what is happening. At other times, the signs and symptoms only confirm that something is wrong, without being clear as to what is wrong. In either case, the signs and symptoms of a sudden illness often are confusing. You may find it difficult to determine if the person's condition is an emergency and whether to call 9-1-1 or the designated emergency number.

Ultimately, if a person looks and feels ill, there could be a medical emergency that requires immediate care. If you have any doubts about the severity of a person's sudden illness, call 9-1-1 or the designated emergency number.

Signs and Symptoms of Sudden Illnesses

When a person becomes suddenly ill, they usually look and feel sick. Common signs and symptoms include:

- Changes in level of consciousness such as drowsiness, confusion or unresponsiveness.

- Numbness, tingling, light-headedness, dizziness or giddiness.

- Breathing problems (i.e., trouble breathing or no breathing).

- Signs and symptoms of a possible heart attack, including persistent chest pain, discomfort or pressure lasting more than a few minutes that goes away and comes back or that spreads to the shoulder, arm, neck, jaw, stomach or back. Refer to Chapter 6 for more about heart attack.

- Signs or symptoms of a stroke, including sudden weakness on one side of the face (facial droop); sudden weakness, often on one side of the body; sudden slurred speech or trouble forming words; or a sudden, severe headache.

- Loss of vision or blurred vision.

- Signs of shock, including rapid breathing, changes in skin appearance and cool, pale or ashen (grayish) skin. Refer to Chapter 9 for more about shock.

- Sweating.

- Persistent abdominal pain or pressure.

- Nausea or vomiting.

- Diarrhea and abdominal cramping.

- Seizures.

Be sure to form an initial impression as part of your scene size-up in the **CHECK—CALL—CARE** emergency action steps, and use the mnemonic SAMPLE to help identify clues that might tell you what is wrong with the person. This may help you to find out what the person was doing when the illness started. For example, if someone suddenly feels ill or acts strangely and is attempting to take medication, the medication may be a clue as to what is wrong.

Care for Sudden Illnesses

Although you may not know the exact cause of the sudden illness, you should still give care based on your level of training and what you observe. Unless you know for sure what is wrong with a person, initially you will care for the signs and symptoms and not for any specific condition. Care for sudden illnesses by following the same general guidelines as you would for any emergency. After checking the scene and then the person for any life-threatening conditions:

- Do no further harm.

- Monitor the person's level of consciousness and breathing. A change in the person's condition may be a sign of a more serious injury or illness. A condition that may not appear serious at first may become serious over time.

- Help the person rest in a comfortable position or the position recommended for a specific condition, such as lying flat on their back for signs and symptoms of shock.

- Keep the person from getting chilled or overheated.

- Comfort and reassure the person, but do not give false hope.

- Give any specific care as needed.

In addition, if the person you are helping is awake and alert, ask them if they have any medical conditions or are taking any medication as part of the SAMPLE questions. If you know the person is having a severe allergic reaction or a diabetic emergency, assist the person with their prescribed medication. Do *not* give the person anything to eat or drink unless they are fully awake, able to swallow and follow simple commands, and are not showing any signs of a stroke (see the section on Stroke later in the chapter). If the person vomits and is unresponsive but breathing normally, position the person on their side in a recovery position so that you can clear the mouth. Finally, remember that depending on the condition in which you find the person, you may be able to do little more than help them rest comfortably and provide comfort and reassurance until emergency medical services (EMS) personnel arrive. However, knowing enough about sudden illness to recognize when to call 9-1-1 or the designated emergency number is your top priority as a trained lay responder.

Specific Sudden Illnesses

Some sudden illnesses may be linked with chronic conditions. These conditions include degenerative diseases, such as heart and lung diseases. There may be a hormone imbalance, such as in diabetes. The person could have epilepsy, a condition that causes seizures. An allergy can cause a sudden and sometimes dangerous reaction to certain substances. When checking a person, remember to look for a medical identification tag, or an app on their mobile phone indicating that the person has a chronic condition or allergy.

Having to deal with a sudden illness can be frightening, especially when you do not know what is wrong. Do not hesitate to give care as trained. Remember, you do not have to know the cause to help; recognizing when to call 9-1-1 or the designated emergency number is just as important. Signs and symptoms for sudden illnesses are similar to those for other conditions, and the care probably involves skills that you already know.

Fainting

One common sign of a sudden illness is temporarily becoming unresponsive. **Fainting** (also known as **syncope** or "passing out") is a temporary loss of consciousness caused by a temporary reduction of blood flow to the brain, such as when blood pools in the legs and lower body. When the brain is suddenly deprived of its normal blood flow, it momentarily shuts down and the person faints.

Fainting usually is not harmful. The person typically recovers quickly with no lasting effects. However, what appears to be a simple case of fainting actually may be a sign of a more serious condition. For example, fainting can be triggered by an emotionally stressful event, such as the sight of blood, or by standing for long periods of time. Some people, such as pregnant women or older adults, are more likely than others to faint when suddenly changing positions, such as moving from sitting or lying down to standing. Yet fainting may also be caused by pain and specific medical conditions such as an irregular or rapid heartbeat. Any time changes inside the body momentarily reduce the blood flow to the brain, fainting may occur. When an older person faints, it is more likely due to a serious cause such as an irregular or rapid heartbeat than something minor. Sometimes the person may note that they can feel their heart beating irregularly, known as palpitations. This is a symptom that there is a more serious cause for the fainting and that advanced medical care should be summoned by calling 9-1-1 or the designated emergency number.

Signs and Symptoms of Fainting

Fainting may occur with or without warning. A person who is about to faint often becomes pale or will have ashen, cool, moist skin; begins to sweat; and then becomes unresponsive and collapses. They may feel a rapid or irregular heartbeat. Sometimes a person may just "feel faint" and complain of feeling light headed, weak, dizzy or clammy. If a person is feeling faint, you may be able to prevent fainting by simply assisting the person to lie down on their back.

Care for Fainting

Usually, fainting is a self-correcting condition. When the person collapses or you assist them to lie down on their back, normal circulation to the brain typically resumes and the person feels better or regains responsiveness within a minute. Fainting itself does not often harm the person, but related injuries, such as those from falling (e.g., striking the head on the ground), may occur. If you can reach the person as they start to collapse, lower them to the ground or other flat surface. Then give care as follows:

- Position the person on their back, lying flat. Raising the legs 12 inches or more with a pillow or folded clothing may improve symptoms of light-headedness, but only do this if there is no evidence of injury and the movement does not cause pain.

- Loosen any tight or restrictive clothing, such as a tie or a collar (Figure 15-1).

- Check that the person is breathing normally.

- If the person vomits, roll them onto their side in a recovery position.

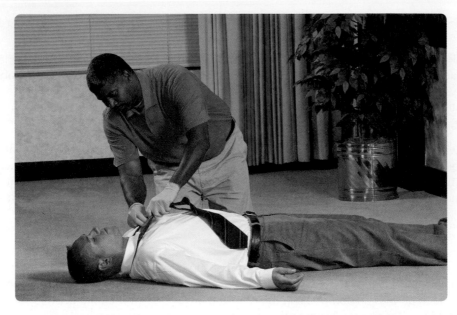

Figure 15-1. To care for a person who has fainted, place the person on their back lying flat and loosen any restrictive clothing, such as a tie or collar.

If you are unsure of the person's condition once they regain responsiveness, or if the person complains of continued light-headedness, palpitations or chest pain, or if moving is painful for the person, keep them lying flat and call 9-1-1 or the designated emergency number. Do *not* give the person anything to eat or drink. Also, do not slap the person or splash water on their face. Splashing water could cause the person to aspirate the water.

As long as the fainting person recovers quickly and has no lasting signs or symptoms, you may not need to call 9-1-1 or the designated emergency number. However, you should make the call if you are in doubt about the condition of the person who has fainted or if they have sustained an injury as a result of the sudden illness. If you do not call for help, it is always appropriate to have a bystander or family member take the person to a healthcare provider or emergency department to determine if the fainting episode is linked to a more serious condition.

Diabetic Emergencies

A total of 29.1 million people in the United States (9.3 percent of the population) have diabetes. Among this group, more than 5 million people are unaware that they have the disease. Overall, the risk for death among people with diabetes is about twice that of people without diabetes.

The American Diabetes Association defines **diabetes** as the inability of the body to change sugar (glucose) from food into energy. This process is regulated by insulin, a hormone produced in the pancreas. Diabetes can lead to other medical conditions such as blindness, periodontal (gum) disease, nerve disease, kidney disease, heart disease and stroke.

The cells in your body need sugar **(glucose)** as a source of energy. The cells receive this energy during digestion or from stored forms of sugar. The sugar is absorbed into the bloodstream with the help of **insulin** (Figure 15-2). Insulin is produced in the pancreas. For the body to function properly, there has to be a balance of insulin and sugar. People who have diabetes may become suddenly ill because there is too much or too little sugar in their bloodstream.

There are two major types of diabetes: type 1 and type 2 diabetes.

Type 1 diabetes, formerly called juvenile diabetes, affects about 1 million Americans. This type of diabetes, which usually begins in childhood, occurs when the body produces little or no insulin. People with type 1

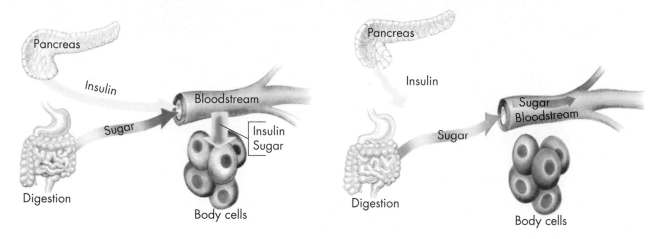

NORMAL   DIABETIC

Pancreas   Pancreas

Insulin   Insulin

Bloodstream   Sugar
                                                          Bloodstream
Sugar   Insulin   Sugar
                         Sugar

Digestion   Body cells   Digestion   Body cells

Figure 15-2. Insulin is needed to take sugar from the bloodstream into the body cells. For the body to function properly, there has to be a balance of insulin and sugar.

diabetes must inject insulin into their bodies daily (Figure 15-3). Type 1 diabetes is a chronic disease that currently has no cure.

The exact cause of type 1 diabetes is not known. Warning signs and symptoms include:

- Frequent urination.

- Increased hunger and thirst.

- Unexpected weight loss.

- Irritability.

- Weakness and fatigue.

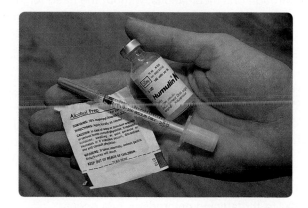

Figure 15-3. People with type 1 diabetes must inject insulin into their bodies daily.

Type 2 diabetes is the most common type, affecting about 90 to 95 percent of people with diabetes. This condition usually occurs in adults but can also occur in children. With type 2 diabetes, the body does not produce enough insulin to meet the body's needs or the body becomes resistant to the insulin it produces. Since type 2 diabetes is a progressive disease, people with this type of diabetes eventually may need to use insulin.

People from certain racial and ethnic backgrounds are known to be at greater risk for diabetes. Type 2 diabetes is more common in people of African-American, Latino and Asian descent, as well as among certain Native American tribes and Pacific Islanders. Although genetics and other factors increase the risk for diabetes, being overweight or obese also is a risk factor for developing the disease in adults and children.

People with type 2 diabetes often do not experience any warning signs or symptoms. Possible warning signs and symptoms of type 2 diabetes include:

- Any signs and symptoms of type 1 diabetes.

- Frequent infections, especially involving the skin, gums and bladder.

- Blurred vision.

- Numbness in the legs, feet and fingers.

- Cuts or bruises that are slow to heal.

- Itching.

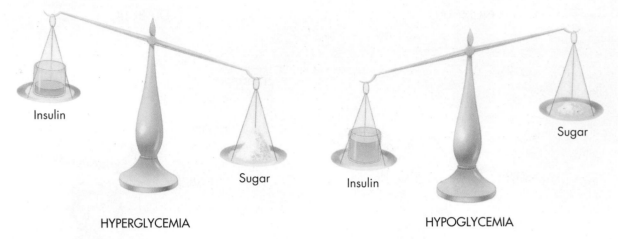

Insulin

Sugar

HYPERGLYCEMIA

Insulin

Sugar

HYPOGLYCEMIA

Figure 15-4. Hyperglycemia and hypoglycemia are diabetic emergencies that result from an imbalance between sugar and insulin within the body.

People with type 2 diabetes can regulate their blood glucose levels sufficiently through diet and sometimes through oral medications, without the need for insulin injections. People must carefully monitor their blood glucose levels, diet and exercise. If insulin-dependent, type 2 diabetics also must monitor their use of insulin. If the person with diabetes does not control these factors, they can have a **diabetic emergency.** A diabetic emergency is caused by an imbalance between sugar and insulin in the body (Figure 15-4).

When the insulin level in the body is too low, the sugar level in the blood begins to rise too high. This condition is called **hyperglycemia.** Sugar is present in the blood, but it cannot be transported from the blood into the cells without insulin. In this condition, body cells become starved for sugar. The body attempts to meet its need for energy by using other stored food and energy sources, such as fats. However, converting fat to energy is less efficient, produces waste products and increases the acidity level in the blood, causing a condition called **diabetic ketoacidosis (DKA).** As this occurs, the person with DKA becomes ill. They may have flushed, hot, dry skin and a sweet, fruity breath odor that can be mistaken for the smell of alcohol. The person also may appear restless or agitated. If the condition is not treated promptly, **diabetic coma,** a life-threatening emergency, can occur.

A person who is experiencing a diabetic emergency may appear to be under the influence of alcohol. For example, the person may slur their words or have difficulty walking. Interviewing the person (or bystanders) using SAMPLE and conducting a head-to-toe check may help you identify the true cause of the person's signs and symptoms.

On the other hand, when the insulin level in the body is too high, the person has a low blood sugar level. This condition is known as **hypoglycemia.** The blood sugar level can become too low if the diabetic:

- Takes too much insulin.

- Fails to eat adequately, or due to sudden illness cannot keep food or liquids down.

- Over-exercises and burns off sugar faster than normal.

- Experiences great emotional stress.

In this situation, sugar is used up rapidly, so not enough sugar is available for the brain to function properly. If left untreated, hypoglycemia may result in a life-threatening condition called **insulin shock.**

Many people who have diabetes have blood glucose monitors that can be used to check their blood sugar level if they are awake. Many hyperglycemic and hypoglycemic episodes are now managed at home because of the rapid information these monitors provide.

Signs and Symptoms of Diabetic Emergencies

Although hyperglycemia and hypoglycemia are different conditions, their major signs and symptoms are similar. These include:

- Changes in level of consciousness.
- Changes in mood.
- Irregular breathing.
- Feeling and looking ill.

- Abnormal skin appearance.
- Dizziness and headache.
- Confusion.

It is not important for you to differentiate between hyperglycemia and hypoglycemia because the basic first aid care for both of these diabetic emergencies is the same.

Care for Diabetic Emergencies

If you know someone experiencing the signs or symptoms listed above, you may know the person is a diabetic. A person who is awake and alert may also tell you they are a diabetic. You can also look for a medical identification tag. Often diabetics know what is wrong and will ask for something with sugar in it. They may carry some form of sugar with them in case they need it.

If the diabetic person is awake, can follow simple commands, is able to swallow and advises you that they need sugar:

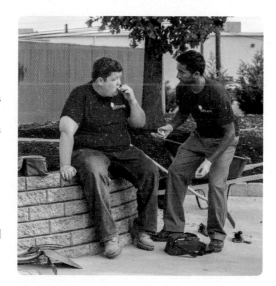

Figure 15-5. If a person having a diabetic emergency is awake and able to swallow, give them 15 to 20 grams of sugar.

- Give 15 to 20 grams of sugar in the form of 3 to 4 glucose tablets (Figure 15-5), a handful of candies containing sucrose or glucose that can be chewed, 8 ounces of milk, a non-diet soft drink, fruit strips or 4 to 5 teaspoons of table sugar dissolved in a glass of water or juice. Most fruit juices and non-diet soft drinks have enough sugar to be effective.

- If the problem is hyperglycemia (too much sugar in the body), this amount of sugar will not cause immediate harm.

- If symptoms persist for more than 10 to 15 minutes, repeat the administration of sugar and call 9-1-1 or the designated emergency number.

Some people with diabetes may have a prescribed glucagon kit that they carry with them to use in case of a severe hypoglycemic emergency. Glucagon is a hormone that stimulates the liver to release glucose into the bloodstream. The glucagon kit is used only when the person is unresponsive or has lost the ability to swallow. Those who spend a significant amount of time with the person (for example, family members, teachers, coaches or co-workers) may receive additional training to learn how to administer a glucagon injection.

Always call 9-1-1 or the designated emergency number if:

- The person is unresponsive and breathing normally or responsive but not fully awake. In this situation, do not give the person anything by mouth. After calling 9-1-1 or the designated emergency number, care for the person in the same way you would care for an unresponsive person. This includes conducting a head-to-toe check and placing the person in a recovery position if no injuries are found, making sure the person's airway is clear of any vomit, checking for breathing and giving care until advanced medical personnel take over.

- The person is awake but unable to swallow or follow simple commands. (In this case, do not put anything, liquid or solid, into the person's mouth.)

- The person does not feel better within about 10 to 15 minutes after taking some form of sugar.

- You cannot find any form of sugar immediately. Do not spend time looking for it.

For more information about diabetes, contact the American Diabetes Association at 800-DIABETES, go to www.diabetes.org or visit the National Diabetes Education Program website at www.ndep.nih.gov. For specific information about type 1 diabetes, contact the Juvenile Diabetes Research Foundation at 800-533-CURE or at jdrf.org.

What if... *I am helping a person having a diabetic emergency, but I do not know whether they have type 1 or type 2 diabetes?*

You do not need to identify what type of diabetes the person has; rather, you simply need to know if the person has diabetes (remember to look for a medical identification tag if the person cannot tell you) and whether or not the person is exhibiting signs and symptoms of a diabetic emergency. A responsive person with a history of diabetes will normally be able to tell you what is wrong and what care or assistance they require. If the person is unresponsive, call 9-1-1 or the designated emergency number and do not *give them anything by mouth, including food, water, or commercially produced glucose (sugar) tablets, gel or paste.*

What if... *A member of a group I am traveling with has diabetes, and the weather service is predicting a major storm event that could strand us for several days? How can I help make sure the person is prepared to avoid a diabetic emergency?*

The American Diabetes Association believes that people with diabetes should always be ready for an emergency that has the potential to cause a major disruption in one's life, such as a hurricane, earthquake, tornado or blizzard. The organization offers the following tips for emergency preparedness: A person with diabetes should always have adequate supplies on hand (the American Diabetes Association recommends storing 3 days' worth), such as oral medication, insulin, insulin delivery supplies, lancets, extra batteries for the person's meter and/or pump, and a quick-acting source of glucose. In addition, there should be a plan in place before a situation such as the ones above arises; and a list of emergency contacts, including physicians and medical supply stores, should be stored with the emergency supplies. Finally, if you are aware that a member of your group has diabetes, ask the person to tell you where you can find their emergency supplies and contact information in case the person needs to rely on you for help.

Seizures

When the normal functions of the brain are disrupted by injury, disease, fever, infection, metabolic disturbances or conditions causing a decreased oxygen level, a seizure may occur. The seizure is a result of abnormal electrical activity in the brain and causes temporary involuntary changes in body movement, function, sensation, awareness or behavior.

Types of Seizures

Generalized Seizures

Generalized tonic-clonic seizures, also called *grand mal seizures,* are the most well-known type of seizure. They involve both hemispheres (halves) of the brain and usually result in loss of consciousness. The seizure activity is known as tonic-clonic, which refers to the initial rigidity (tonic phase) followed by rhythmic muscle contractions (clonic phase), or convulsions.

Before a generalized seizure occurs, the person may experience an unusual sensation or feeling called an **aura.** An aura can include a strange sound, taste or smell, or an urgent need to get to safety. If the person recognizes the aura, there may be time to warn bystanders and to sit or lie down before the seizure occurs.

Generalized seizures usually last 1 to 3 minutes and can produce a wide range of signs. When a seizure occurs, the person becomes unresponsive and can fall, causing injury. The person may become rigid, and then experience sudden, uncontrollable muscular contractions (convulsions), lasting several minutes. Breathing may become irregular and even stop temporarily. The person may drool and the eyes may roll upward. As the seizure subsides and the muscles relax, the person may have a loss of bladder or bowel control.

The stages of most generalized seizures are as follows:

1. *Aura phase:* person may sense something unusual (not all persons will experience an aura)

2. *Tonic phase:* unresponsiveness then muscle rigidity

3. *Clonic phase:* uncontrollable muscular contractions (convulsions)

4. *Post-ictal phase:* diminished responsiveness with gradual recovery and confusion (person may feel confused and want to sleep)

Partial Seizures

Partial seizures may be simple or complex. They usually involve only a very small area of one hemisphere of the brain. Partial seizures are the most common type of seizure experienced by people with epilepsy (see the related section on Epilepsy in this chapter). Partial seizures can spread and become a generalized seizure.

In *simple partial seizures,* the person usually remains aware. There may be involuntary, muscular contractions in one area of the body, such as the arm, leg or face. Some people cannot speak or move during a simple partial seizure, although they may remember everything that occurred. Simple partial seizures may produce a feeling of fear or a sense that something bad is about to happen. Simple partial seizures can also produce odd sensations such as strange smells or hearing voices. Rarely, feelings of anger and rage or joy and happiness can be brought on by the seizure. Auras are a form of simple partial seizure.

Complex partial seizures usually last for 1 to 2 minutes, though they may last longer, and awareness is either impaired or lost while the person remains responsive. Complex partial seizures often begin with a blank stare followed by random movements such as smacking the lips or chewing. The person appears dazed, the movements are clumsy and the person's activities lack direction. They may be unable to follow directions or answer questions. The person cannot remember what happened after the seizure is over, and may be confused. This is called the post-ictal phase.

Absence (Petit Mal) Seizures

Individuals may also experience an *absence seizure,* also known as a petit mal seizure. These are most common in children. During an absence seizure, there is brief, sudden loss of awareness or conscious activity that may be mistaken for daydreaming. There may be minimal or no movement and the person may appear to have a blank stare. Most often these seizures last only a few seconds.

Absence seizures may also be referred to as nonconvulsive seizures, because the body remains relatively still during the episode, though eye fluttering and chewing movements may be seen.

Febrile Seizures

Young children and infants may be at risk for *febrile seizures,* which are seizures brought on by a rapid increase or spike in body temperature. They are most common in children under the age of 5 and typically last from a few minutes to no more than 15 minutes.

Febrile seizures are often caused by ear, throat or digestive system infections and are most likely to occur when a child or an infant runs a rectal temperature of over 103° F (39° C). An individual experiencing a febrile seizure may experience some or all of the following symptoms:

- Sudden rise in body temperature
- Change in consciousness
- Rhythmic jerking of the head and limbs
- Loss of bladder or bowel control
- Confusion

- Drowsiness
- Crying out
- Becoming rigid
- Holding the breath
- Rolling the eyes upward

Epilepsy

Epilepsy is a common neurological disorder, estimated to affect approximately 3 million people in the United States alone. Epilepsy is not a specific disease but a term used to describe a group of disorders in which the individual experiences recurrent seizures as the main symptom. In about one-third of all cases, seizures occur as a result of a brain abnormality or neurological disorder, but in two-thirds of cases there is no known cause.

In young people (up to the age of 20), the risk for having epilepsy is approximately 1 percent, with the greatest likelihood occurring during the first year of life. People ages 20 to 55 may also develop epilepsy but have a somewhat lower risk. The risk increases again after the age of 55 as people in this age group develop strokes, brain tumors or Alzheimer's disease, all of which can cause epilepsy. In fact, the highest rate of new epilepsy diagnoses is in this age group. The prevalence of epilepsy, or the number of individuals suffering with it at any time, is estimated to be approximately 5 to 8 in every 1000 people. By age 75, approximately 3 percent of people will have been diagnosed with epilepsy.

Persons who have epilepsy often can control the seizures with medication. Those with seizures that are difficult to control may also be treated with surgical resection, which can be curative, or with implanted devices, such as the vagus nerve stimulator, that help reduce seizure frequency. While some people require lifelong medical therapy, sometimes medication may be reduced or even eliminated over time. Some childhood epilepsies may resolve with age.

Care for Seizures

Seeing someone have a seizure may be intimidating, but you can easily care for the person. The person cannot control any muscular contractions that may occur and it is important to allow the seizure to run its course, because attempting to stop it or restrain the person can cause musculoskeletal injuries.

Protecting the person from injury and managing the airway are your priorities when caring for a person having a seizure. To help avoid injury, you should move nearby objects, such as furniture, away from the person. People having seizures rarely bite the tongue or cheeks with enough force to cause any significant bleeding. Do *not* place anything in the mouth to prevent this type of injury. Foreign bodies in the mouth may cause airway obstruction. Do *not* put fingers into the mouth of an actively seizing person to clear the airway. Place the person on their side in a recovery position as soon as it is feasible so that fluids (saliva, blood, vomit) can drain from the mouth. Typically, once the muscular convulsion stage passes, the person will remain unresponsive for a period of time and then gradually return to a normal level of responsiveness. Maintain the person in the recovery position until they are once again awake and alert.

In many cases, the seizure will be over by the time you arrive. In this case, the person may be drowsy and disoriented; this is the post-ictal phase. Check to see if the person was injured during the seizure. Offer comfort and reassurance, especially if the seizure occurred in public, as the person may feel embarrassed and self-conscious. If this is the case, keep bystanders well back to provide maximum privacy, and stay with the person until they are fully awake and aware of the surroundings.

Care for a child or an infant who experiences a febrile seizure is similar to the care for any other person experiencing a seizure. Immediately after a febrile seizure, cool the body by removing excess clothing. Contact a healthcare provider before administering any medication, such as acetaminophen, to control fever. Do *not* give aspirin to a feverish child under 18 years of age or to an infant, as this has been linked to **Reye's syndrome,** an illness that affects the brain and other internal organs.

> **Myth-Information.** *Myth: Put something between the teeth of a person who is having a seizure to prevent the person from biting or swallowing their tongue.* This practice is unsafe and unnecessary. It is impossible to swallow one's own tongue. And although the person may bite down on their tongue, causing it to bleed, this is a minor problem compared with the problems that can be caused by attempting to put an object in the mouth of a person who is having a seizure. You could chip a tooth or knock a tooth loose, putting the person at risk for choking. The person may also bite down with enough force to break the object and then choke on a piece of the object. Additionally, attempting to place an object in the person's mouth puts you at risk for getting bitten.

> **What if…** *A person starts having a seizure, and another individual at the scene insists that something should be put between the person's teeth to prevent them from biting the tongue? Should I stop them?*
>
> *Yes! Trying to insert an object into a person's mouth when they are having a seizure is dangerous and, in fact, may cause dental damage or aspiration of foreign materials into the lungs. If the person seems to doubt your stance, let them know you are trained in first aid and explain that there is no current evidence that recommends taking this step to care for a person having a seizure.*

When to Call 9-1-1

The person will usually recover from a seizure in a few minutes. If you discover the person has a medical history of seizures that are medically controlled, there may be no need for medical attention. However, in the following cases, advanced medical care should be provided:

- This is the person's first seizure.

- The seizure lasts more than 5 minutes or the person has repeated seizures with no sign of slowing down **(status epilepticus).**

- The person appears to be injured.

- You are uncertain about the cause of the seizure.

- The person is pregnant.

- The person is known to have diabetes.

- The person is a child or an infant.

- The seizure takes place in water.

- The person fails to regain consciousness after the seizure.

- The person is a young child or an infant who experienced a febrile seizure brought on by a rapid increase in body temperature.

- The person is older and could have suffered a stroke.

Status epilepticus is an epileptic seizure (or repeated seizures) that lasts longer than 5 minutes without any sign of slowing down. A status epilepticus seizure is a true medical emergency that may be fatal. If you suspect the person is experiencing this type of seizure, call 9-1-1 or the designated emergency number immediately.

Stroke

Stroke is one of the leading causes of death and long-term disability in the United States. Nearly 800,000 Americans will have a stroke this year.

A ***stroke*** is caused when there is a disruption of blood flow to part of the brain from an obstruction (a clot) or from bleeding into the brain. A stroke can cause permanent brain damage (if not treated appropriately within several hours), but sometimes the damage can be stopped or reversed.

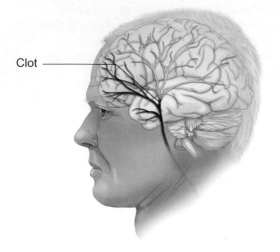

Clot

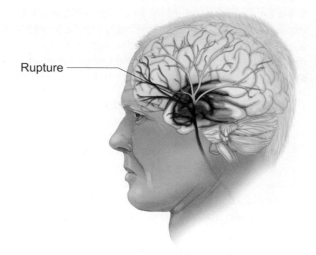

Rupture

Figure 15-6. Strokes are most commonly caused by a blood clot in the arteries that supply blood to the brain.

Figure 15-7. A less common cause of a stroke is bleeding from a ruptured artery in the brain.

Most commonly, a stroke is caused by a blood clot, called a **thrombus** or **embolus,** that forms or lodges in the arteries that supply blood to the brain (Figure 15-6). Another common cause of a stroke is bleeding from a ruptured artery in the brain caused by a head injury, high blood pressure or an **aneurysm**—a weak area in the wall of an artery that balloons out and can rupture (Figure 15-7). Fat deposits lining an artery **(atherosclerosis)** may also cause a stroke. Less commonly, a tumor or swelling from a head injury may compress an artery and cause a stroke.

A *transient ischemic attack (TIA),* often referred to as a "mini-stroke," is a temporary episode that, like a stroke, is caused by a disruption in blood flow to a part of the brain. However, unlike a stroke, the signs and symptoms of TIA disappear within a few minutes or hours of its onset. Although the indicators of TIA disappear quickly, the person is not out of danger at that point. In fact, someone who experiences TIA has a greater chance (10 times) of having a stroke in the future than someone who has not had a TIA. Because you cannot distinguish a stroke from a TIA, remember to call 9-1-1 or the designated emergency number immediately when any signs and symptoms of a stroke appear.

Risk Factors for a Stroke

The risk factors for a stroke are similar to those for heart disease. Some risk factors are beyond one's control, such as age, gender and family history of stroke or cardiovascular disease. Other risk factors can be controlled through diet, changes in lifestyle or medication. The chances of having a stroke are increased in persons with a history of high blood pressure, previous stroke or mini-stroke, diabetes or heart disease.

Uncontrolled high blood pressure is the number one risk factor for a stroke. If you have high blood pressure, you are approximately seven times more likely to have a stroke compared with someone who does not have high blood pressure. High blood pressure puts added pressure on the arteries and makes them stiffer. The excess pressure also damages organs, including the brain, heart and kidneys. Even mildly elevated blood pressure can increase one's risk of a stroke. Diabetes is another major risk factor for a stroke. If uncontrolled, the resulting elevated blood sugar levels can damage blood vessels throughout the body. See Smart Moves: Preventing a Stroke to learn strategies for controlling the risk factors for a stroke.

While some risk factors for a stroke are beyond your control, there are steps that can be taken to decrease the role other risk factors play—and live a healthier lifestyle all around.

- **Control your blood pressure.** This is the most important of the controllable risk factors. Have your blood pressure checked regularly. If it is high, follow the advice of your healthcare provider about how to lower it. Often, high blood pressure can be controlled by losing weight, changing diet, exercising routinely and managing stress. If those measures are not sufficient, your healthcare provider may prescribe medication.

- **Control diabetes.** If you have been diagnosed with diabetes, follow the advice of your healthcare provider about how to control it.

- **Do not smoke.** Smoking increases your blood pressure, damages blood vessels and makes blood more likely to clot. If you smoke and would like to quit, many techniques and support systems are available to help, including seeking help from your healthcare provider or local health department. The benefits of quitting smoking begin as soon as you stop, and some of the damage from smoking actually may be reversible. Approximately 10 years after a person has stopped smoking, their risk for a stroke is about the same as the risk for a person who has never smoked.

- **Avoid secondhand smoke.** Even if you do not smoke, it is important to avoid long-term exposure to secondhand cigarette smoke and to protect children from this danger as well.

- **Eat a healthy diet.** Limiting your intake of foods high in cholesterol and saturated fat can help to prevent a stroke as these can cause fatty materials to build up on the walls of your blood vessels. Foods high in cholesterol include egg yolks and organ meats, such as liver and kidneys. Saturated fats are found in beef, lamb, veal, pork, whole milk and whole-milk products.

- **Exercise regularly.** Regular exercise reduces your chance of having a stroke by strengthening the heart and improving blood circulation. Exercise also helps in weight control. Being overweight increases the chance of developing high blood pressure, heart disease and atherosclerosis.

Signs and Symptoms of a Stroke

By recognizing the signs and symptoms of a stroke and calling 9-1-1 or the designated emergency number, you can prevent damage before it occurs. Experiencing a TIA is the clearest warning that a stroke may occur. Do not ignore its stroke-like signs and symptoms, even if they disappear completely within minutes or hours.

As with other sudden illnesses, looking or feeling ill and behaving in a strange way are common general signs and symptoms of a stroke or mini-stroke. Other specific signs and symptoms of a stroke have a sudden onset, including:

- Facial droop or drooling.

- Weakness or numbness of the face, arm or leg. This usually happens on only one side of the body.

- Trouble with speech. The person may have trouble talking, getting words out or being understood when speaking, and may have trouble understanding.

- Loss of vision or disturbed (blurred or dimmed) vision in one or both eyes. The pupils may be of unequal size.

- Sudden severe headache. The person will not know what caused the headache and may describe it as "the worst headache ever."

- Dizziness, confusion, agitation, unresponsiveness or other severe altered mental status.

- Loss of balance or coordination, trouble walking or ringing in the ears.

- Incontinence.

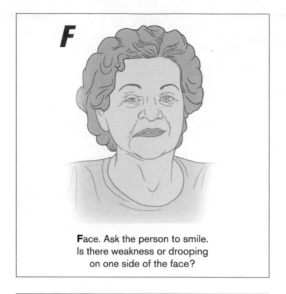

Face. Ask the person to smile. Is there weakness or drooping on one side of the face?

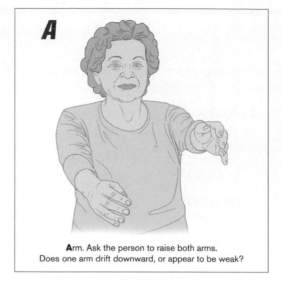

Arm. Ask the person to raise both arms. Does one arm drift downward, or appear to be weak?

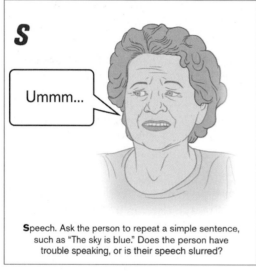

Speech. Ask the person to repeat a simple sentence, such as "The sky is blue." Does the person have trouble speaking, or is their speech slurred?

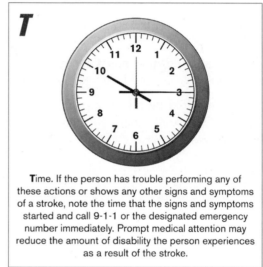

Time. If the person has trouble performing any of these actions or shows any other signs and symptoms of a stroke, note the time that the signs and symptoms started and call 9-1-1 or the designated emergency number immediately. Prompt medical attention may reduce the amount of disability the person experiences as a result of the stroke.

Figure 15-8. The FAST check for a stroke.

The "FAST" check (Figure 15-8) is a quick way of checking for signs and symptoms of a stroke.

See Think FAST for a Stroke to learn more about spotting the signs and symptoms and acting quickly to get the person advanced medical care by calling 9-1-1 or the designated emergency number.

Care for a Stroke

Call 9-1-1 or the designated emergency number immediately if you encounter someone who is having or has had a stroke, or if the person had a mini-stroke (even if the signs and symptoms have gone away). In addition:

- Note the time of onset of the signs and symptoms if witnessed or the last time the person was known to be well, and report it to the 9-1-1 call taker or EMS personnel when they arrive.

- If the person is unresponsive, make sure that they have an open airway and care for any life-threatening conditions:

  - If fluid or vomit is in the person's mouth, position them in a recovery position.

  - You may have to remove some fluids or vomit from the mouth by using one of your fingers (use precautions when possible).

  - Stay with the person and monitor their breathing and for changes in their condition.

- If the person is awake, check for non-life-threatening conditions:

  - Offer comfort and reassurance as a stroke can make the person fearful and anxious. Often, they do not understand what has happened.

  - Have the person rest in a comfortable position.

  - Do not give them anything to eat or drink.

Although a stroke may cause the person to experience difficulty speaking, they can usually understand what you say. If the person is unable to speak, you may have to use nonverbal forms of communication, such as hand squeezing or eye blinking, and communicate in forms that require a yes-or-no response (squeeze or blink once for "yes," twice for "no").

In the past, a stroke almost always caused irreversible brain damage. Today, new medications and medical procedures can limit or reduce the damage caused by a stroke. Many of these new treatments are time-sensitive; therefore, you should immediately call 9-1-1 or the designated emergency number to get the best care for the person. Minutes matter!

Think FAST for a Stroke

For a stroke, think FAST to identify the signs and symptoms, and get the person advanced medical care in the most timely manner possible by calling 9-1-1 or the designated emergency number. FAST stands for:

Face: Weakness, numbness or drooping on one side of the face. Ask the person to smile. Does one side of the face droop?

Arm: Weakness or numbness in one arm. Ask the person to raise both arms. Does one arm drift downward?

Speech: Slurred speech or difficulty speaking. Ask the person to repeat a simple sentence (e.g., ask the person to say something like, "The sky is blue."). Are the words slurred? Can the person repeat the sentence correctly?

Time: Try to determine when the signs and symptoms began. If the person shows any one sign or symptom of a stroke, time is critical. Call 9-1-1 or the designated emergency number right away.

The FAST mnemonic is based on the Cincinnati Pre-Hospital Stroke Scale, which was developed in 1997 to help EMS personnel to identify strokes in the field. The FAST method for public awareness has been in use in the community in Cincinnati, Ohio, since 1999. Researchers at the University of North Carolina validated it in 2003 as an appropriate tool for helping laypersons to recognize and respond quickly to the signs and symptoms of a stroke. In 2015, the International Liaison Committee on Resuscitation (ILCOR) recommended the FAST mnemonic as an effective tool for trained lay responders to use.

What if... *I think a person is having a stroke, but I am not really sure?*

A stroke is a significant medical emergency requiring timely advanced medical care. Even if you are not 100 percent sure a stroke is the cause of a person's sudden illness, always immediately call 9-1-1 or the designated emergency number if you think a person may be having, or may have already experienced, a stroke. The person's greatest chance for recovery from a stroke begins when emergency care is started immediately. The sooner physicians can determine the cause of the stroke, the sooner they can prescribe a plan of care.

Summary

Sudden illness can strike anyone at any time. When a person becomes suddenly ill, it can be frightening to that person, to you and to other bystanders. Unless a person can tell you what is wrong, such as a diabetic who knows they need sugar, or the signs or symptoms seem to clearly indicate a stroke according to the FAST mnemonic, it may be difficult to determine what is causing the sudden illness, and you might not know what care to give. However, even if you do not know the cause of the illness, you can still give proper care. Recognizing the signs and symptoms of sudden illness—such as changes in consciousness; pale, cool or clammy skin; confusion and weakness—will help you determine the necessary care to give the person until EMS personnel arrive.

READY TO RESPOND? ❯

Think back to Paul in the opening scenario, and use what you have learned to respond to these questions:

1. What type of sudden illness does Paul seem to have? Why do you think so?

2. What should you do after making sure the scene in the office is safe?

3. After calling 9-1-1, the receptionist comes in with a glass of juice to offer Paul. Should you allow her to give it to him?

Study Questions

1. **Match each term with the correct definition.**

   a. Diabetic emergency   e. Hypoglycemia   h. Stroke

   b. Epilepsy   f. Insulin   i. Transient ischemic attack (TIA)

   c. Fainting   g. Generalized tonic-clonic seizure

   d. Hyperglycemia

   ____ A hormone produced by the pancreas to help glucose move into cells

   ____ Temporary loss of consciousness; usually related to temporary insufficient blood flow to the brain

   ____ A disruption of blood flow to a part of the brain that may cause permanent damage to brain tissue

   ____ A seizure that affects most or all of the brain

   ____ A condition in which too little sugar is in the bloodstream

   ____ A condition in which too much sugar is in the bloodstream

   ____ A brain disorder characterized by recurrent seizures

   ____ A condition that produces stroke-like symptoms but causes no permanent damage; may be a precursor to a stroke

   ____ A situation in which a person becomes ill because of an imbalance of insulin and sugar (glucose) in the bloodstream

2. **List six general signs and symptoms of a sudden illness.**

3. **List four general guidelines of care that should be applied for any sudden illness.**

4. **Describe how to care for a seizure once the seizure is over.**

In questions 5 through 12, circle the letter of the correct answer.

5. **If you were caring for someone who looked pale, was unresponsive and was breathing normally, what should you do?**

   a. Call 9-1-1 or the designated emergency number.

   b. Inject the person with insulin.

   c. Give sugar to the person.

   d. Let the person rest for a while.

(Continued)

6. A friend who has diabetes is drowsy but is able to answer questions and follow simple commands. They are not sure if they took their insulin today. What should you do?

   a. Suggest they rest for an hour or so.

   b. Tell them to take their insulin.

   c. Have them eat or drink something with sugar in it.

   d. Check for breathing and signs of life.

7. Your father has diabetes. He also suffered a stroke a year ago. You find him lying on the floor, uninjured and unresponsive but breathing normally. What should you do after calling 9-1-1 or the designated emergency number on your mobile phone?

   a. Call his physician.

   b. Lift his head up and try to give him a sugary drink.

   c. Place him in a side-lying recovery position and monitor his breathing.

   d. Inject him with insulin yourself, while waiting for EMS personnel to arrive.

8. In caring for the person having a seizure, you should—

   a. Move any objects that might cause injury.

   b. Try to hold the person still.

   c. Place a spoon between the person's teeth.

   d. Splash the person's face with water.

9. To reduce the risk of aspiration of blood or other fluids in a person who has a seizure—

   a. Place an object between the person's teeth.

   b. Position the person on their side as soon as it is safe to do so.

   c. Place a thick object, such as a rolled blanket, under the person's head.

   d. Move the person into a sitting position.

10. Controlling high blood pressure reduces your risk for—

   a. Heart disease, a stroke and TIA.

   b. Seizure.

   c. Diabetes.

   d. Epilepsy.

(Continued)

Study Questions continued

11. **At the office, your boss complains that they have had a severe headache for several hours. Their speech suddenly becomes slurred, they lose their balance and they fall to the floor. What should you do?**

    a. Give two aspirin.

    b. Help your boss find and take their high blood pressure medication.

    c. Call 9-1-1 or the designated emergency number.

    d. Tell your boss to rest for a while.

12. **Which of the following is (are) included in the care you give for fainting?**

    a. If possible, help to lower the person to the floor or other flat surface.

    b. If possible, elevate the legs.

    c. Give the person something to eat or drink.

    d. a and c

Answers are listed in the Appendix.

16 POISONING

You stop by your cousin's house to drop off some things for a family party later that evening. Your cousin answers the door and explains that they are in the middle of cleaning the bathroom. After directing you to drop the things you've brought in the kitchen, your cousin heads back upstairs to finish. That's when you hear a cry out, "Oh no! Sophia!" Sophia is your cousin's 3-year-old daughter, and when you run up to see what's wrong, your cousin is wiping something from Sophia's mouth and looking distressed. Sophia is seated next to the cleaning supplies that were left on the floor.

Learn and Respond ▶

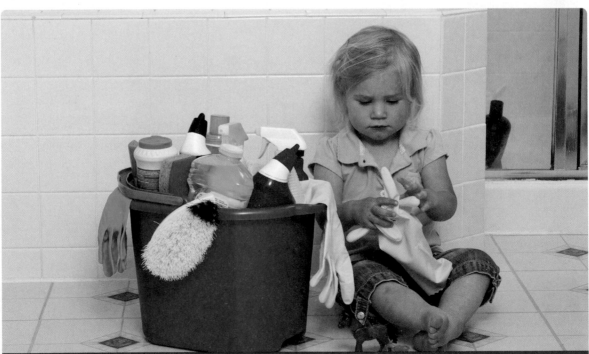

After reading this chapter, you should be able to:

- Understand when to call the Poison Control Center and when to call 9-1-1 or the designated emergency number.

- Identify the general guidelines for care for any poisoning emergency.

- List the four ways poisons enter the body.

- Identify the signs and symptoms of each type of poisoning.

- Describe how to care for a person based on the type of poisoning.

- Identify the signs and symptoms of and care for anaphylaxis.

- List the ways to prevent poisoning.

KEY TERMS

Absorbed poison: A poison that enters the body through the skin.

Anaphylaxis: A form of distributive shock caused by an often sudden severe allergic reaction, in which air passages may swell and restrict breathing; also referred to as anaphylactic shock.

Ingested poison: A poison that is swallowed.

Inhaled poison: A poison that is breathed into the lungs.

Injected poison: A poison that enters the body through a bite, sting or syringe.

Poison: Any substance that can cause injury, illness or death when introduced into the body, especially by chemical means.

Poison Control Center (PCC): A specialized health center that provides information on poisons or suspected poisoning emergencies.

Introduction

A *poison* is any substance that causes injury, illness or death when introduced into the body. In 2014, Poison Control Centers (PCCs) received more than 2.1 million calls from people who had come into contact with a poison. Over 91 percent of these poisonings took place in the home, and 48 percent involved children under age 6. Poisoning deaths in children under age 6 represented about 1.4 percent of the total deaths from poisoning, while the 20- to 59-year-old age group represented about 66 percent of all deaths from poisoning. Child-resistant packaging for medications and preventive actions by parents and others who care for children have resulted in a decline in child poisonings. At the same time, there has been an increase in adult poisoning deaths, which is linked to an increase in both suicides and drug-related poisonings. See Common Causes of Poisoning (by Age Group) for more information.

In this chapter, you will learn about the four ways in which poisons can enter the body—ingestion, inhalation, absorption and injection. You will also learn about the types of poisons that fall into each of these categories, how to recognize the signs and symptoms of each type of poisoning and how to give care for each. You will learn about how and when to contact your local or regional PCC or summon more advanced medical personnel.

Later chapters cover additional types of poisoning emergencies, including bites and stings (Chapter 17) and substance abuse and misuse (Chapter 18).

Common Causes of Poisoning (By Age Group)

Younger than age 6

Analgesic medications ("painkillers")	Insecticides
Cleaning substances	Plants
Cosmetics and personal care products	Topical medications
Cough and cold remedies	Vitamins
Gastrointestinal medications	

Ages 6 to 19

Analgesic medications	Cough and cold remedies
Bites and stings	Food products and food poisoning
Cleaning substances	Plants
Cosmetics	Stimulants and street drugs

Older than age 19

Analgesic medications	Cleaning substances
Antidepressant drugs	Food products and food poisoning
Bites and stings	Fumes and vapors
Cardiovascular drugs	Insecticides
Chemicals	Sedatives and hallucinogenic drugs

Poisoning

Poisonings can be accidental or intentional. Box 16-1 lists common household poisons, and Box 16-2 describes strategies for reducing the risk for unintentional poisoning at home. Some poisons—including many medications—are not deadly or harmful in small doses but become dangerous if taken into the body in larger amounts. The severity of a poisoning depends on three factors:

- The type and amount of the substance
- The time that has elapsed since the poison entered the body
- The person's age, size (build), weight and medical conditions

How will you know if someone who is ill has been poisoned? Look for clues about what has happened. Try to get information from the person or from bystanders. As you check the scene during the scene size-up, be aware of unusual odors, flames, smoke, open or spilled containers, an open medicine cabinet, or an overturned or damaged plant. Also, notice if the person is showing any of the signs and symptoms of poisoning that are described in this chapter.

Box 16-1. **Household Poisons**

Many everyday household items can be poisonous if they are used incorrectly. Young children and older adults with medical conditions that are associated with confusion (e.g., dementia) or who have impaired vision are at particularly high risk for unintentional poisoning. Common causes of unintentional poisonings at home include:

- Alcohol (found in many products, including hand sanitizer, mouthwash, perfume, cologne, aftershave and vanilla extract).

- Medications (over-the-counter and prescription) and vitamins.

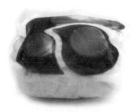

- Cleaning products (detergent "pods" are especially attractive to children).

- Glues and paints.

- Insect and weed killers.

- Car maintenance products (e.g., antifreeze, windshield washer fluid).

- Plants (both houseplants and outdoor plants).

- Oils, lubricants and polishes.

- Personal care products.

- Tobacco.

- Heavy metals, such as lead (often found in old, peeling paint).

PHOTOS: © Scott Rothstein/Shutterstock.com

Box 16-2. **Lowering the Risk for Unintentional Poisoning**

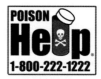

If your household contains members who are at high risk for unintentional poisoning, these are simple steps you can take to help keep them safe:

- Keep all medications and household products well out of reach (preferably up, away and out of sight) of children or older adults with medical conditions that are associated with confusion (e.g., dementia).

- Store potentially poisonous substances in locked cabinets.

- Be aware that purses and bags may contain potential poisons (such as medications or hand sanitizer). Avoid putting bags or purses down where they are within reach of curious children or confused older adults.

- Closely supervise children and confused older adults, especially in areas where potential poisons are commonly stored (such as kitchens, bathrooms and garages).

- Keep medications and products in their original containers with their original labels in place.

- Use poison symbols to identify potentially poisonous substances, and teach children the meaning of the symbols.

- Be aware that a child or confused older adult may try to consume products that feature fruit on the label (e.g., cleaning products), so take care when storing these.

- Never call a medicine "candy" to entice a child to take it, even if the medicine has a pleasant candy-like flavor.

- Use child-resistant safety caps on containers of medication and other potentially dangerous products, but do not assume that children cannot open them. (There is no such thing as "childproof.")

- Dispose of medications and other potentially poisonous substances properly. Check with your local government for procedures for the safe disposal of unused and expired medications and other hazardous materials.

You also may suspect a poisoning based on information from or about the person. If you suspect someone has swallowed a poison, try to find out:

- The type of poison.
- The quantity taken.
- When it was taken.
- How much the person weighs.

This information can help you and others to give the most appropriate care.

General Care for Poisoning

After you have checked the scene and determined that there has been a poisoning, you should follow these general care guidelines:

- Remove the person from the source of poison if the scene is dangerous. Do this only if you are able to do so without endangering yourself or bystanders.

- Check the person's level of consciousness and breathing:

  - For life-threatening conditions, such as if the person is unresponsive or is not breathing, or if a change in the level of consciousness occurs, call 9-1-1 or the designated emergency number immediately.

  - Care for any life-threatening conditions.

- If the person is awake, ask questions to get more information about the current situation.

- Look for any containers and/or packaging and take them with you to the telephone.

- Call the 24-hour national Poison Help line at 800-222-1222 and follow any directions the call taker gives.

Poison Control Centers

Poison Control Centers (PCCs) are specialized health centers that provide information on poisons and suspected poisoning emergencies. A network of PCCs exists throughout the United States. Medical professionals in these centers have access to information about virtually all poisonous substances and can tell you how to care for someone who has been poisoned. The American Association of Poison Control Centers operates a 24-hour national Poison Help line, which is staffed by pharmacists, physicians, nurses and toxicology specialists and can be reached at 800-222-1222.

PCCs answer over 2 million calls about poisoning each year. Since many poisonings can be treated without the help of emergency medical services (EMS) personnel, PCCs help prevent overburdening of the EMS system and hospitals. Approximately 70 percent of poison exposure cases can be managed over the phone without a referral to a healthcare facility. For more information, visit the American Association of Poison Control Centers website at www.aapcc.org.

You should call 9-1-1 or the designated emergency number for a poisoning if you are unsure about what to do, you are unsure about the severity of the problem or it is a life-threatening condition. In general, call 9-1-1 or the designated emergency number instead of the PCC if a person:

- Is unresponsive, confused or responsive but not fully awake.
- Has trouble breathing.
- Has persistent chest pain or pressure.
- Has pressure or pain in the abdomen that does not go away.
- Is vomiting blood or passing blood in their stool or urine.
- Exhibits signs of shock such as pale, ashen or grayish, cool, moist skin.
- Has a seizure, severe headache or slurred speech.
- Acts aggressively or violently.

Types of Poisoning

Poisons are generally placed in four categories based on how they enter the body: ingestion, inhalation, absorption and injection (Figure 16-1, A–D).

Ingested Poisonings

Ingested poisons are poisons that are swallowed and include items such as foods (e.g., certain mushrooms and shellfish), drugs (e.g., alcohol), medications (e.g., aspirin) and household items (e.g., cleaning products, pesticides and even household plants). See The Danger in the Garden later in this chapter for information on poisonous plants.

Young children tend to put almost everything in their mouths, so they are at a higher risk for ingesting poisons, including household cleaners and medications. Older adults may make medication errors if they are prone to forgetfulness or have difficulty reading the small print on medicine container labels.

In addition, in 2011 the Centers for Disease Control and Prevention (CDC) estimated that 48 million people contract foodborne illnesses each year in the United States. Approximately 128,000 people are hospitalized and more than 3000 die from foodborne illness.

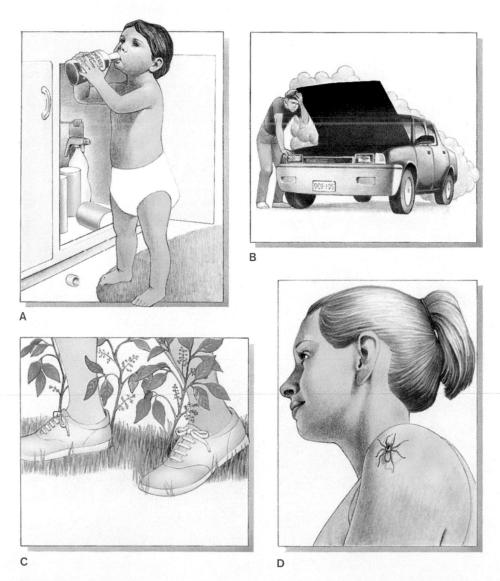

A

B

C

D

Figure 16-1, A–D. A poison can enter the body in four ways: **A,** ingestion; **B,** inhalation; **C,** absorption; and **D,** injection.

Two of the most common categories of food poisoning are bacterial and chemical food poisoning. Bacterial food poisoning typically occurs when bacteria grow on food that is allowed to stand at room temperature after being cooked, which releases toxins into the food. Foods most likely to cause bacterial food poisoning are meats, fish and dairy or dairy-based foods. Chemical food poisoning typically occurs when foods with high acid content, such as fruit juices or sauerkraut, are stored in containers lined with zinc, cadmium or copper or in enameled metal pans. Another primary source of chemical food poisoning is lead, which is sometimes found in older pipes that supply drinking and cooking water. Mercury, a heavy metal, can also be a source of food poisoning. Fish and shellfish, such as shark and swordfish, are a major dietary source of mercury. However, mercury can also come from other dietary items and contact with mercury metal or its compounds (e.g., a mercury thermometer).

Two of the most common causes of food poisoning are *Salmonella* bacteria (most often found in poultry and raw eggs) and *Escherichia coli* (*E. coli*) (most often found in raw meats and unpasteurized milk and juices). The deadliest type of food poisoning is botulism, which is caused by a bacterial toxin usually associated with home canning. See Smart Moves: Preventing Food Poisoning to learn how to avoid foodborne illnesses.

SMART MOVES > PREVENTING FOOD POISONING

By following the steps Clean, Separate, Cook and Chill, you can reduce the likelihood of foodborne illnesses from occurring.

Clean

- Wash hands thoroughly (for 20 seconds) with soap and running water before and after preparing or handling food; between handling raw and cooked foods; and whenever handling food preparation surfaces, dishes and utensils.

- Wash all surfaces and utensils after each use.

- Wash fruits and vegetables, but not meat, poultry or eggs.

Separate

- Use separate cutting boards—one for produce and one for raw meat, poultry, seafood and eggs—as well as separate plates and utensils for cooked and raw foods.

- Keep meat, poultry, seafood and eggs separate from other food in your grocery cart, when bagging and later at home in the refrigerator.

Cook

- Use a food thermometer to make sure food is cooked to the proper temperature (see www.foodsafety.gov for more details). Clean the thermometer after each use.

- Keep food hot after cooking, at a temperature of at least 140° F (60° C).

- Follow microwave directions to cook food thoroughly (to 165° F, or 74° C). If the instructions say to let food sit after microwaving, do so as it allows the food to cook more completely.

Chill

- Refrigerate perishable foods within 2 hours.

- Make sure your refrigerator and freezer are at the right temperature: between 40° F (4° C) and 32° F (0° C) and at 0° F (−18° C) or below, respectively.

- Never thaw or marinate foods on the counter.

- Know when to throw food out.

SOURCE: FoodSafety.gov: *Keep food safe: Check your steps.* http://www.foodsafety.gov/keep/basics/index.html. Accessed December 2016.

Signs and Symptoms of Ingested Poisonings

A person who has ingested poison generally looks ill and displays symptoms common to other sudden illnesses. If you have even a slight suspicion that a person has been poisoned, seek immediate assistance from the PCC or by calling 9-1-1 or the designated emergency number.

Signs and symptoms of ingested poisonings include:

- Nausea, vomiting or diarrhea.
- Chest or abdominal pain.
- Trouble breathing.
- Sweating.
- Changes in level of consciousness.
- Seizures.

- Headache or dizziness.
- Weakness.
- Irregular pupil size.
- Double vision.
- Abnormal skin color.
- Burn injuries around the lips or tongue or on the skin around the mouth.

The symptoms of food poisoning, which can begin between 1 and 48 hours after eating contaminated food, include nausea, vomiting, abdominal pain, diarrhea, fever and dehydration. Severe cases of food poisoning can result in shock or death, particularly in children, older adults and those with an impaired immune system.

> **What if...** *A person has ingested a poison and I have a bottle of syrup of ipecac? Should I give it to the person? That's what my mother used to keep on hand for such an emergency.*
>
> *Although keeping a bottle of syrup of ipecac at home used to be widely recommended, that has changed and it is no longer recommended. In fact, these days there is no situation in which syrup of ipecac should be given for an ingested poison as there is a possibility of significant harm. Ipecac can cause serious complications and excessive and difficult-to-control vomiting, as well as delay care given later in an advanced medical facility if needed. More generally, as taught in this chapter, you should never administer anything by mouth for any poison, or induce vomiting, unless advised to do so by PCC or EMS personnel.*

Care for Ingested Poisonings

For ingested poisons, immediately call the PCC and follow the call taker's directions. Do *not* give the person anything to eat or drink unless you are told to do so.

In rare instances of ingested poisoning, the PCC may instruct you to induce vomiting. Vomiting may prevent the poison from moving to the small intestine, where most absorption takes place. However, vomiting should be induced only if advised by the PCC or a medical professional. The PCC or a medical professional will advise you exactly how to induce vomiting. In most instances, vomiting should not be induced. This includes when the person:

- Is unresponsive.
- Is having a seizure.
- Is pregnant (in the last trimester).

- Has ingested a corrosive substance (such as drain or oven cleaner) or a petroleum product (such as kerosene or gasoline). Vomiting these corrosives could burn the esophagus, throat and mouth.
- Is known to have heart disease.

Some people who have contracted food poisoning may require antibiotic or antitoxin therapy. Fortunately, most cases of food poisoning can be prevented by proper food handling and preparation.

What if... *I suspect a person has food poisoning? Should I call 9-1-1 for that?*

Maybe. It depends on the severity of the person's condition. The great majority of foodborne illnesses are mild and cause symptoms for only a day or two. More severe cases tend to occur in the very old, the very young, those who have an illness already that reduces their immune system function and healthy people exposed to a very high dose of an organism. If a person with food poisoning is unresponsive, not breathing or has changes in their level of consciousness, always call 9-1-1 or the designated emergency number. Otherwise contact a local healthcare provider and/or the board or department of health.

Inhaled Poisonings

Inhaled poisons are those that are breathed into the lungs. Poisoning by inhalation occurs when a person breathes in poisonous gases or fumes. A commonly inhaled poison is carbon monoxide (CO), which is present in substances such as car exhaust and tobacco smoke (Box 16-3). CO can also be produced by fires (gas and natural), defective gas cooking equipment, defective gas furnaces, gas water heaters and kerosene heaters. CO, which is a tasteless, odorless and colorless gas, is highly lethal and can cause death after only a few minutes of exposure.

Other common inhaled poisons include carbon dioxide, chlorine gas, ammonia, sulfur dioxide, nitrous oxide, chloroform, dry cleaning solvents, fire extinguisher gases, industrial gases and hydrogen sulfide. Paints and solvents produce fumes that some people deliberately inhale to get high, as do certain drugs, such as crack cocaine.

Signs and Symptoms of Inhaled Poisonings

Look for a substance (e.g., paint or solvent) around the mouth and nose of the person if you suspect deliberate inhalation. A pale or bluish skin color, which indicates a lack of oxygen, may be a sign of exposure to an inhaled poison. Other signs and symptoms of inhaled poisonings include:

- Trouble breathing or a breathing rate that is faster or slower than normal.
- Chest pain or tightness.
- Burning in the nose or eyes.
- Nausea and vomiting.
- Cyanosis.
- Headaches, dizziness and confusion.
- Coughing, possibly with excessive secretions.
- Seizures.
- Altered mental status with possible unresponsiveness.

Box 16-3. **Carbon Monoxide Poisoning**

Carbon monoxide is a gas that is produced whenever a fuel such as gas, oil, kerosene, diesel, wood or charcoal is burned. When equipment that burns these fuels is ventilated properly, carbon monoxide is not a problem. But if the equipment or ventilation system is faulty, or if equipment that is only supposed to be run outdoors is run inside an enclosed area, toxic levels of carbon monoxide can build up quickly, leading to carbon monoxide poisoning. Carbon monoxide poisoning is often called a "silent killer" because the gas has no smell and you cannot see it. Signs and symptoms of carbon monoxide poisoning include drowsiness, confusion, headache, dizziness, weakness, and nausea or vomiting. A person with signs or symptoms of carbon monoxide poisoning needs fresh air and medical attention immediately. Remove the person from the area if you can do so without endangering yourself, and call 9-1-1 or the designated emergency number.

Care for Inhaled Poisonings

When giving care to a person who may have inhaled poison, follow appropriate safety precautions to ensure that you do not also become poisoned. Toxic fumes may or may not have an odor. If you notice clues during the scene size-up that lead you to suspect toxic fumes are present, such as a strong smell of fuel (sulfur or skunk smell) or a hissing sound (which could indicate gas escaping from a pipe or valve), you may not be able to reach the person without risking your own safety. In cases like this, call 9-1-1 or the designated emergency number instead of entering the scene. Let EMS and public safety professionals know what you discovered, and only enter the scene if you are told it is safe to do so.

Anyone who has inhaled a poison needs fresh air as soon as possible. If you can remove the person from the source of the poison without endangering yourself, then do so. You can help a person who is awake by getting them to fresh air and then calling for more advanced care personnel based on the situation. If you find an unresponsive person, remove the person from the scene if it is safe to do so, and call 9-1-1 or the designated emergency number. Then give care for any life-threatening conditions, including CPR if the person is not breathing normally.

Absorbed Poisonings

Absorbed poisons enter through the skin or the mucous membranes in the eyes, nose and mouth. Absorbed poisons come from plants, as well as from chemicals and medications. Millions of people each year suffer irritating effects after touching or brushing against poisonous plants such as poison ivy, poison oak and poison sumac (Figure 16-2, A–C). Other poisons absorbed through the skin include dry and wet chemicals, such as those used in flea collars for dogs and in yard and garden maintenance products, which may also burn the skin. Some medications, such as topical medications or transdermal patches, can also be absorbed through the skin.

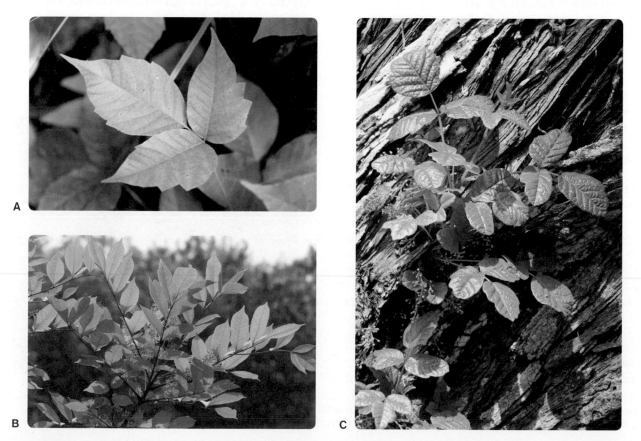

Figure 16-2, A–C. Examples of absorbed poisons include: **A,** poison ivy; **B,** poison oak; and **C,** poison sumac.
*Photos: **A,** Shutterstock.com/Tim Mainiero; **B,** Shutterstock.com/Dwight Smith; and **C,** www.poison-ivy.org*

Signs and Symptoms of Absorbed Poisonings

Some of the signs and symptoms of absorbed poisonings include:

- Traces of the liquid, powder or chemical on the person's skin.
- Skin that looks burned, irritated, red or swollen.
- Blisters that may ooze fluid, or a rash.
- Itchy skin.

> **What if...** *A person has poison ivy? Can they spread it to me while I'm helping care for it?*
>
> *Poison ivy causes a rash when a person who is allergic comes into contact with the plant's urushiol, an oily resin produced by the plant that is responsible for irritating the skin. Urushiol does not dry easily and attaches to one's skin, clothing, tools, equipment or pet's fur. So, yes, if there is still urushiol on a person or anything else you touch, it can spread poison ivy to you even if you do not have direct contact with the plant itself. As with the person you are helping, if you do come into contact with the urushiol, immediately wash the skin with soap and lukewarm water and wash all clothing and everything else that may have the oil on it.*

Care for Absorbed Poisonings

To care for a person who has come into contact with a poisonous plant, follow standard precautions and then immediately rinse the affected area thoroughly with water. Using soap cannot hurt, but soap may not do much to remove the poisonous plant oil that causes the allergic reaction. Before washing the affected area, you may need to have the person remove any jewelry. This is only necessary if the jewelry is contaminated or if it constricts circulation due to swelling. Rinse the affected areas for at least 20 minutes, using a shower or garden hose if possible. If a rash or weeping lesion (an oozing sore) develops, advise the person to seek the opinion of a pharmacist or healthcare provider about possible treatment. Medicated lotions may help soothe the area.

Antihistamines may also help dry up the lesions and help stop or reduce itching. Over-the-counter antihistamines are available at pharmacies and grocery stores and should be used according to the manufacturer's directions. If the condition worsens or if large areas of the body or the face are affected, the person should see a healthcare provider, who may administer anti-inflammatory drugs, such as corticosteroids, or other medications to relieve discomfort.

If the poisoning involves dry chemicals, brush off the chemicals using gloved hands before flushing with tap water (under pressure). Take care not to inhale any of the chemical or get any of the dry chemical on you, your eyes or the eyes of the person or any bystanders. Many dry chemicals are activated by contact with water. However, if continuous running water is available, it will flush the chemical from the skin before the activated chemical can do harm.

If wet chemicals contact the skin, flush the area continuously with large amounts of cool, running water. Running water reduces the threat to you and quickly and easily removes the substance from the person. Continue flushing for at least 20 minutes or until more advanced medical personnel arrive (Figure 16-3).

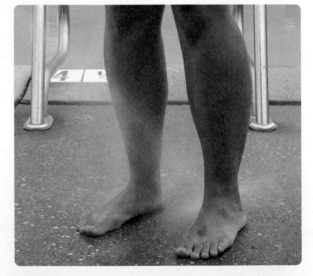

Figure 16-3. If the poisoning involves chemicals, flush the exposed area continuously with cool, running water for at least 20 minutes.

If a poison has been in contact with the person's eye(s), irrigate the affected eye or eyes from the nose side of the eye, not directly onto the middle of the cornea, with clean water for at least 15 minutes. If only one eye is affected, make sure you do not let the water run into the unaffected eye by tilting the head so the water runs from the nose side of the eye downward to the ear side. Continue care as long as advised by the PCC or until EMS personnel take over.

Injected Poisonings

Injected poisons enter the body through the bites or stings of certain insects, spiders, aquatic life, animals and snakes in the form of venom, or as drugs or misused medications injected with a hypodermic needle. Insect and animal bites and stings are among the most common sources of injected poisons. See Chapter 17 for more information about bites and stings, and how to give care for them.

Signs and Symptoms of Injected Poisonings

Some of the signs and symptoms of injected poisonings include:

- A bite or sting mark at the point of entry.

- A stinger, tentacle or venom sac in or near the entry site.

- Redness, pain, tenderness or swelling around the entry site.

- Signs and symptoms of allergic reaction, including localized itching, hives or rash.

- Signs and symptoms of a severe allergic reaction (anaphylaxis), including weakness, nausea, dizziness, shock, swelling of the throat or tongue, constricted airway or trouble breathing.

Care for Injected Poisonings

When caring for injected poisons, check the person for life-threatening conditions and care for any found. If there are no life-threatening conditions, applying a cold pack can reduce pain and swelling in the affected area. To give specific care for certain bites and stings, see Chapter 17. To learn about care for injected drugs, see Chapter 18. Call 9-1-1 or the designated emergency number if the person has signs and symptoms of anaphylaxis, which is discussed in greater detail starting on the next page.

The Danger in the Garden

By the time we are adults, most of us are aware that eating an unidentified mushroom can be a one-way ticket to the hospital. We are rarely aware of the other poisonous plants that are quietly sitting in our gardens and vases.

Lily-of-the-valley, mistletoe, philodendron, oleander, hyacinth, foxglove, mountain laurel and hemlock are just a few of the many common plants that can be highly toxic and even lethal if ingested. Surprisingly, even the seeds or leafy parts of things we eat every day can be poisonous, including seeds from peaches, apricots, cherries, apples and other fruit, and rhubarb and tomato plant leaves.

What precautions can you take to ensure against plant poisoning? First, learn about the plants you have in your home, office, garden and neighborhood. Do not rely on those who sell plants to provide warnings. Keep plants you know are toxic out of reach of infants and small children; remove berries and leaves from the floor; and, if in doubt, consult a PCC. In addition, do not store bulbs where they can be mistaken for onions; do not bite into an unfamiliar seed, no matter where you find it; never eat any plant you cannot positively identify; and clean up, but do not burn, any clippings and leaves from garden work, as smoke from a poisonous plant can become an inhalation hazard as well.

Finally, if you have an urge to forage for wild plant foods, take a field identification course taught by someone credentialed in the subject. Do not rely on field guidebooks. Even the clearest photograph is no proof against mistaking a "safe" plant for an unsafe one.

Anaphylaxis

Severe allergic reactions to poisons are rare, but when one occurs, it is truly a life-threatening medical emergency. This reaction, called **anaphylaxis,** was introduced in Chapter 7. Anaphylaxis is a form of shock. It can be caused by an insect bite or sting, or contact with certain drugs, medications, foods and chemicals. Anaphylaxis can result from any of the four modes of poisoning described in this chapter.

Every year in the United States, fewer than 100 deaths are caused by anaphylaxis. Fortunately, some deaths can be prevented if anaphylaxis is recognized immediately and cared for quickly.

Allergic Reactions

Our immune systems help to keep us healthy by fighting off harmful pathogens that can cause disease. But sometimes our immune systems overreact and try to fight off ordinary things that are not usually harmful, such as certain foods, grass or pet dander (tiny flakes of skin that animals shed). A person can have an allergy to almost anything. Common allergens (allergy triggers) include venomous insect stings, certain foods, animal dander, plant pollen, certain medications (such as penicillin and sulfa drugs) and latex. Over 15 million people in the United States have food allergies. Every year in the United States, there are over 200,000 visits to emergency departments because of food-related allergies. Certain types of food commonly cause an allergic reaction in individuals with sensitivities to those foods. Peanuts and tree nuts cause the most cases of fatal and near-fatal allergic reactions to food. Other common food allergens include cow's milk, eggs, seafood (especially shellfish), soy and wheat.

Signs and Symptoms of Anaphylaxis

An allergic reaction can range from mild to very severe. A person who is having a mild to moderate allergic reaction may develop a skin rash, a stuffy nose, or red, watery eyes. The skin or area of the body that came into contact with the allergen usually swells and turns red.

A person who is having a severe, life-threatening allergic reaction (anaphylaxis) may develop one or more of the following signs and symptoms within seconds or minutes of coming into contact with the allergen:

- Trouble breathing (Figure 16-4)

- Swelling of the face, neck, tongue or lips

- A feeling of tightness in the chest or throat

- Skin reactions (such as hives, itchiness or flushing)

- Stomach cramps, nausea, vomiting or diarrhea

- Dizziness

- Loss of consciousness

- Signs and symptoms of shock (such as excessive thirst; skin that feels cool or moist and looks pale or grayish; an altered level of consciousness; and a rapid, weak heartbeat)

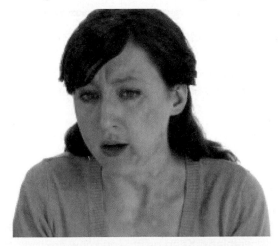

Figure 16-4. In anaphylaxis, air passages can swell, restricting breathing. The person may develop hives.

To determine if a person is having a severe, life-threatening allergic reaction (anaphylaxis), look at the situation as well as the person's signs and symptoms (Table 16-1).

Table 16-1. **How Do I Know If It Is Anaphylaxis?**

Situation	Look For
You do not know if the person has been exposed to an allergen.	■ Any skin reaction (such as hives, itchiness or flushing) **OR** ■ Swelling of the face, neck, tongue or lips **PLUS** ■ Trouble breathing **OR** ■ Signs and symptoms of shock
You think the person may have been exposed to an allergen.	Any **TWO** of the following: ■ Any skin reaction ■ Swelling of the face, neck, tongue or lips ■ Trouble breathing ■ Signs and symptoms of shock ■ Nausea, vomiting, cramping or diarrhea
You know that the person has been exposed to an allergen.	■ Trouble breathing **OR** ■ Signs and symptoms of shock

Care for Anaphylaxis

If you know that the person has had a severe allergic reaction before, and the person is having trouble breathing or is showing signs and symptoms of anaphylaxis, have someone call 9-1-1 or the designated emergency number immediately. If the person carries medication (e.g., epinephrine) used for the emergency treatment of anaphylaxis, offer to help the person use the medication. If you are alone, help the person administer the medication and then call 9-1-1 or the designated emergency number. While you wait for help to arrive, make sure the person is sitting in a comfortable position, or have the person lie down if they are showing signs of shock.

Epinephrine

Epinephrine is a drug that slows or stops the effects of anaphylaxis. If a person is known to have an allergy that could lead to anaphylaxis, they may carry an **epinephrine auto-injector** (a syringe system, available by prescription only, that contains a single dose of epinephrine). Devices are available containing different doses because the dose of epinephrine is based on weight (0.15 mg for children weighing between 33 and 66 pounds, and 0.3 mg for children and adults weighing more than 66 pounds). Many healthcare providers advise that people with a known history of anaphylaxis carry an anaphylaxis kit containing at least two doses of epinephrine (i.e., two auto-injectors) with them at all times (Figure 16-5). This is because more than one dose may be needed to stop the anaphylactic reaction. Have the person administer a second dose only if emergency responders are delayed and the person is still having signs and symptoms of anaphylaxis 5 to 10 minutes after administering the first dose.

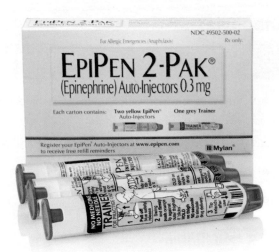
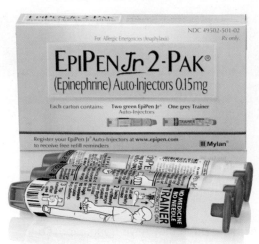

Figure 16-5. It is advisable to carry a kit containing at least two doses of epinephrine because more than one dose may be needed to stop anaphylaxis. *EpiPen® is a registered trademark owned by the Mylan companies.*

It is important to act fast when a person is having an anaphylactic reaction because difficulty breathing and shock are both life-threatening conditions. If the person is unable to self-administer the medication, you may need to help. You may assist a person with using an epinephrine auto-injector when the person has a previous diagnosis of anaphylaxis and has been prescribed an epinephrine auto-injector; the person is having signs and symptoms of anaphylaxis; the person requests your help using an auto-injector; and your state laws permit giving assistance. Where state and local laws allow, some organizations (such as schools) keep a stock epinephrine auto-injector for designated staff members who have received the proper training to use it in an anaphylaxis emergency. If you are using a stock epinephrine auto-injector, follow your organization's emergency action plan, which may include verifying that the person is showing signs and symptoms of anaphylaxis, ensuring that the person has been prescribed epinephrine in the past as appropriate and making sure to use a device containing the correct dose based on the person's weight.

Different brands of epinephrine auto-injectors are available but all work in a similar fashion. Begin by holding the person's leg firmly just above the knee to help prevent injury to the person, and then activate the device by pushing it against the person's mid-outer thigh (Figure 16-6). Once activated, the device injects the epinephrine into the thigh muscle. The device must be held in place for the recommended amount of time (e.g., 3 seconds, although the recommended time may vary by device) to deliver the medication. Some medication may still remain in the auto-injector even after the injection is complete. After removing the auto-injector, massage the injection site for several seconds (or have the person massage the injection site). Handle the used device carefully to prevent accidental needlestick injuries. Place the device in a rigid container, and then give the container to EMS personnel for proper disposal. For step-by-step instructions on helping a person to use an epinephrine auto-injector, see Skill Sheet 16-1.

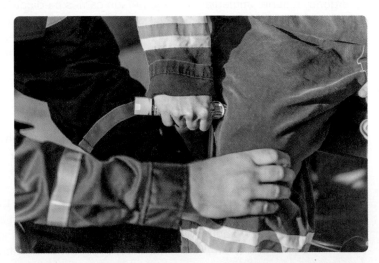

Figure 16-6. Pushing the auto-injector against the leg activates the device. It should be used on the muscular area of the person's mid-outer thigh. *Photo: courtesy of the Canadian Red Cross*

If a person is awake and able to use the auto-injector, help them in any way they ask you to. This might include getting the auto-injector from a purse, car, home or out of a specially designed carrier or belt; taking it out of the plastic tube; or assisting with or administering the injection.

Antihistamines

The person's healthcare provider may recommend that the person carry an antihistamine in their anaphylaxis kit, in addition to epinephrine. An **antihistamine** is a medication that counteracts the effects of histamine, a chemical released by the body during an allergic reaction. Antihistamines are supplied as pills, capsules or liquids and are taken by mouth. The person should take the antihistamine according to the medication label and their healthcare provider's instructions.

Summary

Poisoning can occur in any one of four ways: ingestion, inhalation, absorption and injection. The severity of a poisoning depends on the type and amount of the substance; how and where it entered the body; the time elapsed since the poison entered the body; and the person's size, weight and age. For suspected poisonings, call the 24-hour national Poison Help line at 800-222-1222. PCC personnel are specially trained to handle these types of emergencies. Call 9-1-1 or the designated emergency number instead if the person has any life-threatening conditions. Follow the directions of PCC personnel or the EMS dispatcher. Also, look for any signs and symptoms of anaphylaxis, and help the person with administering an epinephrine auto-injector or antihistamine as needed.

Increasing your awareness and taking steps to reduce the risks is one of the best ways to prevent a poisoning emergency. Identify items in your environment, such as household cleaners, plants, and medications that may pose a danger to you, your family or co-workers. Learn to handle and store these items properly by following the manufacturer's directions.

READY TO RESPOND? ▶

Think back to Sophia in the opening scenario, and use what you have learned to respond to these questions:

1. What clues did you find at the scene to alert you that Sophia may have been poisoned?

2. What should you do to care for Sophia?

Study Questions

1. **Match each term with the correct definition.**

   a. Absorbed poison   c. Ingested poison   e. Injected poison

   b. Anaphylaxis   d. Inhaled poison   f. Poison Control Center

   ____ A poison that enters the body through a bite, sting or syringe

   ____ A form of distributive shock caused by an often sudden severe allergic reaction, in which air passages may swell and restrict breathing

   ____ A specialized health center that provides information on poisons or suspected poisoning emergencies

   ____ A poison that is swallowed

   ____ A poison that enters the body through the skin

   ____ A poison that is breathed into the lungs

2. **List the general steps to care for a poisoning.**

3. **List three factors that determine the severity of poisoning.**

4. **Describe how to care for a person who has spilled a poisonous substance on their skin or has touched a poisonous plant, such as poison ivy.**

5. **List seven reasons to call 9-1-1 or the designated emergency number instead of the national Poison Help line for a poisoning emergency.**

Base your answers for questions 6 and 7 on the scenario below.

Beth was putting fertilizer on her favorite rosebush. She looked down and saw a strange plant that appeared to be a weed. She leaned over and plucked the plant out of the ground with her bare hand. A little while later, her hands started itching and burning. Her fingers became swollen, and red bumps began to appear all over her forearm.

6. **Identify the signs and symptoms that indicate that a poisoning emergency has occurred.**

7. **What could Beth have done to prevent this situation from happening?**

(Continued)

Study Questions continued

In questions 8 through 10, circle the letter of the correct answer.

8. Signs and symptoms of anaphylaxis include—

a. Trouble breathing, wheezing or shortness of breath.

b. Swelling of the face, throat or tongue.

c. Rash or hives.

d. All of the above

9. Your neighbor has accidentally swallowed some pesticide. He is awake and alert. What should you do?

a. Give him something to drink.

b. Induce vomiting.

c. Call the national Poison Help line.

d. Have him lie down.

10. You walk into a room and find an unresponsive child on the floor. There is an empty medicine bottle next to them. What should you do first?

a. Call 9-1-1 or the designated emergency number.

b. Call the national Poison Help line.

c. Give the child something to drink.

d. Check the airway.

Answers are listed in the Appendix.

Skill Sheet 16-1
Administering an Epinephrine Auto-Injector

After conducting a scene size-up, checking the person, and having someone call 9-1-1 or the designated emergency number, check the auto-injector:

- Remove the auto-injector from the carrier tube or package, if necessary.

- If applicable, confirm it is prescribed for the person.

- Check the expiration date of the auto-injector. If it has expired, do not use the auto-injector.

- If the medication is visible, confirm that the liquid is clear and not cloudy. If it is cloudy, do not use it.

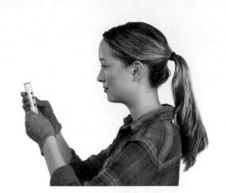

Put on disposable latex-free gloves and make sure the person is sitting or lying down.

Note: These instructions are based on the EpiPen®. If you are using a different device, follow the manufacturer's instructions.

If the person is unable to self-administer the auto-injector, and if state regulations allow and you are authorized by your organization to do so:

1. With the person sitting or lying down, locate the outside middle of one thigh to use as an injection site.

Note: If injecting through clothing, check that there are no obstructions at the injection site (such as a pant seam, keys or a mobile phone).

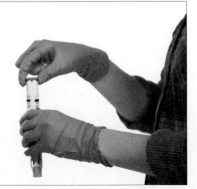

---

2. Grasp the auto-injector firmly in one fist, and pull off the safety cap with your other hand.

Note: Hold the auto-injector with the orange tip (needle end) pointing down; pull straight up on the blue safety cap without bending or twisting it.

Note: Never put your thumb, fingers or hand over the ends of the auto-injector.

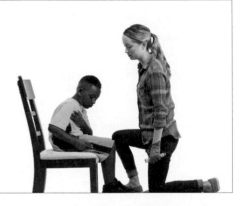

(Continued)

Administering an Epinephrine
Auto-Injector *Continued*

3. Hold the person's leg firmly just above the knee to limit movement during the injection. While you are holding the person's leg, make sure your hands are a safe distance away from the injection site.

4. Hold the auto-injector so that the needle end of the auto-injector is against the person's outer thigh at a 90-degree angle (perpendicular) to the thigh.

5. Quickly and firmly push the tip straight into the outer thigh. You will hear and/or feel a click indicating that the spring mechanism in the auto-injector has been triggered.

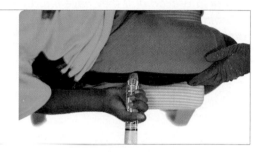

6. Hold the auto-injector firmly in place for 3 seconds (counting "1-1000; 2-1000; 3-1000") to deliver the medication.

7. Remove the auto-injector from the thigh carefully and massage (or have the person massage) the injection area with gloved hands for 10 seconds.

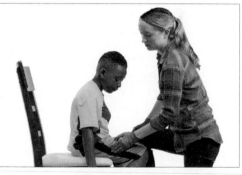

8. Encourage the person to remain seated and to lean forward to make it easier for the person to breathe. If signs and symptoms of shock are present, encourage the person to lie down and provide reassurance to the person that EMS personnel are on the way and you are doing everything you can to help.

9. Handle the auto-injector carefully while placing it in a safe container with one hand, and avoid touching the tip of the auto-injector. Give the auto-injector to EMS personnel when they arrive so the discharged device can be properly disposed of.

(Continued)

Administering an Epinephrine
Auto-Injector *Continued*

10. After administering the injection, ensure 9-1-1 or the designated emergency number has been called if this has not already been done, and monitor the person's response as follows:

   ■ Continue to reassure the person.

   ■ Ask the person how they feel.

   ■ Check the person's breathing.

*If, after 5 to 10 minutes, EMS personnel have not arrived **and** if symptoms of anaphylaxis have not improved or if they have improved but have gotten worse again, administer a second dose of epinephrine in the other thigh.*

17
BITES AND STINGS

You are working as a summer day camp counselor when one of your campers tells you that you need to come see Sara. When you get over to the picnic table where she is sitting, you can see that she has developed a rash that is appearing in spots all over her body. She tells you that last week, she discovered a tick on her leg when she got home one night.

Learn and Respond ❯

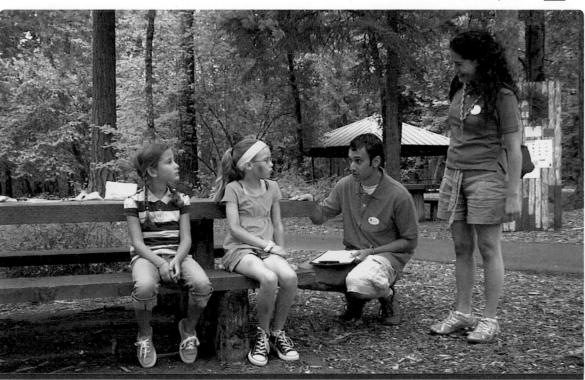

Introduction

Bites and stings are among the most common form of **injected venoms that can enter the human body.** People are bitten and stung every day by insects, spiders, snakes, marine life and animals. Most of the time, these bites and stings do not cause serious problems. However, in rare circumstances, certain bites and stings can cause serious illness or even death in people who are sensitive to the venom. In this chapter, you will learn how to recognize, care for and prevent some of the most common types of bites and stings.

Insect Stings

Between 0.5 and 5 percent of the American population is severely allergic to substances in the venom of bees, wasps, hornets and yellow jackets. For highly allergic people, even one sting can result in anaphylaxis, a life-threatening condition. Such highly allergic reactions account for an average of 34 reported deaths from insect stings each year. For most people, however, insect stings may be painful or uncomfortable but are not life threatening.

Signs and Symptoms of Insect Stings

Signs and symptoms of an insect sting include:

- Presence of a stinger.

- Pain.

- Swelling.

- Redness.

- Signs and symptoms of an allergic reaction.

Care for Insect Stings

If someone is stung by an insect:

- Remove any visible stinger. Scrape it away from the skin with the edge of a plastic card, such as a credit card (Figure 17-1). Do *not* use tweezers, especially for a bee sting, because doing so may cause the venom sac to burst and release more venom into the body.

- Wash the site with soap and water.

- Apply a cold pack to the area to reduce pain and swelling. Place a layer of gauze or cloth between the cold pack and the skin to prevent skin damage from the cold.

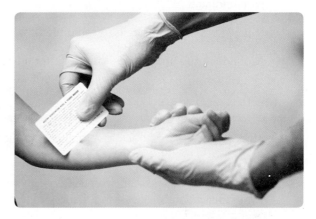

Figure 17-1. If someone is stung and a stinger is present, scrape it away from the skin with the edge of a plastic card.

Ask the person if they have had any prior allergic reactions to insect bites or stings, and observe for signs or symptoms of an allergic reaction, even if there is no known history. An allergic reaction can range from a minor localized skin rash to anaphylaxis. As you learned earlier, signs and symptoms of anaphylaxis include:

- Trouble breathing, wheezing or shortness of breath.

- Tight feeling in the chest and throat.

- Swelling of the face, throat or tongue.

- Weakness, dizziness or confusion.

- Rash or hives.

- Shock.

If you observe any signs and symptoms of anaphylaxis, have someone call 9-1-1 or the designated emergency number immediately, give care for life-threatening emergencies, continue to check the person, and help the person use an epinephrine auto-injector if one is available and you are authorized to do so. See Chapter 16 for all of the care steps you should take for anaphylaxis.

Tick Bites

Ticks can contract, carry and transmit disease to humans. Some of the diseases spread by ticks include Rocky Mountain Spotted Fever and Lyme disease. Box 17-1 describes strategies for limiting exposure to ticks.

Box 17-1. **Lowering the Risk for Tickborne Illnesses**

Ticks are found in wooded, brushy areas; in tall grass; and in leaf litter on the ground. When engaging in activities in environments where ticks are likely to be, lower your risk for picking up a tick by using the following strategies:

- Limit the amount of exposed skin. Wear long-sleeved shirts and long pants. Tuck your shirt into your pants and your pant legs into your socks or boots.

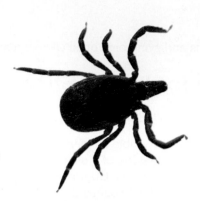

- Wear light-colored clothing to make it easier to see ticks on your clothing.

- Stay in the middle of trails. Avoid underbrush and tall grass.

- Conduct a full-body check for ticks after being outdoors.

  - Check the scalp, under the arms, in and around the ears, inside the navel, around the waist, behind the knees and between the legs. If you are outdoors for an extended period of time, check several times throughout the day.

- Consider using an insect repellent if you will be in a grassy or wooded area for a long period of time or if you know that the tick population in the area is high. Use repellents sparingly. One application will last 4 to 8 hours. Heavier or more frequent applications do not increase effectiveness.

  - DEET is the active ingredient in many insect repellents. The amount of DEET contained in the product can range from less than 10 percent to over 30 percent. The more DEET that a product contains, the longer it will provide protection. Products with 30 percent DEET are as safe as products with 10 percent DEET when used properly.

    - Apply products that contain DEET only once a day, or according to the manufacturer's instructions.

    - Do not use DEET on infants younger than 2 months.

    - Do not use a product that combines a DEET-containing insect repellent with sunscreen. Sunscreens wash off and need to be reapplied often. DEET does not wash off with water. Repeating applications may increase absorption of DEET through the skin, possibly leading to toxicity.

  - To apply repellent to your face, first spray it on your hands and then apply it from your hands to your face. Avoid sensitive areas such as the lips and eyes.

  - Never put repellents on children's hands. They may put them in their eyes or mouth.

  - Never use repellents on an open wound or irritated skin.

PHOTO: iStock.com/Goldfinch4ever

General Care for Tick Bites

If you find an embedded tick, it must be removed as follows:

- With a gloved hand, grasp the tick with fine-tipped, pointed, non-etched, non-rasped tweezers as close to the skin as possible and pull slowly, steadily and firmly upward (Figure 17-2). If you do not have tweezers, use a glove, plastic wrap, a piece of paper or a leaf to protect your fingers.

- Do *not* try to burn the tick off.

- Do *not* apply petroleum jelly or nail polish to the tick.

- Place the tick in jar containing rubbing alcohol to kill it.

- Wash the site with soap and water.

- Apply antiseptic or antibiotic ointment to help prevent infection.

- Wash your hands thoroughly.

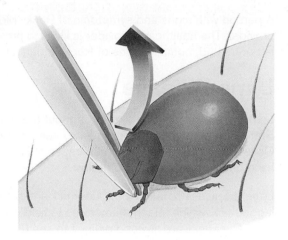

Figure 17-2. Remove a tick by pulling slowly, steadily and firmly with fine-tipped tweezers.

If you cannot remove the tick, have the person seek medical care. Even if you can remove the tick, the person should let their healthcare provider know that a tick has bitten them in case they become ill within the following month or two. The mouth parts of adult ticks may sometimes remain in the skin, but these will not cause disease. The person should check the site periodically thereafter. If a rash, flu-like signs and symptoms or joint pain develop, the person should seek medical care. Redness at the site of a tick bite does not necessarily mean a person is infected with a disease, but they should be evaluated by a healthcare provider as a precaution.

Rocky Mountain Spotted Fever

Rocky Mountain Spotted Fever is caused by the transmission of microscopic bacteria from the wood tick or dog tick host to other warm-blooded animals, including humans. Although the disease was first diagnosed in the western United States, cases of Rocky Mountain Spotted Fever continue to be reported throughout North and South America today. Rocky Mountain Spotted Fever is sometimes known by various regional names, such as black fever, mountain fever, tick fever, spotted fever or pinta fever. It occurs mostly in the spring and summer, and most cases occur in children.

Signs and Symptoms of Rocky Mountain Spotted Fever

Signs and symptoms of Rocky Mountain Spotted Fever usually appear between 2 and 14 days after a tick bite. Initial signs and symptoms include:

- Fever.
- Nausea and vomiting.
- Muscle aches or pain.

- Lack of appetite.
- Severe headache.

Later signs and symptoms include:

- A spotted rash that usually starts a few days after fever develops. The rash first appears as small spots on the wrists and ankles, and then spreads to the rest of the body. However, about one-third of infected persons do not get a rash.

- Abdominal pain.
- Joint pain.
- Diarrhea.

Care for Rocky Mountain Spotted Fever

A person with signs and symptoms of Rocky Mountain Spotted Fever after a tick bite should see a healthcare provider. The healthcare provider is likely to prescribe antibiotics. In most cases, the person will recover fully. If left untreated, complications of Rocky Mountain Spotted Fever can be life threatening.

Lyme Disease

Lyme disease is spreading throughout the United States. Although it is most frequently seen on the East Coast and in the upper Midwest, cases of Lyme disease have been reported in all 50 states.

Lyme disease is spread by the deer tick and black-legged tick, which attach themselves to field mice and deer. Deer ticks are tiny and difficult to see (Figure 17-3). They are much smaller than the common dog tick or wood tick. They can be as small as a poppy seed or the head of a pin. Adult deer ticks are only as large as a grape seed. Because of the tick's tiny size, its bite usually is painless. Many people who develop Lyme disease cannot recall having been bitten.

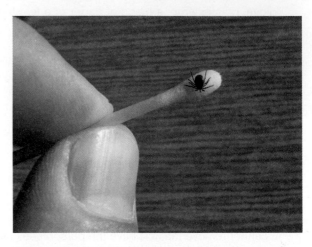

Figure 17-3. Deer ticks are tiny and difficult to see. *Photo: ©iStockphoto.com/Martin Pietak*

The tick is found around branches and in wooded and grassy areas. Like all ticks, it attaches itself to any warm-blooded animal with which it comes into direct contact, including humans. Deer ticks are active any time the temperature is above about 45° F (7° C). However, most cases of infection happen between May and late August, when ticks are most active and people spend more time outdoors. Recent studies indicate that the tick must remain embedded in human skin for about 36 to 48 hours in order to transmit the disease. More information on Lyme disease may be available from your local or state health department, the American Lyme Disease Foundation (aldf.com), or the Centers for Disease Control and Prevention (CDC) (cdc.gov/features/lymedisease).

Signs and Symptoms of Lyme Disease

The first sign of infection may appear a few days or a few weeks after a tick bite. In 80 to 90 percent of all cases of Lyme disease, a rash starts as a small red area at the site of the bite. It may spread up to 7 inches across (Figure 17-4). In fair-skinned people, the center may be a lighter color with the outer edges red and raised. This sometimes gives the rash a bull's-eye appearance. In some individuals, the rash may appear to be solid red. In people with a darker skin tone, the area may look black and blue, like a bruise. The rash may or may not be warm to the touch and usually is not itchy or painful. If a rash does appear, it will do so in about 1 to 2 weeks and may last for about 3 to 5 weeks. Some people with Lyme disease never develop a rash.

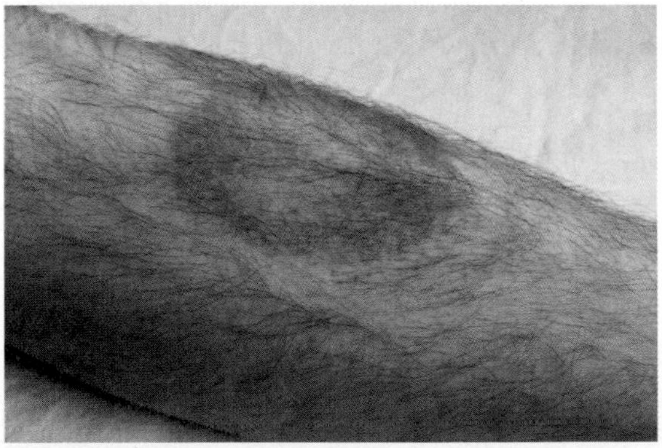

Figure 17-4. A person with Lyme disease may develop a rash. *Photo: ©iStockphoto.com/Heike Kampe*

Other signs and symptoms of Lyme disease include:

- Fever.
- Headache.
- Weakness.
- Joint and muscle pain.

These signs and symptoms are similar to signs and symptoms of flu and can develop slowly. They might not occur at the same time as the rash. Lyme disease can get worse if it is not treated. Signs and symptoms can include severe fatigue; fever; a stiff, aching neck; tingling or numbness in the fingers and toes; and facial paralysis. In its advanced stages Lyme disease may cause painful arthritis; numbness in the arms, hands or legs; severe headaches; long- or short-term memory loss; confusion; dizziness; and problems seeing or hearing. Some of these signs and symptoms could indicate problems with the brain or nervous system. Lyme disease may also cause heart problems such as an irregular or rapid heartbeat.

What if... *A person has a tick bite? With so many potential diseases that can form, should I consider calling 9-1-1 or the designated emergency number?*

Emergency medical services would only need to be contacted if you find an immediate danger, such as a person who is unresponsive or has a change in their level of consciousness. Otherwise, you should just remove the tick as quickly and as carefully as possible, and advise the person to contact their local healthcare provider for follow-up care. Of course, the person should also seek advanced medical care if you cannot successfully remove the tick following the steps described in this chapter.

Care for Lyme Disease

If a rash or flu-like signs or symptoms develop, the person should seek medical care immediately. A healthcare provider usually will prescribe antibiotics to treat Lyme disease. Antibiotics work quickly and effectively if taken as soon as possible. Most people who get treated early make a full recovery. If you suspect Lyme disease, do not delay seeking treatment. Treatment time is longer and less effective when the person has been infected for a long period of time.

Mosquito Bites

Mosquitoes and the viruses they can carry can make a person ill. The best way to prevent illness is to avoid being bitten. To protect yourself from mosquito bites, wear appropriate clothing such as long-sleeved shirts and long pants, avoid areas with standing water or that are known to have virus-carrying mosquitoes, and use insect repellent that contains an active ingredient such as DEET (Box 17-2). These precautions are the best ways to prevent diseases such as Zika, dengue, West Nile virus, eastern equine encephalitis and chikungunya that are spread by mosquitoes.

Box 17-2. **Insect Repellent**

- Repellents containing DEET, Picaridin, IR3535, and some oil of lemon eucalyptus and para-menthane-diol (PMD) products provide long-lasting protection. Choose one insect repellent and use it as directed. Products with higher percentages of active ingredients will provide longer protection.

- The effectiveness of non-Environmental Protection Agency-registered insect repellents, including some natural repellents, is not known.

- Insect repellents should not be used on babies younger than 2 months old, products containing oil of lemon eucalyptus should not be used on children younger than 3 years old, and products containing more than 30 percent DEET should not be used on children.

SOURCE: Centers for Disease Control and Prevention: *Protection against mosquitoes, ticks & other arthropods.* http://wwwnc.cdc.gov/travel/yellowbook/2016/the-pre-travel-consultation/protection-against-mosquitoes-ticks-other-arthropods. Accessed November 2016.

Zika Virus

The Zika virus is spread to people primarily through the bite of an infected *Aedes* species mosquito. These mosquitoes also spread dengue and chikungunya viruses. Mosquitoes that spread Zika, chikungunya and dengue are aggressive daytime biters, prefer to bite people, and live indoors and outdoors near people. They can also bite at night. Mosquitoes become infected when they bite a person already infected with the virus. Infected mosquitoes can then spread the virus to other people through bites.

Signs and Symptoms of the Zika Virus

Common symptoms of the virus include fever, rash, joint pain and conjunctivitis (pinkeye). For pregnant women, Zika virus infection may also cause a birth defect called microcephaly, a condition that affects brain development in the fetus. The virus may also be associated with Guillain-Barré syndrome that causes (usually short-term) paralysis.

West Nile Virus

West Nile virus (WNV) is passed on to humans and other animals by mosquitoes that bite them after feeding on infected birds. WNV has been reported across all the lower 48 states and typically occurs in the summer months. The highest risk for WNV is among people who work outside or participate in outdoor activities because of the greater exposure to mosquitoes.

WNV cannot be passed from one person to another. Also, no evidence supports that humans can acquire the disease by handling live or dead birds infected with WNV. However, it is still a good idea to use disposable latex-free gloves when handling an infected bird. Contact your local health department for instructions on reporting and disposing of the bird's body.

For most people, the risk for infection with WNV is very low. Less than 1 percent of people who are bitten by mosquitoes develop any signs or symptoms of the disease. In addition, relatively few mosquitoes actually carry WNV. Only about 1 in every 150 people who are infected with WNV will become seriously ill.

Signs and Symptoms of West Nile Virus

Most people infected with WNV have no signs or symptoms. Approximately 20 percent develop mild signs and symptoms, such as fever and aches, which pass on their own. The risk for severe disease is higher for people age 50 years and older. People typically develop signs and symptoms of WNV between 3 and 14 days after an infected mosquito bites them. These include:

- High fever.
- Headache.
- Neck stiffness.
- Confusion.
- Coma.
- Tremors.

- Convulsions.
- Muscle weakness.
- Vision loss.
- Numbness.
- Paralysis.

These signs and symptoms may last several weeks. In some cases, WNV can cause fatal encephalitis, which is a swelling of the brain that leads to death.

Care for West Nile Virus

If you suspect a person may have signs and symptoms of severe WNV illness, such as unusually severe headaches or confusion, seek medical attention immediately. Pregnant women and nursing mothers are encouraged to talk to their doctors if they develop signs and symptoms that could indicate WNV. There is no specific treatment for WNV infection or a vaccine to prevent it. In more severe cases, people usually need to go to the hospital, where they will receive intravenous fluids, assistance with breathing and nursing care.

Spider Bites and Scorpion Stings

Few spiders in the United States have venom that causes death. However, the bites of the black widow and brown recluse spiders can make you seriously ill and occasionally cause death. Another dangerous spider is the northwestern brown, or hobo, spider.

Black widow and brown recluse spiders live in most parts of the United States. You can identify them by the unique designs on their bodies. The black widow spider is black with a reddish hourglass shape on its underbody (Figure 17-5, A). The brown recluse spider is light brown with a darker brown, violin-shaped marking on the top of its body (Figure 17-5, B). Both spiders prefer dark, out-of-the-way places where they are seldom disturbed. Bites usually occur on the hands and arms of people reaching into places, such as wood, rock and brush piles or rummaging in dark garages and attics. Often, the person will not know that they have been bitten until signs and symptoms develop.

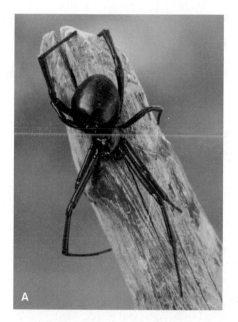

Figure 17-5, A–B. A, Black widow spider. B, Brown recluse spider. *Photos:* **A,** *©iStockphoto.com/Mark Kostich;* **B,** *Department of Entomology, The Ohio State University*

Scorpions typically live in dry regions of the southwestern United States and Mexico, but they are also common in other southern regions of the United States including Florida. They are usually about 3 inches long and have 8 legs and a pair of crablike pincers (Figure 17-6). At the end of the tail is a stinger, used to inject venom. Scorpions live in cool, damp places, such as basements, junk piles, woodpiles and under the bark of living or fallen trees. They are most active in the evening and at night, which is when most stings occur. Like spiders, only a few species of scorpions have a potentially fatal sting, and these are mostly found in the southwest. Scorpions from the southeastern part of the country are usually nonpoisonous. Their sting can cause localized allergic reactions similar to a bee sting and can be cared for in the same way. However, because it is difficult to distinguish highly poisonous

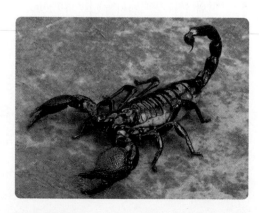

Figure 17-6. A scorpion. *Photo: ©iStockphoto. com/John Bell*

scorpions from nonpoisonous scorpions, all scorpion stings should be treated as medical emergencies. If it is possible and safe to do so, carefully attempt to capture the scorpion so that it could possibly be identified as poisonous or nonpoisonous by the Poison Control Center.

Signs and Symptoms of Spider Bites and Scorpion Stings

Signs and symptoms of spider bites depend on the amount of poison, called venom, injected and the person's sensitivity to the venom. Most spider bites heal with no adverse effects or scarring. Signs and symptoms of venomous spider bites can seem identical to those of other conditions and therefore can be difficult to recognize. The only way to be certain that a spider has bitten a person is to have witnessed it.

The bite of the black widow spider is the most painful and deadly, especially in very young children and older adults. The bite usually causes an immediate sharp pinprick pain, followed by a dull pain in the area of the bite. However, the person often does not know that they have been bitten until they start to feel ill or notice a bite mark or swelling. Other signs and symptoms of a black widow spider bite include:

- Rigid muscles in the shoulders, chest, back and abdomen.
- Restlessness.
- Anxiety.
- Dizziness.
- Headache.
- Excessive sweating.
- Weakness.
- Drooping or swelling of the eyelids.

The bite of the brown recluse spider may produce little or no pain initially. Pain in the area of the bite develops an hour or more later. A blood-filled blister forms under the surface of the skin, sometimes in a target or bull's-eye pattern. Over time, the blister increases in size and eventually ruptures, leading to tissue destruction and a black scab.

The hobo spider also can produce an open, slow-healing wound.

General signs and symptoms of spider bites and scorpion stings may include:

- A mark indicating a possible bite or sting.
- Severe pain in the sting or bite area.
- Redness and itching at the bite or sting site.
- A blister, lesion or swelling at the bite or sting site.
- Hives or other signs or symptoms of anaphylaxis.
- Nausea and vomiting.
- Stiff or painful joints.
- Chills or fever.
- Trouble breathing or swallowing.
- Sweating or salivating profusely.
- Muscle aches or severe abdominal or back pain.
- Dizziness or fainting.
- Chest pain.
- Elevated heart rate.
- Infection at the site of the bite or sting.

Care for Spider Bites and Scorpion Stings

Call 9-1-1 or the designated emergency number immediately if you suspect that someone has been bitten by a black widow or brown recluse spider, stung by a scorpion or if the person has any other life-threatening conditions. Also consider calling the national Poison Help line because Poison Control Centers often have the best information concerning venom toxicity. Healthcare professionals will clean the wound and give medication to reduce the pain and inflammation. An **antivenom,** a substance used to counteract the poisonous effects of the venom, is available for black widow and some scorpion bites. Antivenom is used mostly for children and older adults and is rarely necessary when bites occur in healthy adults.

While waiting for help to arrive:

- Wash the site thoroughly with soap and water.

- Apply a cold pack to the site to reduce pain and swelling. Place a layer of gauze or cloth between the cold pack and the skin to prevent skin damage from the cold.

- If the national Poison Help line, 9-1-1 or the designated emergency number has not been called, the person should seek medical attention.

- If you transport the person to a medical facility, keep the bitten area elevated and as still as possible.

Venomous Snakebites

Snakebites kill few people in the United States. Of the estimated 7000 to 8000 people reported bitten annually, fewer than five die. Most deaths occur because the person has an allergic reaction, is in poor health or because too much time passes before the person receives medical care. Figure 17-7, A–D shows the four kinds of venomous snakes found in the United States. Rattlesnakes account for most snakebites and nearly all deaths from snakebites.

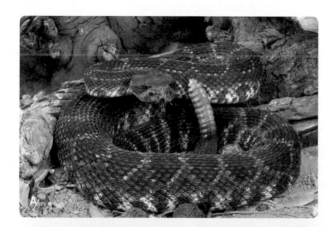
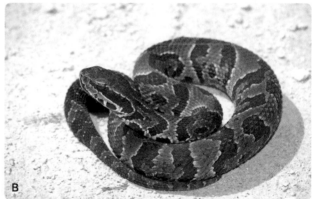
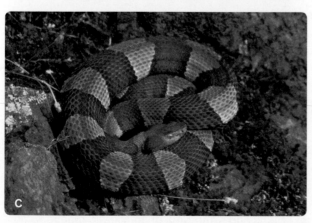
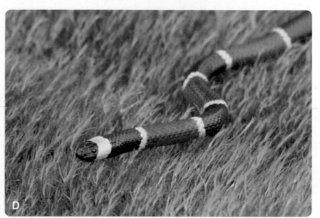

Figure 17-7, A–D. Four kinds of venomous snakes are found in the United States: **A,** rattlesnake; **B,** cottonmouth; **C,** copperhead; **D,** coral snake. *Photos: **A,** ©Audrey Snider-Bell, 2010, Used under license from Shutterstock.com; **B,** ©Leighton Photography & Imaging, 2010, Used under license from Shutterstock.com; **C,** Rauch, Ray/USFWS; **D,** ©iStockphoto.com/Mark Kostich*

Signs and Symptoms of Venomous Snakebites

Signs and symptoms that indicate a venomous snakebite include:

- One or two distinct puncture wounds from the snake's fangs, which may or may not bleed. The exception is the coral snake, whose teeth leave a semicircular mark.

- Severe pain and burning at the wound site immediately after or within 4 hours of the incident.

- Swelling and discoloration at the wound site immediately after or within 4 hours of the incident.

Care for Venomous Snakebites

If the bite is from a venomous snake such as a rattlesnake, copperhead, cottonmouth or coral snake, call 9-1-1 or the designated emergency number immediately. To give care until help arrives:

- Wash the site with soap and water.

  o Keep the injured area still and lower than the heart. The person should walk *only* if absolutely necessary.

- For any snakebite:

  o Do *not* apply ice.

  o Do *not* cut the wound.

  o Do *not* apply suction.

  o Do *not* apply a tourniquet.

  o Do *not* use electric shock, such as from a car battery.

> **Myth-Information.** *Myth: Actions such as applying a tourniquet, cutting the wound, applying suction, applying ice or applying electricity can help to slow the spread of venom throughout the body.* None of these measures are effective for slowing the spread of venom. In fact, they are likely to cause pain and injury. Your time is better spent seeking medical attention as quickly as possible.

Marine-Life Stings

The stings of some forms of marine life are not only painful but can also make you sick and, in some parts of the world, can kill you (Table 17-1). The side effects include allergic reactions that can cause breathing and heart problems, as well as paralysis and death. The lifeguards in your area should know the types of marine life that may be present.

Signs and Symptoms of Marine-Life Stings

Signs and symptoms of marine-life stings include:

- Rash, which may be red, raised or purplish in the shape of tentacles.

- Tentacles stuck to the skin.

- Puncture wounds (from stingrays or sea urchins).

- Pain or itching.

- Swelling.

- Signs and symptoms of an allergic reaction.

Table 17-1. **Venomous Marine Life**

Marine Life	Usually Found
Jellyfish	■ East and west coasts of the continental United States
Portuguese man-of-war (bluebottle jellyfish)	■ Tropical and subtropical waters
Stingray	■ Tropical and subtropical waters
Sea urchin	■ Oceans all over the world (warm and cold water) ■ In rock pools and mud, on wave-exposed rocks, on coral reefs, in kelp forests and in sea grass beds

PHOTOS: jellyfish, iStock.com/Mshake; Portuguese man-of-war (bluebottle jellyfish), Yann Hubert/Shutterstock.com; stingray, iStock.com/naturediver; sea urchin, iStock.com/naturediver

Care for Marine-Life Stings

Call 9-1-1 or the designated emergency number if the person does not know what stung them, has a history of allergic reactions to marine-life stings, is stung on the face or neck, or starts to have trouble breathing. Additional steps to take if you encounter someone who has sustained a marine-life sting include:

- Get a lifeguard to remove the person from the water as soon as possible. If a lifeguard is not available, use a reaching assist, if possible (see Chapter 20). Avoid touching the person with your bare hands, which could expose you to the stinging tentacles.

- Use gloves or a towel when removing any tentacles. A credit card edge or shell can be used to gently scrape away remaining tentacles.

- If you know the sting is from a jellyfish, irrigate the injured part with large amounts of seawater as soon as possible for at least 30 seconds. This can help to remove the tentacles and stop the injection of venom.

- Do *not* rub the wound or apply a pressure immobilization bandage, aluminum sulfate, meat tenderizer or other remedies because these may increase pain.

- Once the stinging action is stopped and tentacles removed, care for pain by hot-water immersion. Have the person take a hot shower if possible for at least 20 minutes. The water temperature should be as hot as can be tolerated (non-scalding) or about 113° F (45° C) if the temperature can be measured.

- Pain from most jellyfish stings in U.S. waters resolves within 20 minutes. If pain persists, consider applying a topical over-the-counter lidocaine gel or cream.

- If you know the sting is from a stingray, sea urchin or spiny fish, flush the wound with tap water. Seawater also may be used. Keep the injured part still and soak the affected area in non-scalding hot water (as hot as the person can stand) for at least 20 minutes or until the pain goes away. If hot water is not available, packing the area in hot sand may have a similar effect if the sand is hot enough. Carefully clean the wound and apply a bandage. Watch for signs and symptoms of infection and check with a healthcare provider to determine if a tetanus shot or additional care is needed.

> **What if...** *I am with a person at the beach who has been stung by a jellyfish? Is it true that urine is effective for controlling the pain?*
>
> *The use of urine to offset the toxin and reduce the pain of a jellyfish sting is not recommended; in fact, urine can actually cause the stingers to release more venom. To inactivate the venom and prevent further envenomation, follow the care steps in this chapter by rinsing with seawater, followed, once tentacles are removed, by a hot-water shower or immersion for at least 20 minutes or for as long as pain persists.*

Domestic and Wild Animal Bites

The bite of a domestic or wild animal carries the risk for infection, as well as soft tissue injury. One of the most serious possible results of a bite is rabies. **Rabies** is an infectious disease that affects the nervous system and is caused by a virus transmitted commonly through the saliva of diseased mammals, such as skunks, bats, raccoons, cats, dogs, cattle and foxes.

Animals with rabies may act in unusual ways. For example, nocturnal animals, such as raccoons, may be active in the daytime. A wild animal that usually tries to avoid humans may not run away when you approach. Rabid animals may salivate; appear partially paralyzed; or act irritable, aggressive or strangely quiet. To reduce your risk of becoming infected with rabies, do not pet or feed wild animals and do not touch the body of a dead wild animal.

If not treated, rabies is fatal. *Anyone bitten by a domestic or wild animal must get professional medical attention as soon as possible.* To prevent rabies from developing, the person receives a series of vaccine injections to build up immunity.

Tetanus is another potentially fatal infection that can result from a bite. Tetanus, caused by the transmission of bacteria that produce a toxin, can occur in wounds created by animal and human bites as well as in other contaminated deep flesh wounds. The toxin associated with tetanus, which attacks the central nervous system, is one of the deadliest poisons known. Wounds to the face, head and neck are the most likely to be fatal because of the proximity of these areas to the brain. If someone is bitten, they may need an immunization to prevent this infection from occurring.

Care for Domestic and Wild Animal Bites

If someone is bitten by a domestic or wild animal, try to get them away from the animal without endangering yourself. Do not try to restrain or capture the animal. Avoid coming into contact with the animal's saliva by wearing some form of protection such as disposable latex-free gloves.

Call 9-1-1 or the designated emergency number if the wound is bleeding seriously or you suspect the animal might have rabies. If possible, try to remember the animal's appearance and where you last saw it. When you call 9-1-1 or the designated emergency number, the dispatcher will direct the proper authorities, such as animal control, to the scene.

To care for an animal bite:

- Control bleeding first if the wound is bleeding seriously.

- Do *not* clean serious wounds. The wound will be cleaned at a medical facility.

- If bleeding is minor:

  - Wash the wound with soap and water, then irrigate with large amounts of clean running tap water to minimize the risk for infection.

  - Control any bleeding.

  - Cover the wound with a dressing. Apply an antibiotic ointment (or wound gel) to the dressing first if the person has no known allergies or sensitivities to the medication.

- Watch for signs and symptoms of infection.

- Advise the person to seek additional care from their healthcare provider or a medical facility, especially for possible tetanus or rabies treatment, for wounds to the hands or face, or for people with diseases such as diabetes, which may lower their resistance to infection.

Human Bites

Human bites are quite common and differ from other bites in that they may be more contaminated, tend to occur in higher-risk areas of the body (especially on the hands) and often receive delayed care. At least 42 different species of bacteria have been reported in human saliva, so it is not surprising that serious infection often follows a human bite. According to the CDC, however, human bites are not considered to carry a risk for transmitting human immunodeficiency virus (HIV), the virus that causes acquired immunodeficiency syndrome (AIDS). Children are often the inflictors and the recipients of human bite wounds.

Care for Human Bites

As with animal bites, it is important to get the person who has been bitten to professional medical care as soon as possible so that antibiotic therapy can be prescribed, if necessary. For a severe bite, call 9-1-1 or the designated emergency number. Other care includes:

- Control bleeding first if the wound is bleeding seriously.

- Do *not* clean serious wounds. The wound will be cleaned at a medical facility.

- If bleeding is minor:

  - Wash the wound with soap and water, then irrigate with large amounts of clean running tap water to minimize the risk for infection.

  - Control any bleeding.

  - Cover the wound with a dressing. Apply an antibiotic ointment (or wound gel) to the dressing first if the person has no known allergies or sensitivities to the medication.

- Watch for signs and symptoms of infection.

- Advise the person to seek additional care from their healthcare provider or a medical facility.

SMART MOVES > PREVENTING BITES AND STINGS

You can prevent bites and stings from insects, ticks, mosquitoes, spiders, scorpions or snakes by following these guidelines when you are in wooded or grassy areas, or around your home:

- Wear long-sleeved shirts and long pants.

- Tuck your pant legs into your socks or boots.

- Use a rubber band or tape to hold pants against socks so that nothing can get under your clothing.

- Tuck your shirt into your pants.

- Wear light-colored clothing to make it easier to see tiny insects or ticks.

- When hiking in woods and fields, stay in the middle of trails. Avoid underbrush and tall grass.

- If you are outdoors for a long time, check yourself several times during the day. Especially check in hairy areas of the body such as the back of the neck and the scalp line.

- Inspect yourself carefully for insects or ticks after being outdoors, or have someone else do it.

- Consider staying indoors at dusk and dawn, when mosquitoes are most active. If you must be outside, follow the clothing suggestions above.

- Get rid of mosquito breeding sites by emptying sources of standing water outside the home, such as from flowerpots, buckets and barrels. Also, change the water in pet dishes and replace the water in bird baths weekly, drill drainage holes in tire swings so that water drains out, and keep children's wading pools empty and on their sides when they are not being used.

- Avoid walking in areas where snakes are known to live.

(Continued)

- If you encounter a snake, look around for others. Turn around and walk away on the same path on which you came.

- Wear sturdy hiking boots.

- If you have pets that go outdoors, spray them with repellent made for that type of pet and use tick prevention remedies such as collars and vaccinations. Apply the repellent according to the label, and check your pet for ticks often.

- If you will be in a grassy or wooded area for a long time or if you know that an area is highly infested with insects or ticks, consider using a repellent. Follow the label instructions carefully:

  ○ Repellents containing DEET can be applied on exposed areas of skin and clothing. However, repellents containing permethrin, another common repellent, should be used only on clothing.

  ○ Keep all repellents out of the reach of children.

  ○ To apply repellent to the face, first spray it on your hands and then apply it from your hands to your face. Avoid sensitive areas, such as the lips, eyes and near the mouth.

  ○ Never spray repellents containing permethrin on your skin or a child's skin.

  ○ Never use repellents on a wound or on irritated skin.

  ○ Never put repellents on children's hands. Children may put their hands in their eyes or mouth.

  ○ Use repellents sparingly. Heavier or more frequent applications will not increase effectiveness and may be toxic.

  ○ Wash treated skin with soap and water, and remove clothes that have been treated after you come indoors.

  ○ If you suspect you are having an allergic reaction to a repellent, wash the treated skin immediately and call your healthcare provider.

To prevent stings from marine animals:

- Consider wearing a wet suit or dry suit and/or protective footwear in the water—especially at times or in areas where there is a high risk for such occurrences. Lightweight "rash guards" are effective at preventing jellyfish stings.

To prevent dog bites, the Humane Society of the United States offers several guidelines. Many of the dog bites that are reported in the United States each year could have been prevented by taking these precautions:

- Do not run past a dog. The dog's natural instinct is to chase and catch prey.

- If a dog threatens you, do not scream. Avoid eye contact; try to remain motionless until the dog leaves, then back away slowly until the dog is out of sight.

- Do not approach a strange dog, especially one that is tied or confined.

- Always let a dog see and sniff you before you pet the animal.

Summary

Bites and stings are among the most common types of venomous poisonings. The good news is that while there are many thousands of species of insects, spiders, scorpions and snakes, only a few are venomous and pose any danger to humans. Taking steps to prevent bites and stings from occurring in the first place is one of the most important actions you can take (see Smart Moves: Preventing Bites and Stings). Recognizing the signs and symptoms of a bite or sting, as well as when a serious allergic reaction may be occurring—and quickly taking steps to give care and summon additional help when needed—will help reduce the effects.

READY TO RESPOND? >

Think back to Sara in the opening scenario, and use what you have learned to respond to these questions:

1. Given the details of the scenario, what do you think is causing Sara's rash?

2. What can you do to help Sara?

Study Questions

1. **Match each term with the correct definition.**

   a. Lyme disease   b. Antivenom   c. Rabies   d. Rocky Mountain Spotted Fever

   ____ A disease transmitted by the deer tick and black-legged tick

   ____ A substance used to counteract the poisonous effects of venom

   ____ A disease caused by the transmission of microscopic bacteria from the wood tick or dog tick host

   ____ An infectious viral disease that affects the nervous system of humans and other mammals

2. **List the steps of care for a tick bite.**

3. **List three general signs or symptoms of insect stings.**

4. **List the steps of care for a snakebite.**

In questions 5 through 10, circle the letter of the correct answer.

5. **In caring for a bee sting, what should you do?**

   a. Remove the remaining stinger by scraping it from the skin.

   b. Leave the stinger in place until more advanced personnel arrive.

   c. Pull the stinger out with your bare hands.

   d. Rub over the stinger with an alcohol swab.

6. **When spending time outdoors in woods or tall grass, what should you do to prevent bites and stings?**

   a. Wear light-colored clothing.

   b. Use insect or tick repellent.

   c. Tuck pant legs into boots or socks.

   d. All of the above

7. **Which of the following are signs and symptoms of Lyme disease?**

   a. Trouble breathing

   b. Headache, fever, weakness, joint and muscle pain

   c. Excessive saliva

   d. Sneezing

(*Continued*)

Study Questions continued

8. **Which of the following should you do to care for a scorpion sting?**

   a. Apply suction to the wound.

   b. Call 9-1-1 or the designated emergency number.

   c. Wash the wound and apply a cold pack.

   d. b and c

9. **Which of the following should you apply to a bluebottle jellyfish/Portuguese man-of-war sting?**

   a. Seawater

   b. Meat tenderizer

   c. Baking soda paste

   d. Vinegar

10. **Which of the following should you do to care for a severe human bite?**

    a. Wash the wound with an antiseptic.

    b. Control bleeding.

    c. Call 9-1-1 or the designated emergency number immediately.

    d. b and c

Answers are listed in the Appendix.

18

SUBSTANCE ABUSE AND MISUSE

You are at an off-campus gathering with friends. You and your friend Julia exchange a glance. Tom, who had been animated and talking loudly, now has an agitated look on his face. "I've got to get some air," Tom mutters to the group as he puts down his drink and wanders toward the door. You and Julia decide to follow, and you find him slumped against the wall outside, limp and seemingly becoming unresponsive.

Learn and Respond ▶

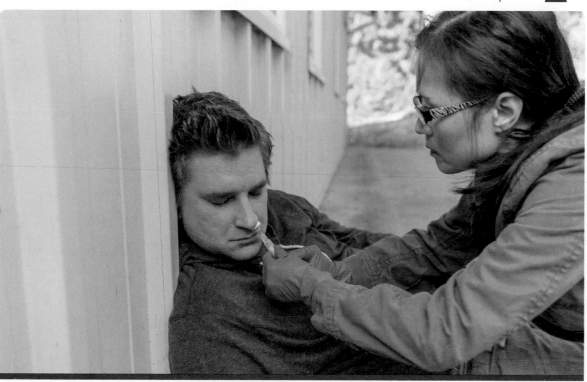

After reading this chapter, you should be able to:

- Identify the main categories of commonly abused or misused substances.

- Identify the signs and symptoms that may indicate substance abuse and misuse.

- Describe how to care for someone who you suspect or know is abusing or misusing a substance.

- Explain how you can help prevent substance abuse and misuse.

KEY TERMS

Addiction: The compulsive need to use a substance; stopping use would cause the user to suffer mental, physical and emotional distress.

Cannabis products: Substances such as marijuana and hashish that are derived from the *Cannabis sativa* plant; can produce feelings of elation, distorted perceptions of time and space, and impaired motor coordination and judgment.

Dependency: The desire or need to continually use a substance.

Depressant: A substance that affects the central nervous system and slows down physical and mental activity; can be used to treat anxiety, tension and high blood pressure.

Drug: Any substance, other than food, intended to affect the functions of the body.

Hallucinogen: A substance that affects mood, sensation, thinking, emotion and self-awareness; alters perception of time and space; and produces hallucinations or delusions.

Inhalant: A substance, such as a medication, that a person inhales to counteract or prevent a specific condition; also a substance inhaled to produce mood-altering effects.

Medication: A drug given therapeutically to prevent or treat the effects of a disease or condition, or otherwise enhance mental or physical well-being.

Opioid narcotic: A drug used to dull the senses or reduce pain; often derived from opium or opium-like compounds.

Overdose: The use of an excessive amount of a substance, resulting in adverse reactions ranging from mania (mental and physical hyperactivity) and hysteria to coma and death.

Stimulant: A substance that affects the central nervous system and speeds up physical and mental activity.

Substance abuse: The deliberate, persistent, excessive use of a substance without regard to health concerns or accepted medical practices.

Substance misuse: The use of a substance for unintended purposes or for intended purposes but in improper amounts or doses.

(Continued)

┌─ KEY TERMS continued

Synergistic effect: The outcome created when two or more drugs are combined; the effects of each may enhance those of the other.

Tolerance: The condition in which the effects of a substance on the body decrease as the result of continued use.

Withdrawal: The condition of mental and physical discomfort produced when a person stops using or abusing a substance to which they are addicted.

Introduction

A **drug** is any substance, other than food, intended to affect body functions. A drug given therapeutically to prevent or treat a disease or otherwise enhance mental or physical well-being is a **medication. Substance abuse** is the deliberate, persistent and excessive use of a substance without regard to health concerns or accepted medical practices. **Substance misuse** refers to the use of a substance for unintended purposes or for appropriate purposes but in improper amounts or doses.

Because of the publicity they receive, we tend to think of illegal (also known as illicit or controlled) drugs when we hear of substance abuse. However, legal substances (also called licit or noncontrolled substances) are among those most often abused or misused. These include nicotine (found in tobacco products), alcohol and over-the-counter (OTC) medications such as sleeping pills and diet pills.

In the United States, substance abuse costs tens of billions of dollars each year in medical care, insurance and lost productivity. Even more important, however, are the lives lost or permanently impaired each year from injuries or medical emergencies related to substance abuse or misuse. In 2014, there were a total of 47,055 drug overdose deaths in the United States. Drug overdose is the leading cause of accidental death in the country, resulting in even more deaths than motor-vehicle collisions. Experts estimate that as many as two-thirds of all homicides and serious assaults occurring annually involve alcohol. Other problems directly or indirectly related to substance abuse include dropping out of school, adolescent pregnancy, suicide, involvement in violent crime and transmission of the human immunodeficiency virus (HIV).

This chapter will address how to recognize common forms of substance abuse and misuse, how to care for people who abuse or misuse substances, and how to prevent substance abuse and misuse from occurring.

Forms of Substance Abuse and Misuse

Many substances that are abused or misused are legal. Other substances are legal only when prescribed by a healthcare provider. Some are illegal only for those under a certain age, such as alcohol.

Any drug can cause **dependency,** or the desire to continually use the substance. Those with drug dependency issues feel that they need the drug to function normally. Persons with a compulsive need for a substance and those who would suffer mental, physical and emotional distress if they stopped taking it are said to have an **addiction** to that substance.

The term **withdrawal** describes the condition produced when people stop using or abusing a substance to which they are addicted. Stopping the use of a substance may occur as a deliberate decision or because the person is unable to obtain the specific drug. Withdrawal from certain substances, such as alcohol, can cause severe mental and physical distress. Because withdrawal may become a serious medical condition, medical professionals often oversee the process.

When someone continually uses a substance, its effects on the body often decrease—a condition called **tolerance.** The person then has to increase the amount and frequency of use to obtain the desired effect.

An **overdose** occurs when someone uses an excessive amount of a substance. Signs and symptoms can vary but may range from mania and hysteria to coma and death. Specific reactions include changes in blood pressure and heart rate, sweating, vomiting and liver failure. An overdose may occur unintentionally if a person takes too much medication at one time. For example, an older person might forget about taking one dose of a medication and thus takes an additional dose. An overdose may also be intentional, as in a suicide attempt. Sometimes the person takes a sufficiently high dose of a substance to be certain to cause death. In other cases, the person may take enough of a substance to need medical attention but not enough to cause death.

> **What if...** *A person has ingested a large amount medication in an attempt to harm themselves? Should I try to induce vomiting?*
>
> *Whether a person ingests a large amount of medication by accident or on purpose, it is treated as an ingested poison emergency. In such a case, your first step would be to assess for scene safety during the scene size-up, then assess for life-threatening conditions. If any are found, you would call 9-1-1 or the designated emergency number and give care as needed for the conditions found. If no life-threatening conditions are found, you would call the national Poison Help line and follow any directions given. As you may recall from Chapter 16, you should* not *induce vomiting unless specifically instructed to do so.*

Abused and Misused Substances

Substances are categorized according to their effects on the body (Table 18-1). The six major categories are stimulants, hallucinogens, depressants, opioid narcotics, inhalants and cannabis products. The category to which a substance belongs depends mostly on the effects it has on the central nervous system or the way the substance is taken. Some substances depress the nervous system, whereas others speed up its activity. Some are not easily categorized because they have various effects or may be taken in a variety of ways. A heightened or exaggerated effect may be produced when two or more substances are used at the same time. This is called a **synergistic effect,** which can be deadly.

Stimulants

Stimulants are drugs that affect the central nervous system by speeding up physical and mental activity. They produce temporary feelings of alertness and prevent fatigue. They are sometimes used for weight reduction because they also suppress appetite, or to enhance exercise routines because they provide bursts of energy.

Many stimulants are ingested as pills, but some can be absorbed or inhaled. Amphetamine, dextroamphetamine and methamphetamine are stimulants. On the street, an extremely addictive, dangerous and smokable form of methamphetamine is often called "crystal meth" or "ice." The street term "speed" usually refers to amphetamine or methamphetamine. Other street terms for amphetamines are "uppers," "bennies," "black beauties," "crystal," "meth" and "crank."

Cocaine is one of the most publicized and powerful stimulants. It can be taken into the body in different ways. The most common way is sniffing it in powder form, known as "snorting." In this method, the drug is absorbed into the blood through capillaries in the nose. Street names for cocaine include "coke," "snow," "blow," "flake," "foot" and "nose candy." A potent and smokable form of cocaine is called "crack." The vapors of crack are inhaled into the lungs, reach the brain and cause almost immediate effects. Crack is highly addictive. Street names for crack include "rock" and "freebase rocks."

Ephedra, also known as "ma huang," is a stimulant plant that has been used in China and India for over 5000 years. Until it was banned by the Food and Drug Administration (FDA) in 2004, it was a common ingredient in dietary supplements sold in the United States. The dried stems and leaves are put into capsules, tablets, extracts, tinctures or teas, and then ingested. It is used for weight loss, increased energy and to enhance athletic performance.

The FDA banned ephedra because it appears to have little effectiveness, along with some substantial health risks. Taking ephedra can cause nausea, anxiety, headache, psychosis, kidney stones, tremors, dry mouth, irregular heart rhythms, high blood pressure, restlessness and sleep problems. It has been found to increase the risk of heart problems, a stroke and even death.

Table 18-1. Commonly Abused and Misused Substances

Category	Substances	Common Names	Possible Effects
Stimulants	Caffeine Cocaine, crack cocaine Amphetamines Methamphetamine Dextroamphetamine Nicotine Ephedra OTC diet aids Asthma treatments Decongestants	Coke, snow, nose candy, blow, flake, Big C, lady, white, snowbirds, powder, foot, crack, rock, cookies, freebase rocks, speed, uppers, ups, bennies, black beauties, crystal, meth, crank, crystal meth, ice, ma huang	Increase mental and physical activity. Produce temporary feelings of alertness. Prevent fatigue. Suppress appetite.
Hallucinogens	Diethyltryptamine (DET) Dimethyltryptamine (DMT) LSD PCP Mescaline Peyote Psilocybin 4-Methyl-2,5-dimethoxyamphetamine (DOM)	Psychedelics, acid, white lightning, sugar cubes, angel dust, hog, loveboat, peyote, buttons, cactus, mesc, mushrooms, magic mushrooms, 'shrooms, STP (serenity, tranquility and peace)	Cause changes in mood, sensation, thought, emotion and self-awareness. Alter perceptions of time and space. Can produce profound depression, tension and anxiety, as well as visual, auditory or tactile hallucinations.
Depressants	Barbiturates Benzodiazepines Narcotics Alcohol Antihistamines Sedatives Tranquilizers OTC sleep aids Ketamine Rohypnol® GHB	Valium®, Xanax®, downers, barbs, goofballs, yellow jackets, reds, Quaaludes, ludes, club drugs, date rape drugs, special K, vitamin K, roofies, roach, rope, liquid ecstasy, soap, vita-G	Decrease mental and physical activity. Alter level of consciousness. Relieve anxiety and pain. Promote sleep. Depress respiration. Relax muscles. Impair coordination and judgment.

(Continued)

Table 18-1. continued

Category	Substances	Common Names	Possible Effects
Opioid Narcotics	Morphine Codeine Heroin Oxycodone Methadone Opium	Pectoral syrup, Oxycontin®, Percodan®, Percocet®, smack, horse, mud, brown sugar, junk, black tar, big H	Relieve pain. Produce stupor or euphoria. Can cause coma or death. Highly addictive.
Inhalants	Medical anesthetics Lacquer and varnish thinners Propane Toluene Butane Acetone Fuel Propellants	Laughing gas, whippets, glue, lighter fluid, nail polish remover, gasoline, kerosene, aerosol sprays	Alter mood. Produce a partial or complete loss of feeling. Produce effects similar to drunkenness, such as slurred speech, lack of inhibitions and impaired motor coordination. Can cause damage to the heart, lungs, brain and liver.
Cannabis Products	Hashish Marijuana THC Synthetic cannabinoids	Hash, pot, grass, weed, reefer, ganja, mary jane, dope K2, spice	Produce feelings of elation. Increase appetite. Distort perceptions of time and space. Impair motor coordination and judgment. Irritate throat. Redden eyes. Increase heart rate. Cause dizziness.
Other	MDMA	Ecstasy, E, XTC, Adam, essence	Elevate blood pressure. Produce euphoria or erratic mood swings, rapid heartbeat, profuse sweating, agitation and sensory distortions.

(Continued)

Table 18-1. continued

Category	Substances	Common Names	Possible Effects
	Anabolic steroids	Androgens, hormones, juice, roids, vitamins	Enhance physical performance. Increase muscle mass. Stimulate appetite and weight gain. Chronic use can cause sterility, disruption of normal growth, liver cancer, personality changes and aggressive behavior.
	Aspirin		Relieves minor pain. Reduces fever. Impairs normal blood clotting. Can cause inflammation of the stomach and small intestine.
	Laxatives and emetics	Ipecac syrup, Senna	Relieve constipation or induce vomiting. Can cause dehydration, uncontrolled diarrhea and other serious health problems.
	Decongestant nasal sprays		Relieve congestion and swelling of nasal passages. Chronic use can cause nosebleeds and changes in the lining of the nose, making it difficult to breathe without sprays.

Interestingly, the most common stimulants in America are legal. Leading the list is caffeine, present in coffee, tea, high-energy drinks, many kinds of sodas, chocolate, diet pills and pills used to combat fatigue. The next most common stimulant is nicotine, found in tobacco products. Other stimulants used for medical purposes are asthma medications or decongestants that can be taken by mouth or inhaled.

Hallucinogens

Hallucinogens, also known as psychedelics, are substances that cause changes in mood, sensation, thought, emotion and self-awareness. They alter one's perception of time and space and produce visual, auditory and tactile (relating to the sense of touch) delusions.

Among the most widely abused hallucinogens are lysergic acid diethylamide (LSD), called "acid"; psilocybin, called "mushrooms"; phencyclidine (PCP), called "angel dust"; mescaline, called "peyote," "buttons" or "mesc"; and ketamine, called "special K" or "vitamin K." These substances are usually ingested, but PCP is also often inhaled.

Hallucinogens often have physical effects similar to stimulants but are classified differently because of the other effects they produce. Hallucinogens sometimes cause what is called a "bad trip." A bad trip can involve intense fear, panic, paranoid delusions, vivid hallucinations, profound depression, tension and anxiety. The person may be irrational and feel threatened by any attempt others make to help.

Depressants

Depressants are substances that affect the central nervous system by slowing down physical and mental activity. Depressants are commonly used for medical purposes. All depressants alter consciousness to some degree. They relieve anxiety, promote sleep, depress respiration, relieve pain, relax muscles, and impair coordination and judgment. Like other substances, the larger the dose or the stronger the substance, the greater its effects.

Common depressants are barbiturates, benzodiazepines (e.g., Valium®, Xanax®), narcotics and alcohol. Most depressants are ingested or injected. Their street names include "downers," "barbs," "goofballs," "yellow jackets," "reds" or "ludes."

Two depressants that have gained popularity as club drugs (so called because they are used at all-night dance parties) include Rohypnol® (also referred to as "roofies," "roach" or "rope"), a benzodiazepine that is illegal in the United States; and gamma-hydroxybutyrate (GHB) (also referred to as "liquid ecstasy," "soap" or "vita-G"), an illicit drug that has depressant, euphoric and body-building effects. These drugs are particularly dangerous because they are often used in combination or with other depressants (including alcohol), which can have deadly effects, and because they are the "date rape drugs" of choice. As such, they are sometimes slipped to others unnoticed.

Alcohol is the most widely used and abused substance in the United States. In small amounts, its effects may be fairly mild. In higher doses, its effects can be toxic. Alcohol is like other depressants in its effects and risks for overdose. Frequent drinkers may become dependent on the effects of alcohol and increasingly tolerant of those effects. Alcohol poisoning occurs when a large amount of alcohol is consumed in a short period of time and can result in unresponsiveness and, if untreated, death.

Drinking alcohol in large or frequent amounts can have many unhealthy consequences. Alcohol can irritate the digestive system and even cause the esophagus to rupture, or it can injure the stomach lining. Chronic drinking can also affect the brain and cause memory loss, apathy and a lack of coordination. Other problems include liver disease, such as cirrhosis (Figure 18-1, A–B). In addition, many psychological, family, social and work problems are related to chronic drinking. See The Incalculable Cost of Alcohol Use.

Opioid Narcotics

While they have a depressant effect, *opioid narcotics* (which are often derived from opium) are used mainly to relieve pain. Opioid narcotics are so powerful and highly addictive that all are illegal without a prescription, and some are not prescribed at all. When taken in large doses, narcotics can produce

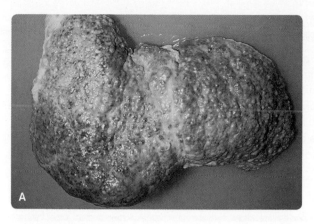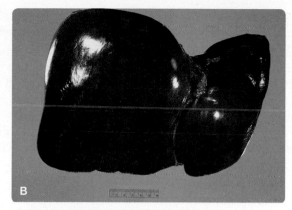

Figure 18-1, A–B. A, Chronic drinking can result in cirrhosis, a disease of the liver. B, A healthy liver.

euphoria, stupor, coma or death. The most common natural opioid narcotics are morphine and codeine. Most other opioid narcotics, including heroin, are synthetic or semi-synthetic. Oxycodone, also known by the trade names Oxycontin® or Percocet®, is a powerful semi-synthetic opioid narcotic that has recently gained popularity as a street drug.

Opioid narcotic abuse has become a major health concern in the United States and throughout the world. Of the 47,055 deaths in the United States in 2014 attributed to drug overdose, 28,647 (61 percent) involved some type of opioid narcotic.

While there are many factors in treating this epidemic, including increased awareness and education, a medication that can reverse the effects of opioid narcotics is becoming increasingly available. This medication, called naloxone, is commonly used by EMS personnel to reverse the effects of opioid drugs. Recent legislation has allowed individuals in some states who are being prescribed opioids by their doctor to also be given a prescription for naloxone. In fact, in some states this medication can even be obtained directly from the pharmacist without a prescription.

Naloxone typically comes as a nasal spray or injectable. Auto-injectors, similar to those used to deliver epinephrine, are even being manufactured for use in the treatment of opioid poisoning. Before using naloxone, it is important to be trained how to recognize when to administer it and how to give it using the different methods of administration. Signs and symptoms of opioid overdose include:

- Slowed and/or shallow breathing (or no breathing).
- Extreme drowsiness or becoming unresponsive.
- Small pupils.

Severe opioid poisoning is a life-threatening emergency; in severe cases the person may be unresponsive, not breathing, have bluish skin (cyanosis) and a faint or absent heartbeat. If you suspect opioid overdose in a person, the most important thing to do is to call 9-1-1 or the designated emergency number immediately. If used appropriately, as allowed by local rules and laws, naloxone can reverse all of the effects of opioid poisoning, including unresponsiveness and breathing difficulties.

What if... *I know a person is suffering from alcohol poisoning? Should I use activated charcoal as I have seen them do on TV?*

Alcohol poisoning is a serious and possibly deadly condition occurring as consequence of drinking large amounts of alcohol in a short period of time. Excessive drinking can affect breathing, heart rate and gag reflex, and potentially lead to coma and death. While treating a person right away might seem like the best thing to do, as with any ingested poison, initial treatment would be to call 9-1-1 or the designated emergency number, or the national Poison Help line depending on the condition of the person. Activated charcoal should never be administered to a person who has ingested a poisonous substance unless you are advised to do so by the Poison Control Center or emergency medical personnel.

Inhalants

Substances inhaled to produce mood-altering effects are called ***inhalants.*** Inhalants also depress the central nervous system. In addition, inhalant use can damage the heart, lungs, brain and liver. Inhalants include medical anesthetics, such as amyl nitrite and nitrous oxide (also known as "laughing gas"), as well as hydrocarbons, known as solvents. The effects of solvents are similar to those of alcohol. People who use solvents may appear to be drunk. Other effects of inhalant use include swollen mucous membranes in the nose and mouth, hallucinations, erratic blood pressure and seizures. Solvents include toluene, found in glues; butane, found in lighter fluids; acetone, found in nail polish removers; fuels, such as gasoline and kerosene; and propellants, found in aerosol sprays.

The Incalculable Cost of Alcohol Use

According to the CDC, some 88,000 people die each year as a result of excessive alcohol use (defined as heavy drinking or binge drinking). Deaths from excessive alcohol use add up to 2.5 million years of potential life lost annually—or an average of about 30 years of potential life lost for every death.

What defines heavy drinking and binge drinking?

For women, it is drinking more than 1 drink per day on average, or 4 or more drinks on a single occasion; for men, it is more than 2 drinks per day on average or 5 or more drinks on a single occasion. Most people who binge drink, incidentally, are not alcoholics or alcohol-dependent.

Among some of the other striking statistics: according to the National Council on Alcoholism and Drug Dependence (NCADD), an estimated 32 percent of fatal car crashes involve an intoxicated driver or pedestrian. And while there are over 1.2 million arrests for drunk driving annually, that is less than 5 percent of the 29 million self-reported incidences of alcohol-impaired driving. In addition, some 40 percent of all violent crimes and two-thirds of intimate partner violence involve alcohol. The CDC reports that alcohol use is involved in up to 70 percent of adolescent and adult deaths associated with water activities.

Motor vehicle crashes, violence and water accidents are just some of the immediate risks of excessive alcohol use. Alcohol use also puts you at increased risk for unintentional injury due to falls, burns and firearm injuries; as well as risky sexual behaviors that can lead to sexually transmitted infections and unintended pregnancy; alcohol poisoning; and in the case of pregnant women, stillbirth, miscarriage and birth defects.

Over the long term, excessive alcohol use can cause a whole host of chronic diseases, neurological impairments and social problems, including dementia, stroke, cardiovascular problems, liver disease, depression, anxiety and suicide, along with loss of employment, lost productivity and family problems. Again according to the CDC, up to 40 percent of all hospital beds (not including maternity and ICU beds) are occupied by someone with a health condition related to alcohol use.

SOURCES: Centers for Disease Control and Prevention: *Fact sheets—Alcohol use and your health.* www.cdc.gov/alcohol/fact-sheets/alcohol-use.htm. Accessed September 2016.

Centers for Disease Control and Prevention: *Unintentional drowning: Get the facts.* www.cdc.gov/homeandrecreationalsafety/water-safety/waterinjuries-factsheet.htm. Accessed September 2016.

National Council on Alcoholism and Drug Dependence: https://www.ncadd.org/about-addiction/addiction-update/driving-while-impaired-alcohol-and-drugs. Accessed September 2016.

Cannabis Products

Cannabis products, including hash oil, tetrahydrocannabinol (THC) and hashish, are all derived from the plant *Cannabis sativa.* Marijuana is the most widely used illicit drug in the United States. Street names include "pot," "grass," "weed," "reefer," "ganja" and "dope." It is typically smoked in cigarette form or in a pipe, but it can also be ingested. The effects include feelings of elation, distorted perceptions of time and space, and impaired judgment and motor coordination. Marijuana irritates the throat, reddens the eyes and causes dizziness and often an increased appetite. Depending on the dose, the person and many other factors, cannabis products can produce effects similar to those of substances in any of the other major substance categories.

Marijuana, although still illegal throughout much of the United States, has been legalized in some states and is available in others for limited medical use to help alleviate symptoms of certain conditions such as multiple sclerosis. Marijuana and its legal synthetic versions are used as an anti-nausea medication for people undergoing chemotherapy for cancer, for treating glaucoma, for treating muscular weakness caused by multiple sclerosis and to combat the weight loss caused by cancer and acquired immunodeficiency syndrome (AIDS).

Newer, more potent synthetic marijuana-like products have been available in the United States since the early 2000s. These products are known as synthetic marijuana or synthetic cannabinoids. Street names include "K2" and "spice." These products are typically smoked or taken orally. They are not a safe alternative to marijuana and, in fact, have more side effects than marijuana and can cause hallucinations, seizures, stupor, coma or death.

Other Substances

Some other substances do not fit neatly into these categories. These substances include **designer drugs,** steroids and OTC substances, which can be purchased without a prescription.

Designer Drugs

Designer drugs are variations of other substances, such as narcotics and amphetamines. Through simple and inexpensive methods, the molecular structure of substances produced for medicinal purposes can be modified into extremely potent and dangerous street drugs; hence the term "designer drug." When the chemical makeup of a drug is altered, the user can experience a variety of unpredictable and dangerous effects. The people who modify these drugs may have no knowledge of the effects a new designer drug might produce.

One of the more commonly used designer drugs is methylenedioxymethamphetamine (MDMA). Another popular club drug, it is often called "ecstasy" or "E." Although ecstasy is structurally related to stimulants and hallucinogens, its effects are somewhat different from either category. Ecstasy can evoke a euphoric high that makes it popular. Other signs and symptoms of ecstasy use range from the stimulant-like effects of high blood pressure, rapid heartbeat, profuse sweating and agitation to the hallucinogenic-like effects of paranoia, sensory distortion and erratic mood swings.

Anabolic Steroids

Anabolic steroids are drugs sometimes used by athletes to enhance performance and increase muscle mass. Their medical uses include stimulating weight gain for persons unable to gain weight naturally. They should not be confused with corticosteroids, which are used to counteract toxic effects and allergic reactions. Chronic use of anabolic steroids can lead to sterility, liver cancer and personality changes, such as aggressive behavior. Steroid use by younger people may also disrupt normal growth. Street names for anabolic steroids include "androgens," "hormones," "juice," "roids" and "vitamins." See Steroids: Body Meltdown for more information.

Steroids: Body Meltdown

If you think using steroids is the way to get those sculpted, muscular bodies that are typical of bodybuilders and many professional athletes, think again. These drugs may build up bodies on the outside, but they can cause a body meltdown on the inside. Physicians and other public health officials warn of the dangers of steroid abuse and are particularly concerned about the long-term effects of high doses.

Anabolic steroids are synthetic chemicals that mimic the naturally occurring hormone testosterone. They are designed to promote the growth of skeletal muscles as well as the development of male sexual characteristics. While there are several legitimate, legal uses of prescribed steroids, when anabolic steroids are used illegally, most often by people looking to improve their athletic performance or enhance their physical appearance, they can have devastating effects on the body. These effects, some of which are permanent even if steroid use is stopped, include:

- Hormonal changes causing breast development, shrinking of the testicles, male-pattern baldness and infertility in men; and excessive growth of body hair, male-pattern baldness, deepening of the voice, a decrease in breast size, and enlargement of the clitoris in women.

- Permanent stunting of growth when taken by adolescents.

- Development of cardiovascular disease (including heart attack and strokes) as well as liver disease (including tumors and cysts) and some cancers.

- Skin changes including severe acne, oily scalp, jaundice and fluid retention.

- Psychiatric effects including rage, aggression, mania and delusions.

- Increased risk for viruses such as HIV and hepatitis from sharing needles to inject steroids.

SOURCE: National Institutes of Health, National Institute on Drug Abuse: *NIDA infofacts: Steroids (anabolic-androgenic).* www.drugabuse.gov/infofacts/steroids.html. Accessed September 2016.

Over-the-Counter Substances

Aspirin, nasal sprays, laxatives and emetics (agents to induce vomiting) are among the most commonly abused or misused OTC substances. Aspirin is an effective minor pain reliever and fever reducer that is found in a variety of medicines. People use aspirin for many reasons and conditions. In recent years, cardiologists have praised the benefits of low-dose aspirin for the treatment of heart disease and prevention of a stroke. As useful as aspirin is, misuse can have toxic effects on the body. Typically, aspirin can cause inflammation of the stomach and small intestine that can result in bleeding ulcers. Aspirin can also impair normal blood clotting.

Decongestant nasal sprays can help relieve the congestion of colds or hay fever. If misused, they can cause a physical dependency. Using the spray over a long period can cause nosebleeds and changes in the lining of the nose that make it difficult to breathe without the spray.

Laxatives are used to relieve constipation. They come in a variety of forms and strengths. If used improperly, laxatives can cause uncontrolled diarrhea that may result in dehydration, which is the excessive loss of water from the body tissues. The very young and older adults are particularly susceptible to dehydration.

Emetics are drugs that induce vomiting. Ipecac syrup is an emetic that has been used in the past to induce vomiting following the ingestion of some toxic substances. The administration of ipecac syrup for ingested poisons is *not* recommended. Use of ipecac can be quite dangerous and may cause recurrent vomiting, diarrhea, dehydration, pain and weakness in the muscles, abdominal pain and heart problems. Over time, the recurrent vomiting can erode tooth enamel, causing dental problems. For these reasons, it is no longer widely available in the United States, and the American Academy of Pediatrics and the American Association of Poison Control Centers do *not* recommend that ipecac syrup be stocked at home.

The abuse of laxatives and emetics is frequently associated with attempted weight loss and eating disorders, such as anorexia nervosa or bulimia. **Anorexia nervosa** is a disorder that most often affects young women and is characterized by a long-term refusal to eat food with sufficient nutrients and calories. People with anorexia typically use laxatives and emetics to keep from gaining weight. **Bulimia** is a condition in which people gorge themselves with food, then purge by vomiting (sometimes with the aid of emetics) or using laxatives. For this reason, the behavior associated with bulimia is often referred to as "binging and purging." Anorexia nervosa and bulimia have underlying psychological factors that contribute to their onset. The effect of both of these eating disorders can be severe malnutrition, which can result in death.

Signs and Symptoms of Substance Abuse and Misuse

Many of the signs and symptoms of substance abuse and misuse are similar to those of other medical emergencies. For example, you should not necessarily assume that someone who is stumbling, is disoriented or has a fruity, alcohol-like odor on the breath is intoxicated by alcohol or other drugs as this may also be a sign of a diabetic emergency (see Chapter 15).

In general, signs and symptoms of possible substance abuse and misuse include:

- Behavioral changes not otherwise explained.

- Sudden mood changes.

- Restlessness, talkativeness or irritability.

- Changes in level of consciousness, including becoming unresponsive.

- Slurred speech or poor coordination.

- Moist or flushed skin.

- Chills, nausea or vomiting.

- Dizziness or confusion.

- Abnormal breathing.

The misuse or abuse of stimulants can have many unhealthy effects on the body that mimic other conditions. For example, a stimulant overdose can cause moist or flushed skin, sweating, chills, nausea, vomiting, fever, headache, dizziness, rapid heart rate, rapid breathing, high blood pressure and chest pain. In some instances, a stimulant overdose can cause respiratory distress, disrupt normal heart rhythms or cause death. The person may appear very excited, restless, talkative or irritable or the person may suddenly lose responsiveness. Stimulant abuse can lead to addiction and can cause a heart attack or a stroke.

Specific signs and symptoms of hallucinogen abuse, as well as abuse of some designer drugs, may include sudden mood changes and a flushed face. Their pupils may be markedly dilated. The person may claim to see or hear something not present. They may be anxious and frightened.

Specific signs and symptoms of depressant abuse may include drowsiness, confusion, slurred speech, slowed heart and breathing rates, and poor coordination. A person who abuses alcohol may smell of alcohol. A person who has consumed a great deal of alcohol in a short time may be unresponsive or hard to arouse. The person may vomit violently.

Specific signs and symptoms of alcohol withdrawal, a potentially dangerous condition, include confusion and restlessness, trembling, hallucinations and seizures.

A telltale sign of cannabis use is red, bloodshot eyes and a pungent odor, while those abusing inhalants may appear drunk or disoriented in a similar manner to a person abusing hallucinogens.

Care for Substance Abuse and Misuse

Your initial care for substance abuse or misuse does not require that you know the specific substance taken. Follow these general principles as you would for any poisoning, normally an ingested poison:

- Check the scene to be sure it is safe to help the person. Do not approach the person if they are behaving in a threatening manner.

- Call 9-1-1 or the designated emergency number immediately if the person:

  o Is unresponsive, confused or responsive but not fully awake.

  o Has trouble breathing or is breathing irregularly.

  o Has persistent chest pain or pressure.

  o Has pain or pressure in the abdomen that does not go away.

  o Is vomiting blood or passing blood.

  o Has a seizure, a severe headache or slurred speech.

  o Acts violently.

- If none of the above conditions are present, and you have good reason to suspect a substance was taken, call the national Poison Help line at 800-222-1222 and follow the call taker's directions.

- Try to learn from the person or others what substances may have been taken.

- Calm and reassure the person.

- Keep the person from getting chilled or overheated.

Because many of the physical signs and symptoms of substance abuse and misuse mimic other conditions, you should not assume that a person has overdosed on a substance. Always check for life-threatening conditions and give care as you would for any person with an injury or sudden illness.

If possible, interview the person or bystanders to try to find out what substance was taken, how much was taken and when it was taken. You may also be able to find clues at the scene that suggest the nature of the problem. Such clues may help you provide more complete information to emergency medical services (EMS) personnel. Look for containers, pill bottles, drug paraphernalia, and signs and symptoms of other medical problems. If you suspect that someone has used a designer drug, tell EMS personnel. Telling EMS personnel your suspicions is important because a person who has overdosed on a designer drug frequently may not respond to usual medical treatment.

See Smart Moves: Preventing Substance Abuse and Smart Moves: Preventing Substance Misuse for more information.

SMART MOVES > PREVENTING SUBSTANCE ABUSE

Experts in the field of substance abuse generally agree that prevention efforts are far more cost effective than treatment. Yet preventing substance abuse is a complex process that involves many underlying factors. These include:

- A lack of parental supervision.

- The breakdown of traditional family structures.

- A wish to escape unpleasant surroundings and stressful situations.

- The widespread availability of substances.

- Peer pressure and the basic need to belong.

- Low self-esteem, including feelings of guilt or shame.

- Media glamorization, especially of alcohol and tobacco, promoting the idea that using substances enhances fun and popularity.

- A history of substance abuse in the home or community environment.

Various approaches—including educating people about substances and their effects on health, and attempting to instill fear of penalties—have not by themselves proved particularly effective. To be effective, prevention efforts must address the various underlying factors of and approaches to substance abuse.

SMART MOVES > PREVENTING SUBSTANCE MISUSE

Many poisonings from medicinal substances are not intentional. The following guidelines can help prevent unintentional misuse or overdose:

- Read the product information and use products only as directed.

- Ask your physician or pharmacist about the intended use and side effects of prescription and OTC medications. If you are taking more than one medication, check for possible interaction effects.

- Never use another person's prescribed medications; what is right for one person is seldom right for another.

- Always keep medications in their appropriate, marked containers.

- Destroy all out-of-date medications by dropping them off at local medication disposal sites. Time can alter the chemical composition of medications, causing them to be less effective and possibly even toxic.

- Always keep medications out of the reach of children.

Summary

There are six major categories of substances that, when abused or misused, can produce a variety of signs and symptoms, some of which are indistinguishable from those of other medical emergencies. Remember, you do not have to diagnose the condition to give care. If you suspect that the person's condition is caused by substance abuse or misuse, give care for a poisoning emergency. Call 9-1-1 or the designated emergency number or the national Poison Help line and follow their directions. If the person becomes violent or threatening, go to a safe place and call 9-1-1 or the designated emergency number. Do not return to the scene until EMS personnel and the police arrive.

READY TO RESPOND? ❯

Think back to Tom in the opening scenario, and use what you have learned to respond to these questions:

1. What are the signs and symptoms of Tom's condition?

2. What do you think is the cause of Tom's condition? Can you be sure?

3. Should you call 9-1-1 or the designated emergency number for Tom? Why or why not?

Study Questions

1. **Match each term with the correct definition.**

   a. Addiction　　　　c. Medication　　　　e. Overdose　　　　g. Tolerance

   b. Dependency　　　d. Drug　　　　　　f. Substance abuse　　h. Withdrawal

   ____ Deliberate, persistent, excessive use of a substance

   ____ A drug given therapeutically to prevent or treat the effects of a disease or condition, or otherwise enhance mental or physical well-being

   ____ Any substance other than food intended to affect the functions of the body

   ____ The use of an excessive amount of a substance, resulting in adverse reactions ranging from mania (mental and physical hyperactivity) and hysteria to coma and death

   ____ The compulsive need to use a substance

   ____ The condition of mental and physical discomfort produced when a person stops using or abusing a substance to which they are addicted

   ____ The desire or need to continually use a substance

   ____ The condition in which the effects of a substance on the body decrease as the result of continued use

2. **List four general signs and symptoms that might indicate substance abuse or misuse.**

3. **List the six major categories of abused or misused legal substances.**

4. **List four things you can do to prevent unintentional substance misuse.**

5. **Describe the care for a person suspected of substance abuse or misuse.**

(Continued)

Study Questions continued

6. Match each type of substance with the effects it has on the body.

    a. Depressants   c. Inhalants   e. Opioid narcotics

    b. Hallucinogens   d. Stimulants   f. Cannabis products

_____ Affect mood, sensation, thought, emotion and self-awareness; alter perception of time and space; and produce hallucinations and delusions

_____ Produce mood-altering effects similar to those of alcohol; found in glues and solvents

_____ Slow down the physical activities of the brain, producing temporary feelings of relaxation

_____ Speed up the physical and mental activity of the brain, producing temporary feelings of alertness and improved task performance

_____ Relieve pain

_____ Produce feelings of elation, disoriented perceptions of time and space, and impaired judgment

In questions 7 and 8, circle the letter of the correct answer.

7. Which of the following is true of substance abuse?

| a. It occurs only among older adults who are forgetful and may have poor eyesight. | b. It is the use of a substance for intended purposes but in improper amounts or doses. | c. It is the use of a substance without regard to health concerns or accepted medical practices. | d. Its effects are minor and rarely result in medical complications. |

8. The effects of designer drugs are—

    a. Well known.   b. Unpredictable.   c. Harmless.   d. Easily controlled.

Answers are listed in the Appendix.

19

HEAT-RELATED ILLNESSES AND COLD-RELATED EMERGENCIES

You are hiking in the woods on a fall day that starts out warm but is quickly getting cooler as gray clouds move in overhead. Although the exertion is still making you sweat, you feel cold as the wind picks up and a steady rain begins to fall. Your hiking partner, Kelly, is shivering and complaining that she cannot get warm, despite having put on all the layers of clothing she brought along. She states that everything she is wearing is soaked through anyway, and asks if you can just stop walking for a while as she does not feel like fighting the wind and rain anymore.

Learn and Respond ▶

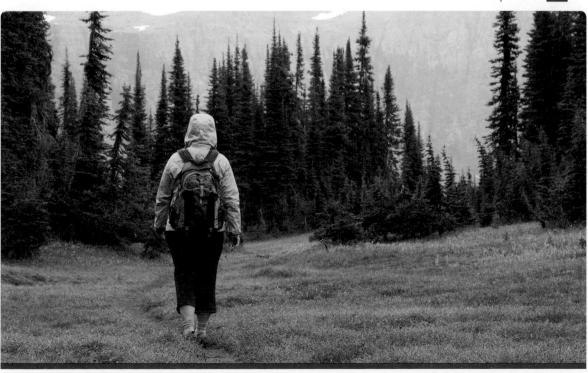

After reading this chapter, you should be able to:

- Describe how body temperature is controlled.

- Identify the factors that influence how well the body maintains its temperature.

- Identify the risk factors that increase a person's susceptibility to heat-related illnesses and cold-related emergencies.

- List the signs and symptoms of dehydration, exercise-associated muscle cramps, exertional heat exhaustion and heat stroke.

- Describe the care for dehydration, exercise-associated muscle cramps, exertional heat exhaustion and heat stroke.

- List the signs and symptoms of frostbite and hypothermia.

- Describe the care for frostbite and hypothermia.

- Describe the ways to help prevent heat-related illnesses and cold-related emergencies.

KEY TERMS

Exercise-associated muscle cramps: Formerly known as heat cramps, these muscle spasms can be intense and debilitating and occur typically in the legs, arms and abdomen; painful involuntary muscle spasms occur during or after physical exertion, particularly in high heat and humidity, possibly due to loss of electrolytes and water from perspiration; not associated with an increase in body temperature.

Exertional heat exhaustion (EHA): An inability to cope with heat and characterized by fatigue, nausea and/or vomiting, loss of appetite, dehydration, exercise-associated muscle cramps, dizziness with possible fainting, elevated heart and respiratory rate, and skin that is pale, cool and clammy or slightly flushed; if a core body temperature can be obtained, it is typically higher than 104° F (40° C). The person may be weak and unable to stand but has *normal mental status;* often results from strenuous work or wearing too much clothing in a hot, humid environment, and may or may not occur with dehydration and electrolyte imbalance.

Exertional heat stroke (EHS): The most serious form of heat-related illness; life threatening and develops when the body's cooling mechanisms are overwhelmed and body systems begin to fail. People with EHS have exaggerated heat production and an inability to cool themselves.

Frostbite: A condition in which body tissues freeze; most commonly occurs in the fingers, toes, ears and nose.

Hypothalamus: Control center of the body's temperature; located in the brain.

Hypothermia: The state of the body being colder than the usual core temperature, caused by either excessive loss of body heat and/or the body's inability to produce heat.

Introduction

The human body is equipped to withstand extremes in temperature. Under normal circumstances, its mechanisms for regulating body temperature work very well. However, when the body is overwhelmed, heat-related illnesses and cold-related emergencies can occur.

Heat-related illnesses and cold-related emergencies can happen anywhere—indoors or outdoors, and under a variety of conditions. The signs and symptoms of heat-related illnesses and cold-related emergencies are progressive and can quickly become life threatening. A person can develop heat-related illnesses and cold-related emergencies even when temperatures are not extreme. The effects of humidity, wind, clothing, living and working environments, physical activity, age and health all play a role in determining an individual's susceptibility. In this chapter, you will learn how to recognize and give care for heat-related illnesses and cold-related emergencies.

How Body Temperature Is Controlled

In order to work efficiently, the human body must maintain a constant core temperature. Normal body temperature is 98.6° F (37° C). The control center of body temperature is in the brain and is called the **hypothalamus.** The hypothalamus receives information that triggers physiological responses that adjust the body temperature accordingly. The body needs to be kept within a specific range of temperatures for the cells to stay alive and healthy (97.8° F to 99° F, or 36.5° C to 37.2° C). It is vital that the body responds properly to temperature signals.

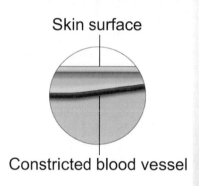

Skin surface

Constricted blood vessel

How the Body Stays Warm

Heat is a byproduct of metabolism, the conversion of food and drink into energy. The body also gains heat with any kind of physical activity. If the body starts to become too cold, it responds by constricting (closing up) the blood vessels close to the skin so it can keep the warmer blood near the center of the body (Figure 19-1). This helps keep the organs warm. If this does not work, the body then begins to shiver. The shivering motion increases body heat because it is a form of movement.

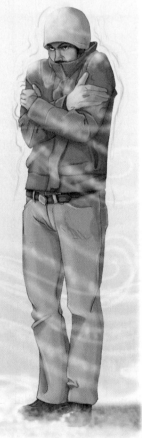

Figure 19-1. The body stays warm by constricting blood vessels close to the skin. If this does not work, it begins to shiver.

How the Body Stays Cool

In a warm or hot environment, the hypothalamus detects an increase in blood temperature. Blood vessels near the skin dilate (widen) to bring more blood to the surface, which allows heat to escape (Figure 19-2).

There are five general ways in which the body can be cooled:

- **Radiation:** This process involves the transfer of heat from one object to another without physical contact. The body loses heat through radiation, mostly from the head, hands and feet.

- **Convection:** This process occurs when air moves over the skin and carries the skin's heat away. The faster the air is moving, the faster the body will be cooled. Convection is what makes warm skin feel cooler in a breeze. Convection also assists in the evaporation process.

- **Conduction:** This occurs when the body is in direct contact with a substance that is cooler than the body's temperature. Through conduction, the body's heat is transferred to the cooler substance (e.g., if you are swimming in cold water or sitting on a cool rock in the shade, body heat is transferred to the water or to the rock).

- **Evaporation:** This is the process by which a liquid becomes a vapor. When body heat causes one to perspire and the perspiration evaporates, the heat that was absorbed into sweat dissipates into the air, which cools off the skin.

- **Respiration:** Heat is also lost through respiration, another term for breathing. Before air is exhaled, it is warmed by the lungs and airway.

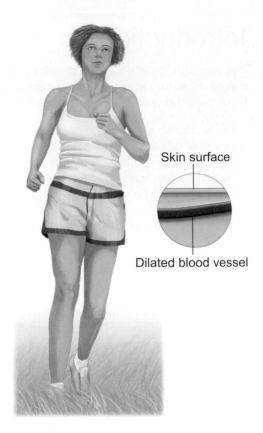

Skin surface

Dilated blood vessel

Figure 19-2. The body stays cool by dilating blood vessels near the skin so heat can escape.

Factors Affecting Body Temperature Regulation

Three main factors affect how well the body maintains its temperature: the air temperature, the humidity level and wind (e.g., wind-chill factor). Extreme heat or cold accompanied by high humidity or high wind speed reduces the body's ability to maintain temperature effectively (Figure 19-3).

Other factors, such as the clothing you wear, how often you take breaks from exposure to extreme temperature, how much and how often you drink water and how intense your activity is, also affect how well the body manages temperature extremes. These are all factors you can control to prevent heat-related illnesses and cold-related emergencies.

People at Increased Risk

Although anyone can be at risk for heat-related illnesses and cold-related emergencies, some people are at greater risk than others. People more susceptible to heat-related illnesses and cold-related emergencies include those who:

- Work (e.g., roofers, construction workers) or exercise (e.g., athletes) strenuously in a warm or hot and humid environment or a cold environment.

- Have a pre-existing health problem, such as diabetes or heart disease. Pre-existing health problems can increase a patient's susceptibility to heat-related illness. Medications taken for these conditions can also cause dehydration.

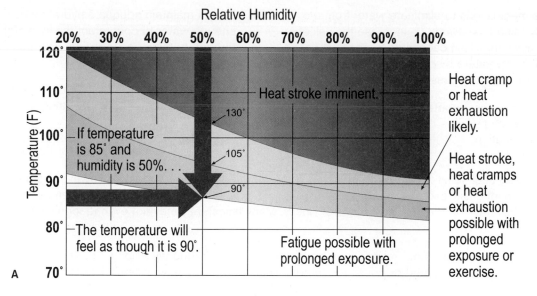

Relative Humidity

Heat stroke imminent.

If temperature is 85° and humidity is 50%...

The temperature will feel as though it is 90°.

Fatigue possible with prolonged exposure.

Heat cramp or heat exhaustion likely.

Heat stroke, heat cramps or heat exhaustion possible with prolonged exposure or exercise.

A

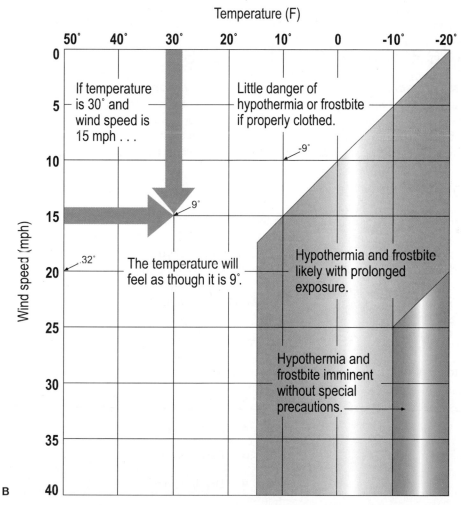

Temperature (F)

If temperature is 30° and wind speed is 15 mph...

Little danger of hypothermia or frostbite if properly clothed.

The temperature will feel as though it is 9°.

Hypothermia and frostbite likely with prolonged exposure.

Hypothermia and frostbite imminent without special precautions.

B

Figure 19-3. Temperature, humidity and wind are the three main factors affecting body temperature.

- Take medications to eliminate water from the body (diuretics). Diuretics increase the risk of dehydration, which causes an increase in core body temperature by preventing adequate blood flow to remove excess heat.

- Consume other substances that have a diuretic effect, such as fluids containing caffeine, alcohol or carbonation.

- Do not maintain adequate hydration by drinking enough water to counteract the loss of fluids through perspiration, exertion, or exposure to heat and humidity.

- Live in a situation or environment that does not provide them with enough heating or cooling, depending on the season.

- Wear clothing inappropriate for the weather.

People usually seek relief from an extreme temperature before they begin to feel ill. However, some people do not or cannot easily escape these extremes. Athletes and those who work outdoors often keep working even after they develop the first indications of illness. Many times, they may not even recognize the signs and symptoms.

Heat-related illnesses and cold-related emergencies occur more frequently among older adults, especially those living in poorly ventilated or poorly insulated buildings or buildings with poor heating or cooling systems. Young children and people with health problems are also at risk because their bodies do not respond as effectively to temperature extremes.

Types of Heat-Related Illnesses

Exercise-associated muscle cramps, exertional heat exhaustion and **heat stroke** are conditions caused by overexposure to heat and/or loss of fluids and electrolytes. Dehydration is another condition often related to heat-related illnesses. Heat-related illness, if not cared for promptly, can get progressively worse in a very short period of time. By recognizing the signs and symptoms of the early stages of heat-related illness and responding appropriately, you may be able to prevent the condition from becoming life threatening.

Dehydration

Dehydration refers to inadequate fluids in the body's tissues and is often caused by inadequate fluid intake, vomiting, diarrhea, certain medications, and alcohol or caffeine use. Dehydration can be a serious and even life-threatening situation. The people at highest risk for dying from dehydration are the very young and the very old. Lay responders can measure dehydration levels by monitoring urine color before, during and after a period of heavy work or exercise. Dark, amber urine or complete lack of urine output suggests a dehydrated state. Fluid loss that is not regained increases the risk for a heat-related illness.

Signs and Symptoms of Dehydration

The signs and symptoms of dehydration worsen as the body becomes drier. Initial signs and symptoms include:

- Fatigue.
- Weakness.
- Headache.
- Irritability.

- Nausea.
- Dizziness.
- Excessive thirst.
- Dry lips and mouth.

As dehydration worsens, signs and symptoms can include:

- Disorientation or delirium.
- Loss of appetite.
- Severe thirst.

- Dry mucous membranes.
- Sunken eyes.

- Dry skin that does not spring back if pinched, creating a "tenting" effect.

- Lack of tears (particularly important among young children).

- Decrease in perspiration.

- Dark, amber urine or complete lack of urine output.

- Unresponsiveness.

Care for Dehydration

To care for a person who is dehydrated, you need to help them replace the lost fluid. If the person is still awake and able to swallow, encourage them to drink small amounts of a commercial sports drink or, if not available, water. The person should be allowed to drink until their thirst sensation is quenched. However, do not let the person gulp the fluid down; instead, have them sip it at a slow pace. If the person drinks too quickly, vomiting may occur. If dehydration is severe, the person will likely need more advanced medical care to receive fluids intravenously.

Exercise-Associated Muscle Cramps

The exact cause of exercise-associated muscle cramps is not known, although it is believed to be a combination of loss of fluid and salt from heavy sweating. Exercise-associated muscle cramps develop fairly rapidly and usually occur after heavy exercise or work in warm or even moderate temperatures.

Signs and Symptoms of Exercise-Associated Muscle Cramps

Exercise-associated muscle cramps are painful spasms of skeletal muscles. While they usually affect the legs, arms and abdomen, they can occur in any voluntary muscle. The person's body temperature is usually normal and the skin moist.

Care for Exercise-Associated Muscle Cramps

To care for exercise-associated muscle cramps:

- Help the person move to a cool place to rest.

- Give an electrolyte- and carbohydrate-containing fluid such as a commercial sports drink, fruit juice or milk. Water also may be given if the drinks are not available.

- Lightly stretch the muscle and gently massage the area (Figure 19-4).

- Do *not* give the person salt tablets. They can worsen the situation.

When cramps stop, the person usually can start activity again if there are no other signs or symptoms of illness. They should keep drinking plenty of fluids. Watch the person carefully for further signs or symptoms of dehydration.

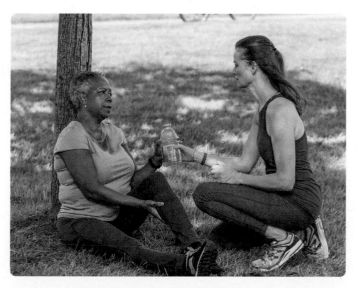

Figure 19-4. Resting, lightly stretching and massaging the affected muscle, and replenishing fluids are usually enough for the body to recover from exercise-associated muscle cramps.

What if... *A person has exercise-associated muscle cramps? I've heard that eating salty food such as cured meat helps to prevent the cramps from recurring.*

Rest, cooling off and drinking an electrolyte-carbohydrate fluid, such as a commercial sports drink, fruit juice or milk, is typically the only care needed for exercise-associated muscle cramps. When exercising heavily in hot and humid conditions in which a person is losing a lot of salt through sweat, however, extra sodium from food intake or rehydration beverages (or both) may be required. Cured meat is not the best option though. Hydrating in advance of planned exercise with a 3 to 8 percent carbohydrate-electrolyte sports drink can help prevent dehydration and loss of electrolytes. Consider consulting with a dietician or medical professional to identify a safe and healthy strategy to increase sodium in the event of excessive exercise-associated muscle cramping.

Exertional Heat Exhaustion

Exertional heat exhaustion (EHA) is a form of heat-related illness. EHA results when fluid lost through perspiration is not replaced by other fluids. This results in the body pulling the blood away from the surface areas of the body to protect the vital organs, such as the heart and brain.

Anyone can be at risk for developing EHA from exposure to a hot or humid environment. However, it happens most often to those engaged in intense physical activity—such as firefighters, construction or factory workers and athletes. Simply being in a hot and humid environment while overdressed with heavy clothes can also cause EHA.

Signs and Symptoms of Exertional Heat Exhaustion

The signs and symptoms of exertional heat exhaustion include:

- Cool, pale, clammy or slightly flushed skin.
- Fatigue.
- Nausea and/or vomiting.
- Loss of appetite.

- Dehydration.
- Dizziness with possible fainting.
- Elevated heart and respiratory rate.
- Muscle cramps.

Care for Exertional Heat Exhaustion

When a heat-related illness is recognized in its early stages, it usually can be reversed. To give care:

- Move the person from the hot environment to a cooler environment with circulating air.

- Loosen or remove as much clothing as possible.

- Apply cool, wet cloths, such as towels or sheets, taking care to remoisten the cloths periodically. Spraying the person with water and fanning also can help increase the evaporative cooling (Figure 19-5).

- If the person is awake and able to swallow, give them small amounts of a cool fluid such as a commercial sports drink or fruit juice to restore fluids and electrolytes. Milk or water also may be given. Do not let the person drink too quickly.

- Let the person rest in a comfortable position and watch carefully for changes in their condition. The person should not resume normal activities the same day.

- If the person's condition does not improve, or they refuse fluids, have a change in level of consciousness or vomit, call 9-1-1 or the designated emergency number, as these are indications that the person's condition is getting worse. Stop giving fluids and place the person on their side in a recovery position if needed. Watch for signs and symptoms of breathing problems. Keep the person lying down and continue to cool the body any way you can (see Care for Heat Stroke for methods).

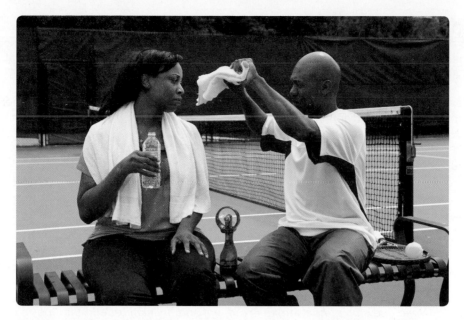

Figure 19-5. Spraying a person with water and fanning a person can be effective at cooling them down.

Heat Stroke

The most serious of heat-related illnesses is heat stroke. Heat stroke is a life-threatening condition that most often occurs when people ignore the signs and symptoms of exertional heat exhaustion or do not act quickly enough to give care. Heat stroke develops when the body systems are overwhelmed by heat and begin to stop functioning. Sweating may stop when body fluid levels are low (i.e., dehydration) but may also still be present for a person suffering heat stroke. The body's exaggerated heat production, combined with an inability to cool itself, causes body temperature to rise quickly, soon reaching a level at which the brain and other vital organs, such as the heart and kidneys, begin to fail. If the body is not cooled, convulsions, coma and death will result.

Two types of heat stroke are typically reported—classic heat stroke and exertional heat stroke.

Classic heat stroke is normally caused by environmental changes and often occurs during the summer months. Classic heat stroke most often occurs in infants, children, older adults, those with chronic medical illnesses and those who suffer from inefficient body heat-regulation mechanisms—such as those in poor socioeconomic settings with limited access to air conditioning and those on certain medications (e.g., antihistamines, amphetamines, diuretics, and blood pressure and heart medicines). Typically, classic heat stroke develops slowly, over a period of several days, with persons presenting with minimally elevated core temperatures.

Exertional heat stroke is the opposite of classic heat stroke and is experienced more frequently than classic heat stroke. Exertional heat stroke—which primarily affects younger, active individuals, such as athletes (recreational and competitive), military recruits and heavy laborers—occurs when excess heat is generated through exercise and exceeds the body's ability to cool off. Exposure to factors such as high air temperature, high relative humidity and dehydration increases the risk for developing exertional heat stroke.

Signs and Symptoms of Heat Stroke

Heat stroke is a serious medical emergency. You must recognize the signs and symptoms of heat stroke and give care immediately. The signs and symptoms include:

- Changes in level of consciousness, including confusion, agitation, disorientation or unresponsiveness.

- Trouble seeing.

- Seizures.

- Extremely high body temperature (above 104° F, or 40° C).

- Flushed or red skin that can be either dry or moist.

- Rapid, shallow breathing.

- Throbbing headache.

- Dizziness, nausea or vomiting.

> **What if...** *A person has signs or symptoms of heat stroke but still seems to be sweating? Should I give care for exertional heat exhaustion instead?*
>
> *Not necessarily. While one sign of heat stroke is red, hot and dry skin (due to the body's lack of fluid and therefore sweat), it is possible for a person with heat stroke to still be sweating in earlier stages, or to appear to be sweating, with wet skin and sweat-soaked clothing. Therefore, if a person has other signs or symptoms of heat stroke, such as an extremely high body temperature, change in level of consciousness, rapid shallow breathing, confusion, trouble seeing, vomiting or seizures, assume heat stroke and call 9-1-1 or the designated emergency number immediately. Then, cool the person as rapidly as possible.*

Care for Heat Stroke

Call 9-1-1 or the designated emergency number immediately for heat stroke as it is a life-threatening emergency. While waiting for help to arrive, you will need to immediately cool the person by following these steps:

- Remove the person from the hot environment.

- Remove excess clothing.

- Rapidly cool the body by immersing the person up to the neck in cold water (preferred); douse the person with ice-water-soaked towels over the entire body, frequently rotating the cold, wet towels, spraying with cold water, fanning the person, or covering the person with ice towels or bags of ice placed over the body.

- If you are not able to measure and monitor the person's temperature, apply rapid cooling methods for 20 minutes or until the person's level of consciousness improves.

- Give care according to other conditions found.

A person having a heat stroke may experience respiratory or cardiac arrest. Be prepared to perform CPR, if needed.

Cold-Related Emergencies

Frostbite and **hypothermia** are two types of cold-related emergencies. Frostbite occurs in body parts exposed to the cold. Hypothermia develops when the body can no longer generate sufficient heat to maintain normal temperature.

Frostbite

Frostbite is the freezing of body tissues, usually the nose, ears, fingers or toes. It usually occurs in exposed areas of the body, depending on the air temperature, length of exposure and the wind. Frostbite can be superficial or deep. In superficial frostbite, the skin is frozen but the tissues below are not. In deep frostbite, both the skin and underlying tissues are frozen. Both types of frostbite are serious and may be accompanied by hypothermia. The water in and between the body's cells freezes and swells. The ice crystals and swelling damage or destroy the cells. Frostbite can cause the eventual loss of the affected body part.

Signs and Symptoms of Frostbite

The signs and symptoms of frostbite include:

- Lack of feeling in the affected area.

- Swelling.

- Skin that appears waxy, is cold to the touch and is discolored (flushed, white, yellow or blue) (Figure 19-6).

- In more serious cases, blisters may form and the affected part may turn black and show signs and symptoms of deep tissue damage.

Care for Frostbite

When giving care for frostbite, the priority is to get the person out of the cold. Once the person is removed from the cold, follow these steps:

- Handle the area gently. Rough handling can damage the body part. *Never* rub the affected area, as this can cause skin damage.

- If there is a chance that the body part may refreeze or if you are close to a medical facility, do *not* attempt to rewarm the frostbitten area.

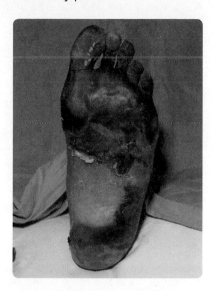

Figure 19-6. In serious cases of frostbite, the affected part may turn black and show deep tissue damage. *Photo: courtesy of Nigel Vardy and Nottingham University Hospitals NHS Trust*

- For minor frostbite, rapidly rewarm the affected part using skin-to-skin contact such as with a warm hand.

- For more serious frostbite, rewarm the affected area by gently soaking it in water between 100° F (38° C) and 105° F (40.5° C) (Figure 19-7, A). If you do not have a thermometer, test the water temperature yourself. If the temperature is uncomfortable to your touch, it is too warm. Keep the frostbitten part in the water until normal color returns and it feels warm (about 20 to 30 minutes). Check the water temperature frequently to ensure it does not cool to less than normal body temperature.

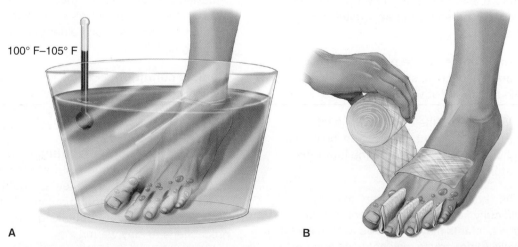

100° F–105° F

A

B

Figure 19-7, A–B. A, Rewarm the frostbitten area by gently soaking it in water between 100° (38° C) and 105° F (40.5° C). **B,** If the fingers or toes are frostbitten, place dry, sterile gauze between them to keep them separated before bandaging.

- Do not use chemical heat packs, such as commercial hand warmers, to rewarm the frostbitten area as they can reach temperatures that will cause further (heat) injury to the damaged tissue.

- Loosely bandage the area with dry, sterile dressings.

- If the fingers or toes are frostbitten, place dry, sterile gauze between them to keep them separated (Figure 19-7, B). If the damage is to the feet, do *not* allow the person to walk.

- *Avoid* breaking any blisters.

- Assess for hypothermia and, if it is suspected, rewarm the person. Otherwise, take precautions to prevent hypothermia.

- Monitor the person and care for shock.

- Do not give any ibuprofen or other nonsteroidal anti-inflammatory drugs.

Call 9-1-1 or the designated emergency number or seek emergency medical care as soon as possible.

Hypothermia

Hypothermia is the state of the body being colder than the usual core temperature. It is caused by either excessive loss of body heat and/or the body's inability to produce heat. Hypothermia can come on gradually or it can develop very quickly. In hypothermia, body temperature drops below 95° F (35° C). Shivering occurs initially as a physiological response to maintain body temperature. As cooling continues, shivering ceases and the person becomes clumsy, slow to respond or unresponsive. The heart rate becomes slow and/or irregular. With severe hypothermia (82° F, or 27.7° C), an abnormal heart rhythm (ventricular fibrillation) may develop. If this happens, the heart will eventually stop and the person will die if not given care.

The air temperature does not have to be below freezing for people to develop hypothermia. This is especially true if the person is wet or if it is windy.

Contributing Factors

As with heat-related emergencies, anyone can develop hypothermia, but predisposing factors place some people at a higher risk. These factors include:

- **A cold environment.** Even if the ambient temperature is not extremely low, hypothermia can occur if a person is not adequately protected from the cold.

- **A wet environment.** The presence of moisture (e.g., perspiration, rain, snow or water) will increase the speed at which body heat is lost.

- **Wind.** Wind makes the environment a lot colder than the ambient temperature indicates. The higher the wind chill effect, the lower the temperature actually is.

- **Age.** The very young and the very old may have difficulty keeping warm in cool or cold conditions. Infants may not yet be able to shiver effectively. Older adults may not have enough body mass to retain body heat. Both age groups may be unable to help themselves stay warm by removing themselves from the cold environment or by protecting themselves with warmer clothing. In addition, many older people have impaired circulation.

- **Medical conditions.** People with certain medical conditions, such as generalized infection, hypoglycemia, shock and head injury, may be at higher risk for developing hypothermia.

- **Alcohol, drugs and poisoning.** Alcohol and certain types of drugs or poisons can reduce a person's ability to feel the cold, or can cloud judgment and impede rational thought, preventing the patient from taking proper precautions to stay warm.

Signs and Symptoms of Hypothermia

The signs and symptoms of hypothermia include:

- Shivering (may be absent in later stages of hypothermia).
- Numbness.
- Glassy stare.
- Apathy or decreasing level of consciousness.
- Weakness.
- Impaired judgment.
- Changes in level of consciousness, unresponsiveness.

Shivering that stops without rewarming is a sign that the person's condition is worsening. They need immediate medical care.

Care for Hypothermia

Call 9-1-1 or the designated emergency number immediately for any suspected case of hypothermia. Your priority is to move the person into a warmer environment if possible. Be careful to move the person gently, as any sudden movement can cause a heart arrhythmia and possibly cardiac arrest.

Layer Your Way to Warmth

When the weather is cold, but you need or want to be outdoors, the best way to ensure your comfort and warmth is to layer your clothing.

The first layer, called the base layer, is next to your skin. The base layer helps to regulate your body temperature by moving perspiration away from your skin. This is important because if perspiration gets trapped inside your clothes, you can become chilled rapidly, which can lead to hypothermia. Thermal underwear makes a good base layer for cold weather. The fabrics that are best at moving sweat away from the skin (also called wicking) are silk, merino wool and certain synthetics. Cotton is not a good choice because it traps moisture rather than wicking it away.

The job of the middle layer is insulation. This layer keeps you warm; it helps you retain heat by trapping air close to your body. Natural fibers, such as wool and goose down, are excellent insulators. So is synthetic fleece. Vests, jackets and tights are examples of clothing that can be worn for insulation.

The shell or outer layer protects you from wind, rain or snow. For cold weather, the shell layer should be both waterproof and "breathable." This will keep wind and water from getting inside of the other two layers while allowing perspiration to evaporate. The shell also should be roomy enough to fit easily over the other layers without restricting your movement.

One of the other advantages of layering is that you can make quick adjustments if the weather changes or you change your activity level. You can take clothes off when you become too warm and put them back on if you get cold.

In addition to layering your clothes, to stay warm in cold weather you also should wear:

- A hat.
- A scarf or knit mask that covers your face and mouth.
- Long-sleeved tops with cuffs that are snug but not too tight at the wrist.
- Mittens (they are warmer than gloves).
- Water-resistant boots.

Then, give care as follows:

- In cases of severe hypothermia, the person may appear to be unresponsive. Breathing may have slowed or stopped. The body may feel stiff because the muscles became rigid. If the person is unresponsive and not breathing normally, perform CPR. Continue to take steps to warm the person until emergency medical services (EMS) personnel take over.

- Make the person comfortable. Remove any wet clothing and dry the person off. Put on dry clothing if available.

- Warm the body gradually by wrapping the person in blankets and plastic sheeting to hold in body heat (Figure 19-8). Also, keep the head covered to further retain body heat.

- If you are far from medical care, position the person near a heat source or apply heating pads or other heat sources to the body, such as containers filled with warm water. Carefully monitor any heat source to avoid burning the person. Keep a barrier, such as a blanket, towel or clothing, between the heat source and the person.

- If the person is alert and can swallow, give warm, not hot, liquids that do not contain alcohol or caffeine. Alcohol can cause heat loss, and caffeine can cause dehydration.

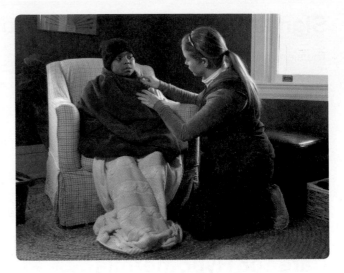

Figure 19-8. For hypothermia, rewarm the body gradually by wrapping the person in blankets and keeping the head covered.

- Do *not* warm the person too quickly, such as by immersing the person in warm water.

- Do *not* rub or massage the extremities.

- Check breathing and monitor for any changes in the person's condition, and care for shock.

- Be prepared to perform CPR or use an automated external defibrillator (AED).

What if... *I am sure a person I am helping has signs or symptoms of hypothermia, but they are insisting on undressing? Could I be wrong that the person is cold?*

In some cases, people who have died from the cold have been discovered in an undressed state known as paradoxical undressing. As unusual as this may sound, individuals in a hypothermic state do often exhibit signs and symptoms of an altered mental status, including judgment, which helps to explain why a person might remove warm clothing even though they are essentially freezing to death. Paradoxical undressing varies from complete stripping of clothes to unzipping of trousers. If you encounter a situation such as this, remember your basic care steps: begin rewarming the person immediately by moving them to a warm environment, and wrap all exposed body surfaces with anything at hand, such as blankets, clothing and newspapers, to increase the body's core temperature. Of course, you should also call 9-1-1 or the designated emergency number immediately for any case of hypothermia.

SMART MOVES > PREVENTING HEAT-RELATED ILLNESSES AND COLD-RELATED EMERGENCIES

Generally, illnesses and emergencies caused by overexposure to extreme temperatures are preventable. Follow these guidelines:

- Avoid being outdoors in the hottest or coldest part of the day. If you plan to work outdoors in hot weather, plan your activity for the early morning and evening hours when the sun is not as strong. Likewise, if you must be outdoors on cold days, plan your activities for the warmest part of the day.

(Continued)

- Dress appropriately for the environment and your activity level. When possible, wear light-colored clothing in the heat as it reflects the sun's rays. When you are in the cold, wear layers to stay warm (see Layer Your Way to Warmth for more information). Wear a head covering in both heat and cold. A hat protects the head from the sun's rays in the summer and prevents heat from escaping in the winter.

- Change your activity level according to the temperature and take frequent breaks. In very hot conditions, exercise only for brief periods, then rest in a cool, shaded area. Frequent breaks allow your body to readjust to normal body temperature, enabling it to better withstand brief periods of exposure to temperature extremes. Avoid heavy exercise during the hottest or coldest part of the day. Extremes of temperature promote fatigue, which hampers the body's ability to adjust to changes in the environment.

- Whether it is hot or cold, drink large amounts of nonalcoholic, non-caffeinated fluids before, during and after activity. Drinking at least six 8-ounce glasses of fluids is the most important way to prevent heat-related illnesses or cold-related emergencies. *Never* restrict fluid intake as a form of punishment.

- Plan to drink fluids when you take a break. Just as you would drink cool fluids in the summer, drink warm fluids in the winter. Cool and warm fluids help the body maintain a normal temperature. If cold or hot drinks are not available, drink plenty of plain water.

- Do not drink beverages containing caffeine or alcohol. Caffeine and alcohol hinder the body's temperature-regulating mechanism.

Summary

Overexposure to extreme heat or cold may cause a person to develop a heat-related illness or cold-related emergency. The likelihood of this also depends on factors such as physical activity, clothing, wind, humidity, working and living conditions, and a person's age and physical condition (see Smart Moves: Preventing Heat-Related Illnesses and Cold-Related Emergencies).

In warm conditions, dehydration is a danger that can be related to heat-related illnesses. Exercise-associated muscle cramps are an early indication that the body's normal temperature-regulating mechanism is not working efficiently. They may signal that the person is in the early stage of a heat-related illness. For heat-related illness, it is important for the person to stop physical activity and be removed from the hot environment. Begin immediate, aggressive cooling for heat stroke and call 9-1-1 or the designated emergency number if life-threatening conditions are found. Heat stroke can rapidly lead to death if it is left untreated.

Both hypothermia and frostbite are serious cold-related emergencies that require professional medical care. Hypothermia can be life threatening. For both hypothermia and frostbite, the immediate goal is to move the person to a warmer place as quickly as possible, then give care based on the conditions found. Always handle a person with a cold-related emergency with care to avoid causing further damage or a dangerous heart arrhythmia. Call 9-1-1 or the designated emergency number for any case of hypothermia.

READY TO RESPOND? ▶

Think back to Kelly in the opening scenario, and use what you have learned to respond to these questions:

1. What cold-related emergency is Kelly showing signs of?

2. What risk factors are present that increase the likelihood of hypothermia?

3. What should be your priority in caring for Kelly?

Study Questions

1. **Match each term with the correct definition.**

   a. Frostbite   b. Exercise-associated muscle cramps   c. Exertional heat exhaustion   d. Heat stroke   e. Hypothermia

   ____ The early stage and most common form of heat-related illness

   ____ A life-threatening condition that develops when the body's warming mechanisms fail to maintain normal body temperature

   ____ A life-threatening condition that develops when the body's cooling mechanism fails

   ____ The freezing of body tissues caused by overexposure to the cold

   ____ Painful spasms of skeletal muscles that develop after heavy exercise or work outdoors in warm or moderate temperatures

2. **List the three main factors that affect body temperature.**

3. **List two conditions that can result from overexposure to heat.**

4. **List the signs and symptoms of exertional heat exhaustion.**

5. **List two reasons why EMS personnel should be called for exertional heat exhaustion.**

6. **List two ways to cool a person with heat stroke.**

7. **List two conditions that result from overexposure to the cold.**

8. **List four ways to prevent heat-related illnesses and cold-related emergencies.**

In questions 9 and 10, circle the letter of the correct answer.

9. **To care for exercise-associated muscle cramps—**

   a. Have the person rest comfortably in a cool place.   b. Call 9-1-1 or the designated emergency number.   c. Give salt tablets.   d. All of the above

(Continued)

Study Questions continued

10. To care for dehydration—

a. Cool the body using wet sheets and towels or cold packs.

b. Cool the body by applying rubbing alcohol.

c. Call 9-1-1 or the designated emergency number.

d. Replace lost fluids.

Use the following scenario to answer questions 11 and 12.

You and a friend have been cross-country skiing all morning. The snow is great, but it is really cold. Your buddy has complained for the past half hour or so that his hands are freezing. Now he says he cannot feel his fingers at all. You decide to return to the ski chalet you are renting. Once inside where it is warm, your friend has trouble removing his mittens. You help him take them off and notice that his fingers look waxy and white and feel cold. You recognize the signs and symptoms of minor frostbite.

11. Circle the signs and symptoms of frostbite you find in the scenario above.

12. How would you care for your friend's hands?

Use the following scenario to answer questions 13 and 14.

You are working on a community service project delivering meals to older, homebound individuals. It is a blustery winter day that has you running from the van to each front door. As you enter the last home, you notice that it is not much warmer inside the house than it is outside. An older woman, bundled in blankets, is sitting as close as possible to a small electric space heater. You speak to her, introducing yourself and asking how things are, but you get no response. The woman's eyes are glassy as she makes an effort to look at you. She seems weak and exhausted, barely able to keep her head up. You touch her arm, but she does not seem to feel it.

13. Circle the signs and symptoms in the scenario above that would lead you to suspect a cold-related emergency.

14. Describe the actions you would take to care for the woman in the scenario.

Answers are listed in the Appendix.

PART SIX

Special Situations

20

WATER-RELATED EMERGENCIES

You are at a backyard pool party at your uncle's house. Once food is put out, everyone climbs out of the pool, ready to dig in. As the family sits around complimenting your uncle on his barbecue skills, one of the younger children quietly wanders off to play by the pool's edge. There is barely a sound when the child falls into the pool while going after a toy that is floating by. Luckily, you happen to look up just in time to see the child struggling to stay at the water's surface.

Learn and Respond ▶

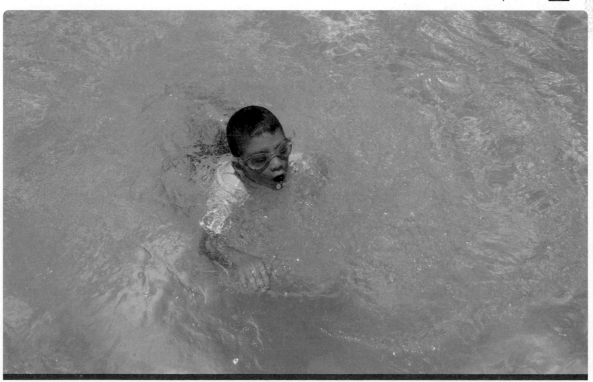

After reading this chapter, you should be able to:

- Describe how to recognize a water emergency involving a distressed swimmer or a drowning victim.

- Understand what actions you can safely take to assist a person who is in distress or is drowning.

- Describe three nonswimming rescues and assists that you can use to help someone who is in trouble in the water.

Distressed swimmer: A swimmer showing anxiety or panic; often identified as a swimmer who has gone beyond their swimming abilities.

Drowning: An event in which a person experiences respiratory impairment due to submersion in water. Drowning may or may not result in death.

Reaching assist: A method of rescuing someone in the water by using an object to extend the responder's reach or reaching with an arm or leg.

Throwing assist: A method of rescuing someone in the water by throwing the person a floating object, with or without a line attached.

Wading assist: A method of rescuing someone in the water by wading out to the person in distress, but to a depth that is no deeper than the responder's chest.

Introduction

One of the most common water-related emergencies is *drowning.* Drowning occurs when a person experiences respiratory impairment due to submersion in water. Drowning may or may not result in death; however, it is the fifth most common cause of death from unintentional injury in the United States among all ages, and it rises to the second leading cause of death among those 1 to 14 years of age. Approximately 4000 Americans die annually from drowning, and more than 50 percent of drowning victims treated in emergency departments require hospitalization or transfer for further care. Children younger than 5 years of age have the highest rate of drowning.

In this chapter, you will learn how to recognize a water-related emergency including how to recognize a distressed swimmer before they become a drowning victim. You will also learn several methods to *safely* reach and assist a person in the water who is in distress or drowning without becoming a drowning victim yourself. Most importantly, you will learn ways to prevent water-related emergencies from happening.

Water-Related Emergencies

An emergency can happen to anyone in, on or around the water, regardless of how good a swimmer the person is or what they are doing at the time. Some people who drown never intended to be in the water. They may have slipped in and then did not know what do. A strong swimmer can get into trouble in the water because of sudden injury or illness. A nonswimmer playing in shallow ocean water can be knocked down by a wave or pulled into deeper water by a rip current. Someone can fall through the ice while skating on a pond.

A child can drown at home in the bathtub, even in as little as an inch of water, or in a large bucket, the toilet or an irrigation ditch.

The key to recognizing an emergency is staying alert and knowing the signs that indicate an emergency. Use all your senses when observing others in and around the water. A swimmer may be acting oddly, or you may hear a scream or sudden splash. Watch for anything that may seem unusual.

> **What if…** *I live in a home that has a swimming pool? What types of information and skills do you think I need to know?*
>
> *When you own a pool, you—and everyone in your home—should first know how to swim. Likewise, everyone in the home should be prepared for an emergency, including knowing how to call for emergency help; having first aid, CPR and automated external defibrillator (AED) skills; learning water rescue skills; and knowing where the emergency equipment is located and how to use it. Finally, it is important that everyone in the home take responsibility for securing the pool area and keeping the pool well maintained.*

Contributing Factors

There are certain factors that increase the likelihood of a drowning incident occurring. These factors include:

- Young children left alone or unsupervised around water (e.g., tubs, pools, lakes).

- Use of alcohol and recreational drugs, which may lead people to make bad decisions and do things they otherwise would not do.

- Traumatic injury, such as from diving into a shallow body of water.

- Condition or disability, such as heart disease, seizure disorder or neuromuscular disorder, that may cause sudden weakness or unresponsiveness while in the water.

Severity

Whether a person survives a drowning incident depends on how long they have been submerged and unable to breathe. Brain damage or death can begin to occur in as little as 4 to 6 minutes when the body is deprived of oxygen. The sooner the drowning process is stopped, the better the person's chances for survival without permanent brain damage. If the submersion lasts any longer, often the result is death. These times are only estimates; brain damage and/or death can occur more or less quickly depending on a variety of factors.

Recognizing a Water-Related Emergency

Being able to recognize that a person is having trouble in the water may help save that person's life. Most people who are drowning cannot or do not call out for help. They spend their energy trying to keep their mouth and nose above water to breathe. They may slip underwater quickly and never resurface. There are three kinds of water emergency situations: a distressed swimmer, a drowning victim—active and a drowning victim—passive. Each kind can be recognized by different behaviors.

A ***distressed swimmer*** may be too tired to get to shore or to the side of the pool but is able to stay afloat and breathe and may be calling for help (Figure 20-1). The person may be floating, treading water, or clinging to an

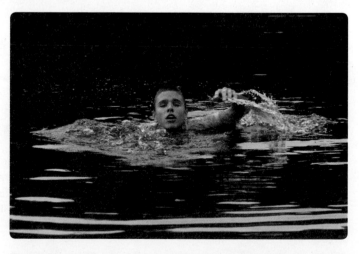

Figure 20-1. A distressed swimmer is able to stay afloat and breathe but may be too tired to get to shore or to the side of the pool.

object or a line for support. Someone who is trying to swim but making little or no forward progress may be in distress. If not helped, a person in distress may lose the ability to float and may start to drown.

A drowning victim—active could be at the surface of the water or sinking. They may be positioned vertically in the water and leaning back slightly. This person may not have a supporting kick or the ability to move forward. The person's arms could be at the side pressing down in an instinctive attempt to keep the head above water to breathe. All energy is going into the struggle to breathe, and the person may not be able to call out for help.

A drowning victim—passive may have a limp body or convulsive-like movements. They could be floating face-up or face-down on or near the surface of the water, or may be submerged (Figure 20-2). Table 20-1 compares the behaviors of distressed swimmers and drowning victims with those of swimmers.

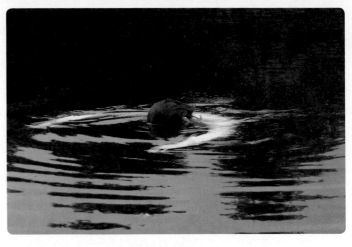

Figure 20-2. A drowning victim may be floating face-up or face-down on or near the surface of the water, or may be submerged.

Table 20-1. **Behaviors of Distressed Swimmers and Drowning Victims Compared with Swimmers**

	Swimmer	Distressed Swimmer	Drowning Victim—Active	Drowning Victim—Passive
Breathing	Rhythmic breathing	Can continue breathing and might call for help	Struggles to breathe; cannot call out for help	Is not breathing
Arm and Leg Action	Relatively coordinated	Floating, sculling or treading water; might wave for help	Holds arms to sides, alternately moving up and pressing down; has no supporting kick	None
Body Position	Horizontal	Horizontal, vertical or diagonal, depending on means of support	Vertical, leaning back slightly	Horizontal or vertical; face-up, face-down or submerged
Locomotion (ability to move from place to place)	Recognizable	Makes little or no forward progress; less and less able to support self	None; has only 20–60 seconds before submerging	None

Taking Action in a Water-Related Emergency

Submersion situations are not always easy to manage. *Consider your own safety above all else when faced with a water-related emergency.* You should not attempt a swimming rescue unless you are trained to do so. In the absence of such training, following these steps will help reduce your risk of drowning:

- Look for a lifeguard to help you before attempting any water rescue.

- If a lifeguard or other professional responder is not present, make sure you have appropriate equipment for your own safety and that of the drowning person.

- Call for help immediately if proper equipment is not available.

- Never swim out to a person unless you have the proper training, skills and equipment.

As in any emergency situation, proceed safely. Make sure the scene is safe. If the person is in the water, decide first whether help is needed in order for the person to get out, and then act based on your training. In addition, you should quickly consider the following factors:

- The condition of the person:

  ○ Is the person responsive and able to cooperate with the rescue or respond to your commands?

  ○ Is the person submerged? If the person is submerged, they will need immediate care once on dry land. Submersion may also make it difficult to find the person in murky or cloudy water.

  ○ Does the person seem injured? If so, you may have to remove the person from the water before giving care.

  ○ Is the person alone? Do others around the person also seem in distress? Are there multiple people who may need to be rescued? A situation involving multiple people can be much more dangerous for a responder.

- The condition of the water:

  ○ Is the water clear enough for you to see the person and any hazards in the water?

  ○ How cold is the water? Is there potential for the person to also have hypothermia? What are the risks for the responder developing hypothermia?

  ○ How fast is the water moving? Fast-flowing water is very strong. If it is above your knees, do *not* attempt to wade through it without being harnessed; otherwise, you could be swept away. In addition, a person's location can change very quickly in fast-moving water.

  ○ How deep is the water? Will you be able to securely stand if you need to do a wading assist?

  ○ Are there additional hazards (e.g., debris, such as from a flood) or a situation in which a motor vehicle is submerged? Be aware of the potential for exposure to a hazardous material such as oil or gas.

- The resources available:

  ○ Are you the only other person on the scene?

  ○ Are there other qualified responders on-site to assist with the rescue?

  ○ Is there anyone available to call for help or to help give care once the person is on dry land?

  ○ Do you have the proper training, skills and equipment for the rescue that needs to be attempted?

  ○ Are you wearing a personal flotation device?

Remember, your first goal is to stay safe. Rushing into the water to help someone may put you at risk for drowning, too. A panicking person could grab and submerge a nontrained responder thus putting both in danger. Once you ensure your own safety, your goal is to help the person out of the water. If the person is unresponsive, send someone to call 9-1-1 or the designated emergency number while you start the rescue if possible.

Nonswimming Rescues and Assists

You should make every effort to assist a person without entering the water. Whenever possible, start the rescue by talking to the person. Let the person know that help is coming. If it is too noisy or if the person is too far away, use nonverbal communication such as hand gestures to direct them to land. Direct the person in what to do to help with the rescue, such as grasping a line, ring buoy or other object that floats. Ask the person to move toward you such as by using the back float with slight leg movements or small strokes. Some people reach safety by themselves with the calm and encouraging assistance of someone calling to them.

If talking the person to safety does not help, there are several nonswimming rescues and assists that you can try for a distressed swimmer or drowning person.

Reaching Assists

If the person is close enough, you can use a **reaching assist** to help them out of the water. Firmly brace yourself on a pool deck, pier or shoreline and reach out to the person with any object that will extend your reach, such as a pole, oar or paddle, tree branch, shirt, belt or towel (Figure 20-3). If equipment is not available, you can still perform a reaching assist by lying down and extending your arm or leg for the person to grab, while making sure that you are stable and cannot be inadvertently pulled into the water.

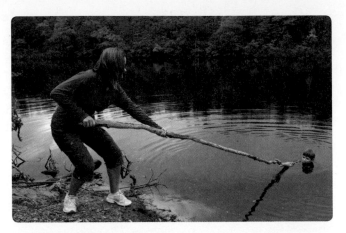

Figure 20-3. To perform a reaching assist, firmly brace yourself on solid ground and reach out to the person with an object that extends your reach.

Throwing Assists

You can rescue a swimmer in distress or a drowning victim who is out of reach by using a **throwing assist.** To do so, throw a floating object with a line attached, aiming so it lands just beyond the person, with the line lying across the person's shoulder if possible (Figure 20-4). The person can grasp the object and then be pulled to safety. Throwing equipment includes heavy lines, ring buoys, throw bags or any floating object available such as a picnic jug, small cooler, buoyant cushion, kickboard or extra life jacket.

Wading Assists

If the water is safe and shallow enough (not over your chest), you can use a **wading assist** to reach the person. If there is a current or the bottom is soft or the depth unknown, making it dangerous to wade, do *not* enter the water. If possible, wear a life jacket and take something with you to extend your reach such as a ring buoy, buoyant cushion, kickboard, life jacket, tree branch, pole, air mattress, plastic cooler, picnic jug, paddle or water exercise belt.

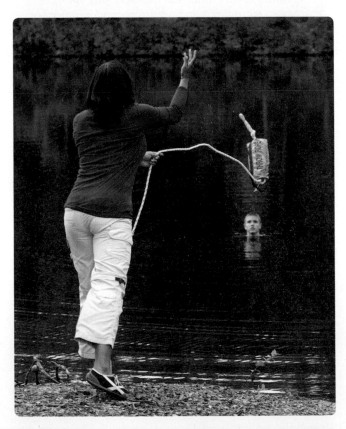

Figure 20-4. To perform a throwing assist, throw a floating object with a line just beyond a person in the water and pull the person to safety once they have grasped the object.

Assisting a Submerged Drowning Person

If a drowning victim is submerged in deep water, and a responder trained in water rescue is not on the scene, call 9-1-1 or the designated emergency number for help immediately. If the person is in shallow water (less than chest deep), you can reach down and grab the person to pull them to the surface. Once at the surface, turn the person face-up, remove the person from the water and give care as described in the following sections.

Care for Drowning

A distressed swimmer or drowning victim should be removed from the water as soon as possible, however, how and when to remove the person depends on their overall condition (i.e., is the person awake or unresponsive; is a head, neck or spinal injury suspected), the person's size, how soon help is expected to arrive and whether anyone else can help. The priorities when giving care in a water emergency are: ensuring the person's face (mouth and nose) is out of the water, maintaining an open airway and beginning resuscitation (when required) as soon as possible.

> **What if...** *I am at the beach and I see someone who is caught in a rip current? How can I help?*
>
> *Currents flowing away from the coast are called rip currents. They are dangerous because strong rip currents can be very fast—much faster than any human can swim—and are capable of taking a person a frightening distance from shore. If you see someone caught in a rip current, first tell the lifeguard or, if no lifeguard is available, call 9-1-1 or the designated emergency number. Second, remember the rule: Reach or Throw, Don't Go. Do not enter the water to help a person who is in trouble unless you are trained to do so. Many people die when attempting to help someone caught in a rip current or otherwise in trouble in the water. While waiting for trained help, the best actions to take are to throw the person something that floats, if possible, such as a life jacket. You should also talk to the person, directing them to try to swim out of the rip current in a direction parallel to shore. When the person is out of the current, they can head back to shore and away from the current at an angle.*

Care for an Unresponsive Person

- Check for responsiveness and breathing for no more than 10 seconds:

  ○ If the person is unresponsive and breathing normally, and you suspect a head, neck or spinal injury, hold the person steady in the water until additional advanced help arrives. Do not lift the person or attempt to remove them from the water if additional help is anticipated.

  ○ If the person is unresponsive and there is no normal breathing or only gasping, immediately remove the person from the water and begin performing CPR, starting with chest compressions as described in Chapter 6. If the chest does not clearly rise with the first rescue breath, retilt the head and ensure a proper seal before giving the second rescue breath. If the second breath does not make the chest rise, an object may be blocking the airway. After the next set of chest compressions and before attempting rescue breaths, open the mouth, look for an object and, if seen, remove it using a finger sweep. Continue to check the person's mouth for an object after each set of compressions until the rescue breaths go in.

If the person needs CPR, they must be removed from the water first (see Moving an Unresponsive Person to Dry Land). If a head, neck or spinal injury is suspected, care should be taken to minimize movement to the spine, but priority must be given to performing CPR.

When giving care, remember that many persons who have been submerged vomit because water has filled the stomach or air has been forced into the stomach during rescue breaths. If the person vomits and is on dry land, roll them into a side-lying recovery position to prevent aspiration (or choking). Use a finger to remove the vomit from the mouth. If possible, use a protective barrier, such as disposable latex-free gloves, gauze or even a handkerchief. Then, roll the person on their back again and continue giving care as necessary. If the person is still in the water, gently roll the person partially while maintaining stabilization and clear the vomit. Be sure to keep the person's face out of the water.

Moving an Unresponsive Person to Dry Land

If you are on a sloping shore or beach, you can use a beach drag to remove an unresponsive person from the water for the purpose of giving care. To perform the beach drag:

- Stand behind the person, and grasp them under the armpits, supporting the person's head, when possible, with your forearms.

- While walking backward slowly, drag the person toward the shore.

- Remove the person completely from the water or at least to a point where the person's head and shoulders are out of the water and on firm ground.

Care for a Responsive Person

If the person you rescue is responsive and a head, neck or spinal injury is not suspected, help them to dry land (use a walking assist as taught in Chapter 3 if needed) and follow the **CHECK—CALL—CARE** steps to determine what care is needed.

Always call 9-1-1 or the designated emergency number when a person has been involved in a drowning incident, even if the person is responsive and you think the danger has passed. Complications can develop as long as 72 hours after the incident and may be fatal.

Helping Someone Who Has Fallen Through Ice

If a person falls through the ice, do *not* go onto the ice to attempt a rescue, as the ice may be too thin to support you. It is your responsibility as a trained lay responder to call 9-1-1 or the designated emergency number immediately. In the case of a drowning person, always attempt to rescue the person using reaching and throwing assists (Figure 20-5) if you can safely do so. Continue talking to the person until help arrives. If you are able to safely pull the person from the water, give care for hypothermia as you learned in Chapter 19.

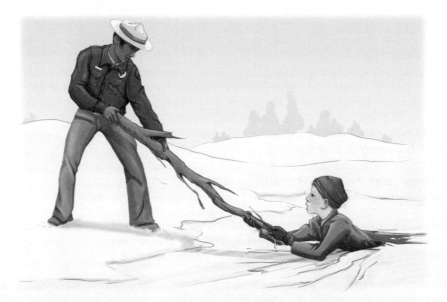

Figure 20-5. Use reaching and throwing assists to rescue a drowning person who has fallen through the ice.

As frightening as the risk of drowning is, it can usually be prevented by following good common sense around water, including steps to prevent injuries that could lead to drowning. Guidelines include:

- Learn to swim. The American Red Cross has swimming courses for people of any age and swimming ability. To find classes, visit redcross.org.

- Never leave children unattended or unsupervised around water, including bathtubs, toilets, wading pools or buckets of water. Proper supervision should be provided by an adult who is able to swim. Full attention must be given to the child/children in and around water. A child should always be within arm's reach of an adult, whether in the bathtub or around some other body of water.

- Always swim with a buddy; never swim alone.

- Read and obey all rules and posted signs, including "no diving" signs.

- Swim in areas supervised by a lifeguard.

- Children or inexperienced swimmers should take extra precautions, such as wearing a U.S. Coast Guard-approved life jacket when around the water.

- Watch out for the "dangerous too's"—too tired, too cold, too far away from safety, too much sun, too much strenuous activity.

- Be knowledgeable of the water environment and the potential hazards (deep and shallow areas, currents, depth changes, obstructions, and where the entry and exit points are located). Use feetfirst entry if you are unsure of any of these things.

- Do not mix alcohol with swimming, diving or boating. Alcohol impairs judgment, balance and coordination; affects swimming and diving skills; and reduces the body's ability to stay warm.

- Learn how to dive safely from a qualified instructor.

- Never dive into an aboveground pool, the shallow end of any inground pool or headfirst into breaking waves at the beach.

- Never dive into cloudy or murky water.

- Do not run on a diving board or attempt to dive a long way through the air. The water might not be deep enough at the point of entry.

- If you are bodysurfing, always keep your arms out in front of you to protect your head and neck.

Summary

Many drownings can be prevented by following simple precautions when in, on or around water (see Smart Moves: Preventing Water-Related Emergencies). Use the basic methods of reaching, throwing or wading to rescue or assist a person in the water without endangering yourself. Always remember to stay safe. If there is any chance that you cannot safely and easily help the person in trouble, call 9-1-1 or the designated emergency number immediately.

When giving care in a water emergency, your priority is ensuring that the person's face (mouth and nose) is out of the water and then giving appropriate care. If the person is unresponsive and not breathing normally, remove the person from the water and immediately begin CPR, starting with chest compressions. If the person is responsive and no head, neck or spinal injury is suspected, help the person to dry land and use the emergency action steps **CHECK—CALL—CARE** to determine what care to give. *Always* call 9-1-1 or the designated emergency number for a person involved in a drowning incident as potentially fatal complications can develop later. Further training in water safety and lifeguarding is available through the American Red Cross.

READY TO RESPOND? ❯

Think back to the water emergency in the opening scenario, and use what you have learned to respond to this question:

1. Knowing that the pool is deep where the child fell in, what is the best way to try to rescue the child?

Study Questions

1. List three nonswimming rescues and assists.

2. List four characteristics of a drowning victim—active.

In questions 3 and 4, circle the letter of the correct answer.

3. **In which of the following situations would a wading assist be appropriate?**

   a. You can reach the person by extending a branch from the shore.

   b. You suspect or see strong currents.

   c. The bottom is not firm.

   d. The water is shallow, and you can stand firmly with your chest out of the water.

4. **You see a man struggling in the rushing waters of a flooded creek. Which is the best way to try to rescue him without endangering yourself?**

   a. Dive into the water and grab him.

   b. Wade in and reach out to him with an object.

   c. From the shoreline, extend an object for him to reach.

   d. Yell to him to kick forcefully.

5. **List the general care steps for a drowning victim who is unresponsive and breathing normally in shallow water.**

Answers are listed in the Appendix.

21

PEDIATRIC, OLDER ADULT AND SPECIAL SITUATIONS

You go with a friend to visit her Grandma Mary for a nice home-cooked meal. When you arrive, her grandmother does not come to the door when you knock. Figuring she did not hear you—after all, her hearing is not the best and she does not always wear her hearing aid—your friend uses the spare key she has to go inside. In the living room, you discover the real reason Grandma Mary did not come to the door. She has fallen and cannot put weight on her leg to get back up. She tells you, "I just don't know how this happened."

Learn and Respond ▶

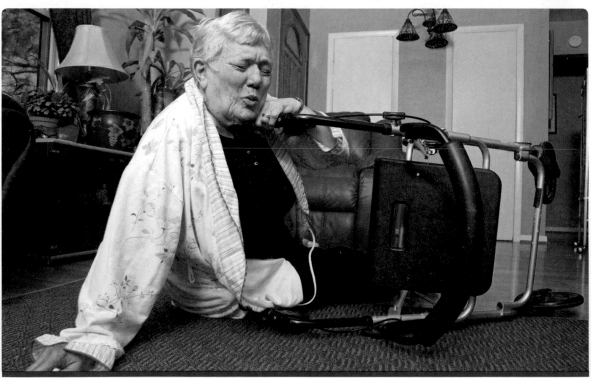

After reading this chapter, you should be able to:

- Describe considerations for checking an infant, a toddler, a preschooler, a school-age child and an adolescent.

- Explain how to observe an injured or ill child or infant, and how to communicate with the parents or guardian.

- Describe the signs and symptoms and care for common childhood illnesses and injuries.

- Describe how to check an older adult.

- Describe four issues that can affect older adults and their implications for care.

- Explain how to communicate with and assist a person with a physical disability or mental impairment.

- Explain the options available when trying to communicate with a person when there is a language barrier.

- Explain what you should do if you encounter a crime scene or hostile person.

Alzheimer's disease: The most common type of dementia in older people, in which thought, memory and language are impaired.

Child abuse: Action that results in the physical or psychological harm of a child; can be physical, sexual, verbal and/or emotional.

Child neglect: The most frequently reported type of child abuse in which a parent or guardian fails to provide the necessary, age-appropriate care to a child; insufficient medical or emotional attention or respect given to a child.

Disability: The absence or impairment of motor, sensory or mental function.

Hearing loss: Partial or total loss of hearing.

Impairment: Damage or reduction in quality, quantity, value or strength of a function.

Mental (cognitive) function: The brain's capacity to reason and to process information.

Motor function: The ability to move the body or a body part.

Motor impairment: The total or partial inability to move or to use a body part.

Sensory function: The ability to see, hear, touch, taste and smell.

Sudden infant death syndrome (SIDS): The sudden death of an infant younger than 1 year that remains unexplained after the performance of a complete postmortem investigation (autopsy).

Vision loss: Partial or total loss of sight.

Introduction

In any emergency, you should be aware of the unique needs and considerations of the person involved. For example, children and infants, older adults, persons with disabilities and persons who speak a different language than your own have special needs and considerations that affect your approach to giving care. It is also important to know what to do if you find yourself in a crime scene or hostile situation.

In any case, there are steps you can take to ensure you respond appropriately. This chapter includes information to help you better understand the nature of an emergency and give appropriate, effective care.

Children and Infants

Children and infants have unique needs that require special care. As you learned in Chapter 5, assessing a responsive child's or infant's condition can be difficult, especially if the child or infant does not know you and their parents or guardians are not readily available. At certain ages, children and infants do not readily accept strangers and may be very apprehensive. Very young children and infants also cannot tell you what is wrong and have difficulty expressing their feelings.

Communicating with Injured or Ill Children or Infants

We tend to react more strongly and emotionally to a child who is in pain or scared. You will need to try exceptionally hard to control your emotions and your facial expressions. Doing so will be helpful to both the child and any concerned adults. To help an injured or ill child or infant, you also need to try to imagine how the person feels. For example, a child may be afraid of the unknown. This includes being injured or ill, being touched by strangers, and being separated from their parents or guardian.

How you interact with an injured or ill child or infant is very important. You need to reduce the child's anxiety and panic, and gain the child's trust and cooperation if possible. Approach the child slowly. The sudden appearance of a stranger may upset the child. Get as close to the child's or infant's eye level as you can, and keep your voice calm. Smile at the child. Ask the child's name, and use it when you talk with them. Talk slowly and distinctly, and use words the child will easily understand. Ask questions the child will be able to answer easily. Depending on the age of the child, it may be necessary to direct questions about the situation to the parents or guardian. Explain to the child and the parents or guardian what you are going to do. Reassure the child that you are there to help and will not leave them. However, do not make promises that you cannot control, such as telling them something will not hurt or that they will be OK. It is important that the child, parent or guardian trust you, and making a promise that you cannot control can jeopardize your ability to care for the child's injury or illness.

Communicating with Children Who Have Special Healthcare or Functional Needs

When communicating with children and parents or guardians, remember to observe the whole situation and ask questions to determine if the child has special physical, developmental or functional needs. If the child has any needs, ask the parent or guardian if there is a list summarizing vital emergency information, such as any unique or specific care procedures associated with the child's condition, or allergies and other medical problems or issues. Generally, the parents and guardians can give you the best information since they are the most familiar with any medical equipment needed by the child.

When you attempt to communicate with children who have a developmental disability, the child's age and developmental level may not be obvious. Do not assume the child has a mental disability because they are unable to express thoughts or words. Ask the parents or guardian what the child is capable of understanding. Speak directly to the child. Do not speak to the parents or guardian as if the child is not in the room.

Communicating with Parents and Guardians

If parents or guardians are excited or agitated during the emergency, the child is likely to be, too. When you can calm the parents or guardians, the child will often calm down as well. Remember to get consent to give care from the parent or guardian of the child when possible. Any concerned adults need your support, so behave as calmly as possible, explaining what you intend to do at each step.

Characteristics of Children and Infants

To be able to effectively check children and infants, it is helpful to be aware of certain characteristics of children and infants in specific age groups.

Children up to 1 year of age are commonly referred to as infants. Infants less than 6 months old are relatively easy to approach and are unlikely to be afraid of you. Older infants, however, often show "stranger anxiety." They may turn away from you and cry and cling to their parent or guardian. If a parent or the guardian is calm and cooperative, ask them to help you. Try to check the infant in the parent's or guardian's lap or arms if possible and the situation allows this.

Children between 1 and 2 years old are often referred to as toddlers. Toddlers may not cooperate with your attempts to check them. They are usually very concerned about being separated from a parent or guardian. If you reassure the toddler that they will not be separated from a parent or guardian, the toddler may be comforted. If possible, give the toddler a few minutes to get used to you before attempting to check them, and check the toddler in the parent's or guardian's lap. A toddler may also respond to praise or be comforted by holding a special toy or blanket.

Children between the ages of 3 and 5 are commonly referred to as preschoolers. Children in this age group are usually easy to check if you use their natural curiosity. Allow them to inspect items such as bandages. Opportunities to explore can reduce many fears and anxiety about the situation and provide distraction. Reassure the child that you are going to help and will not leave them. Sometimes, you can show what you are going to do on a stuffed animal or doll (Figure 21-1). If a child is injured, they may be upset by seeing the cut or other injury, so cover it with a dressing as soon as appropriate.

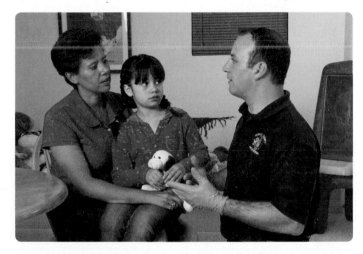

Figure 21-1. Demonstrating first aid steps on a stuffed animal or doll helps a child understand how you will care for them.

School-age children are between 6 and 12 years of age. They are usually cooperative and can be a good source of information about what happened. You can usually talk readily with school-age children. Do not let the child's chronological age influence you to expect an injured or ill child to behave in a way consistent with that age. An injured 11 year old, for example, may behave more like a 7 year old during the emergency. Be especially careful not to talk down to these children. Let them know if you are going to do anything that may be painful. Children in this age group are becoming conscious of their bodies and may not like exposure. Respect their modesty.

Adolescents are between 13 and 18 years of age and are typically more adult than child physically, but developmentally they can make rash decisions and be impulsive. Direct your questions to the adolescent rather than to a parent or guardian. Allow input from a parent or guardian, however. Occasionally, if a parent or guardian is present, you may not be able to get an accurate idea of what happened or what is wrong. Adolescents are modest and often respond better to a first aid responder of the same gender or a gender of their choosing.

Observing Children and Infants

You can obtain a lot of information by observing the child or infant before actually touching them. Look for signs that indicate changes in the level of consciousness, any trouble breathing, and any apparent injuries and conditions. Realize that the situation may change as soon as you touch the child or infant because they may become anxious or upset. Do not separate the child or infant from loved ones. Often, a parent or guardian will be holding a crying child or infant. In this case, you can check the child or infant while the adult continues to comfort them. Unlike some injured or ill adults, a child or an infant is unlikely to try to cover up or deny how they feel. A child in pain, for example, will generally let you know what hurts and what caused the pain.

Whenever necessary (e.g., when the child is agitated), begin your check at the toes rather than at the head if a child or infant is awake and no life-threatening conditions have been found. Checking this way is less threatening to the child or infant and allows them to watch what is going on and take part in it. Ask a young child to point to any place that hurts. An older child can often tell you the exact location of painful areas. If you need to hold an infant, always support the head when you pick them up.

Common Childhood Injuries and Illnesses

Abdominal Conditions

Abdominal pain in children can be the sign of a large range of conditions. Fortunately, most are not serious and usually go away on their own.

Signs and Symptoms of Abdominal Conditions

Abdominal pain accompanied by any of the following signs or symptoms could indicate that the child is suffering from a serious condition or illness:

- A sudden onset of severe abdominal pain or pain that becomes worse with time

- Excessive vomiting or diarrhea

- Blood in the vomit or stool

- A bloated or swollen abdomen

- A change in the child's level of consciousness, such as drowsiness or confusion

- Signs and symptoms of shock, which include abdominal pain or vomiting as well as signs of dehydration such as not drinking or urinating

Care for Abdominal Conditions

Call 9-1-1 or the designated emergency number if you think the child has a life-threatening condition. While you are waiting for help to arrive, help the child rest in a comfortable position, keep the child from becoming chilled or overheated, comfort and reassure the child, and give care based on any conditions found.

Child Abuse and Neglect

At some point, you may encounter a situation involving an injured child or infant in which you have reason to suspect child abuse or neglect. **Child abuse** is the physical, psychological or sexual assault of a child resulting in injury or emotional trauma. Child abuse involves an injury or a pattern of injuries that do not result from an accident. **Child neglect** is a type of child abuse in which the parent or guardian fails to provide the necessary age-appropriate care to a child, or provides insufficient medical care or emotional attention to a child.

Signs of Child Abuse and Neglect

The signs of *child abuse* include:

- An injury whose cause does not fit the parent's, guardian's or caregiver's description.

- Obvious or suspected fractures in a child younger than 2 years of age; any unexplained fractures.

- Injuries in various stages of healing, especially bruises and burns.

- Bruises and burns in unusual shapes, such as bruises shaped like belt buckles, burns the size of a cigarette tip, and burn rings around ankles or buttocks (from dipping in hot water).

- Unexplained lacerations or abrasions, especially to the mouth, lips and eyes.

- Injuries to the genitalia; pain when the child sits down.

- A larger number of injuries than is common for a child of the same age.

The signs of *child neglect* include:

- Lack of adult supervision.

- A child who looks malnourished.

- A child with poor hygiene (e.g., old, dirty diaper on).

- An unsafe living environment.

- Untreated chronic illness (e.g., a child with asthma who has no medications).

Care for Child Abuse or Neglect

When caring for a child or an infant whom you suspect may have been abused or neglected, your first priority is to care for the child's or infant's injuries or illnesses. An abused child may be frightened, hysterical or withdrawn. They may be unwilling to talk about the incident in an attempt to protect the abuser. Do not confront the suspected parent, guardian or child care provider. Instead, continue to treat them with the same respect you would give to any other person. If you suspect abuse, explain your concerns to responding police officers or emergency medical services (EMS) personnel if possible.

If you think you have reasonable cause to believe that abuse has occurred, report your suspicions to a community or state agency, such as the Department of Social Services, the Department of Child and Family Services or Child Protective Services. You may be afraid to report suspected child abuse because you do not wish to get involved or are afraid of getting sued. However, in most states, when you make a report in good faith, you are immune from any civil or criminal liability or penalty, even if you made a mistake. In this instance, "good faith" means that you honestly believe that abuse has occurred or the potential for abuse exists, and a prudent and reasonable person in the same position would also honestly believe the abuse has occurred or the potential for abuse exists. You do not need to identify yourself when you report child abuse, although your report will have more credibility if you do.

In some areas, certain professions are legally obligated to report suspicions of child abuse, such as day care workers or school employees. For more information on reporting child abuse at your workplace, contact your supervisor or mandated reporter.

Diarrhea and Vomiting

Diarrhea, or loose stools, often accompanies an infection or other gastrointestinal issues in children. Vomiting can be frightening for a young child, but it is rarely a serious problem. However, diarrhea and vomiting both can lead to dehydration and shock. This is more likely to occur in young children.

Signs and Symptoms of Serious Diarrhea and Vomiting

A healthcare provider should be contacted if:

- Diarrhea or vomiting persists for more than a few days (in an infant, less than a day).

- The child is not replacing lost liquids or cannot retain liquids.

- An infant has not had a wet diaper in more than 4 to 6 hours, or a child has not urinated for more than 6 to 8 hours.

- The child has a high fever.

- The child has bloody or black stools.

- The child is unusually sleepy, drowsy, unresponsive or irritable.

- The child cries without tears or has a dry mouth.

- The child has a sunken appearance to the abdomen, eyes or cheeks, or, in a very young infant, has a sunken soft spot at the top of the head.

- The child has skin that remains "tented" if pinched and released.

Care for Diarrhea and Vomiting

Remember the following when caring for children and infants with diarrhea:

- If the infant will not tolerate their normal feedings or if a child is drinking less fluid than normal, add a commercially available oral rehydration solution specially designed for children and infants.

- Do not give over-the-counter anti-diarrhea medications to children younger than 2 years old. Use these with the guidance of the healthcare provider in older children.

- Try to limit sugar and artificial sweeteners. Focus on a low-fiber diet. For a child in gastrointestinal distress, think "B.R.A.T.": bananas, rice, applesauce and toast. Tea and yogurt may also be considered.

Remember the following when caring for children and infants who are vomiting:

- For a very young child or infant, lay the child on their side so that the child does not swallow or inhale the vomit.

- Halt solid foods for 24 hours during an illness involving vomiting and replace with clear fluids, such as water, popsicles, gelatin or an oral rehydration solution specially designed for children and infants.

- Introduce liquids slowly. For instance, wait 2 to 3 hours after a vomiting episode to offer the child some cool water. Offer 1 to 2 ounces every half hour, four times. Then, alternate 2 ounces of rehydration solution with 2 ounces of water every 2 hours.

- After 12 to 24 hours with no vomiting, gradually reintroduce the child's normal diet.

Ear Infections

Ear infections are common in young children. Nearly 90 percent of young children have an ear infection at some time before they reach school age.

Signs and Symptoms of Ear Infections

Common signs and symptoms of an ear infection include:

- Pain. Older children can tell you that their ears hurt, but younger children may only cry or be irritable or rub or tug on the affected ear.

- Fever.

- Ear drainage.

- Trouble hearing.

- Loss of appetite.

- Trouble sleeping.

Care for Ear Infections

A healthcare provider should be contacted if:

- The child's signs and symptoms last longer than a day.

- You see a discharge of blood or pus from the ear. This could indicate a ruptured eardrum.

- The child is having hearing problems.

- The child's signs or symptoms do not improve or they worsen after the child has been diagnosed by a healthcare provider.

Pain symptoms may be treated with ibuprofen or acetaminophen. In children younger than 2 years, watch for sleeplessness and irritability during or after an upper respiratory infection, such as a cold. Always consult the child's healthcare provider before giving any over-the-counter pain relievers.

Fever

Fever is an elevated body temperature of 100.4° F (38° C) or greater. Fever indicates a problem, and in a child or an infant, it often means there is a specific problem. Usually these problems are not life threatening, but some can be. A high fever in a child or an infant often indicates some form of infection. In a young child, even a minor infection can result in a high fever, usually defined as of 103° F (39.4° C) and above.

A rapid rise in body temperature can result in seizures. A febrile seizure is a convulsion brought on by a fever in infants or small children. It is the most common type of seizure in children. Most febrile seizures last less than 5 minutes and are not normally life threatening. However, there are conditions in which the child may require additional care. To review care after a febrile seizure, go to Chapter 15.

Signs and Symptoms of Fever

Aside from discovering a fever when checking a child's temperature, other signs and symptoms may indicate a fever is present.

Older children with fever will often:

- Feel hot to the touch.

- Complain of being cold or chilled.

- Complain of body aches.

- Have a headache.

- Have trouble sleeping or sleep more than usual.

- Appear drowsy.

- Have no appetite.

Infants with fever will often:

- Be upset or fussy, with frequent crying.

- Be unusually quiet.

- Feel warm or hot.

- Breathe rapidly and have a rapid heart rate.

- Stop eating or sleeping normally.

When to Call 9-1-1

Call 9-1-1 or the designated emergency number if the child or infant has signs or symptoms of a life-threatening condition, such as unresponsiveness or trouble breathing. Also, call if this is the first time that a child has had a febrile seizure, the seizure lasts longer than 5 minutes or is repeated, or the seizure is followed by a quick rise in the temperature of the child or infant. Child care providers should follow state or local regulations regarding emergency care and contact procedures whenever a child in their care becomes injured or ill.

When to Seek Professional Medical Care

A healthcare provider should be contacted for:

- Any infant younger than 3 months with a fever (100.4° F/38° C or greater).

- Any child younger than 2 years with a high fever (103° F/39.4° C or greater).

- Any child or infant who has a febrile seizure.

Care for Fever

If the child or infant has a fever, make them as comfortable as possible. Encourage the child to rest. Make sure that the child or infant is not overdressed or covered with too many blankets. A single layer of clothing and a light blanket usually is all that is necessary. To prevent dehydration, make sure that the child or infant drinks clear fluids (e.g., water or juice) or continues nursing or bottle-feeding.

Do not give the child or infant aspirin for fever or other signs or symptoms of flu-like or other viral illness. For a child or infant, taking aspirin can result in an extremely serious medical condition called **Reye's syndrome.** Reye's syndrome is an illness that affects the brain and other internal organs. Acetaminophen or ibuprofen may be given for a fever, but always consult the child's healthcare provider before giving any over-the-counter pain relievers.

If the child has a *high fever,* it is important to gently cool the child. Never rush cooling down a child. If the fever caused a febrile seizure, rapid cooling could bring on other complications. Instead, remove any excessive clothing or blankets. Do not use an ice water bath or rubbing alcohol to cool down the body. Both of these approaches are dangerous. Continue caring for the child or infant with a high fever as described above.

Foreign Objects in the Nose

If a child has an object in the nose, *do not* try to remove the object. Special lighting and instruments are necessary to remove objects. It is important to go to a healthcare provider for removal of the object. Also, try to calm the child and parents or guardians as best as possible.

Injuries

Injury is the number one cause of death for children over 6 months of age in the United States. Many of these deaths are the result of motor vehicle crashes. The greatest dangers to a child or infant involved in a motor vehicle incident are airway obstruction and bleeding. Severe bleeding must be controlled as quickly as possible. A relatively small amount of blood lost by an adult is a large amount for a child or an infant.

Because a child's head is large and heavy in proportion to the rest of the body, the head is the most often injured area. A child or an infant injured as the result of force or a blow may also have damage to the organs in the abdominal and chest cavities. Such damage can cause severe internal bleeding. A child secured only by a lap belt may have serious abdominal or spinal injuries in a car crash. Try to find out what happened, because a severely injured child or infant may not immediately show signs of an injury.

To avoid needless deaths of children and infants caused by motor vehicle crashes, laws have been enacted requiring that children and infants ride in the backseat of cars in approved safety seats or wear safety belts. As a result, more children's lives are saved. You may have to check and care for an injured child or infant while they are in a safety seat. A safety seat does not normally pose any problems while you are checking a child or an infant. Leave the child or infant in the seat if the seat has not been damaged. If the child or infant is to be transported to a medical facility for examination, they can often be safely secured in an undamaged safety seat for transport.

Poisoning

Poisoning is one of the top 10 causes of unintentional death in the United States for adolescents, children and infants. Children younger than 6 years account for half of all exposures to poisonous substances in the United States. Children in this age group often become poisoned by ingesting household products or medications (typically those intended for adults). Although children in this age group are exposed more often than any other, only 3 percent of these cases result in death.

There has been a decrease in child poisonings in recent years due in part to child-resistant packaging for medications. This packaging makes it harder for children to get into these substances. The decrease also is a result of preventive actions taken by parents and others who care for children. Care and prevention for poisoning is discussed in Chapter 16.

SIDS

Sudden infant death syndrome (SIDS) is the sudden, unexpected and unexplained death of an apparently healthy baby. In the United States, approximately 2300 infants die every year of SIDS. SIDS is the third leading cause of death for infants between 1 month and 1 year of age. It occurs most often in infants between 4 weeks and 7 months of age. SIDS usually occurs while the infant is sleeping.

The condition does not seem to be linked to a disease. In addition, the cause(s) of SIDS are not yet understood. It is not thought to be hereditary, but it does tend to recur in families. Because of these factors, there is no way of knowing if an infant is at risk for SIDS. Sometimes, it is mistaken for child abuse because of the unexplained death in an apparently healthy infant. In addition, SIDS sometimes causes bruise-like blotches to appear on the infant's body. However, SIDS is not related to child abuse.

Care for SIDS

By the time the infant's condition has been discovered, they will be in cardiac arrest. Make sure someone has called 9-1-1 or the designated emergency number, or make the call yourself. Perform CPR on the infant until EMS personnel take over, an automated external defibrillator (AED) becomes available or you see an obvious sign of life, such as normal breathing.

An incident involving a severely injured or ill child or infant or one who has died can be emotionally upsetting. After such an episode, find someone you trust with whom you can talk about the experience and express your feelings. If you continue to be distressed, seek professional counseling. The feelings engendered by such incidents need to be dealt with and understood, otherwise they can result in serious stress reactions.

See Lowering the Risk for SIDS for ways you can lessen the chance of SIDS occurring.

Lowering the Risk for SIDS

Because it cannot be predicted or prevented, SIDS makes many new parents feel anxious. However, there are several things you can do to lower the risk for SIDS. The American Academy of Pediatrics has guidelines for safe sleep, which include the following for the first year of an infant's life:

- Always place your infant on their back for every sleep time including naps.

- Always use a firm sleep surface. Car seats and other sitting devices are not recommended for routine sleep.

- The infant should sleep in the same room as the parents, but not in the same bed.

- Bed sharing is not recommended for any infants.

- Keep all soft objects or loose bedding out of the crib. This includes pillows, blankets and bumper pads.

- Wedges and positioners should not be used.

- Do not smoke during pregnancy or after birth.

- Offer a pacifier at nap time and bedtime.

- Avoid covering the infant's head or allowing the infant to become overheated.

- Do not use home monitors or commercial devices marketed to reduce the risk of SIDS.

- Supervised, awake tummy time is recommended daily to facilitate development and minimize the occurrence of positional plagiocephaly (flat head).

- Make sure your infant has received all recommended vaccinations. Evidence suggests that immunization reduces the risk for SIDS by 50 percent.

- Breastfeeding is associated with a reduced risk for SIDS and is recommended.

For more information on the new guidelines for sleep position for infants and reducing the risk for SIDS, visit *www.healthychildren.org/safesleep.* Additional information can be found on the National Institutes of Health website at *www.nichd.nih.gov/sids/.*

SOURCE: American Academy of Pediatrics: *Ages & stages: Reduce the risk of SIDS.* http://www.healthychildren.org/safesleep. Accessed December 2016.

Older Adults

Older adults are generally considered those older than 65 years. They are quickly becoming the fastest-growing age group in the United States. Since 1900, life expectancy has increased by over 60 percent. For example, in 1900 the average life expectancy was 46 years for men and 48 years for women. Today, the average life expectancy is greater than 75 years for men and 80 years for women. The main explanations for the increase in life expectancy are medical advancements and improvements in healthcare.

Normal aging brings about changes. People age at different rates, however, and so do their organs and body parts. For example, a person with wrinkled, fragile skin may have strong bones or excellent respiratory function.

Overall, body function generally declines as we age, with some changes beginning as early as age 30. The lungs become less efficient, so older adults are at higher risk for developing pneumonia and other lung diseases. The amount of blood pumped by the heart with each beat decreases, and the heart rate slows. The blood vessels harden, causing increased work for the heart. Hearing and vision usually decline, often causing some degree of sight and hearing loss. Reflexes become slower, and arthritis may affect joints, causing movement to become painful.

Checking an Older Adult

The physical and mental changes associated with aging may require you to adapt your way of communicating and to be aware of certain potential age-related conditions, such as hearing loss.

As you learned in Chapter 5, to check an injured or ill older adult, attempt to learn the person's name and use it when you speak to them. Consider using Mrs., Mr. or Ms. as a sign of respect. Move to the person's eye level so that they can see and hear you more clearly. If the person seems confused at first, the confusion may be the result of impaired vision or hearing. If they usually wear eyeglasses and cannot find them, try to locate them. Speak slowly and clearly, and look at the person's face while you talk. Notice if they have a hearing aid. Someone who needs glasses to see or a hearing aid to hear is likely to be very anxious without them. If the person is truly confused, try to find out if the confusion is the result of the injury, sudden illness or a condition they already have. Information from family members or bystanders is frequently helpful. The person may be afraid of falling, so if they are standing, offer an arm or hand. Remember that an older adult may need to move slowly.

As part of your SAMPLE questions, try to find out what medications the person is taking and if they have any medical conditions so that you can tell EMS personnel. Look for a medical identification tag that will give you the person's name and address and information about any specific condition the person has.

Common Injuries and Illnesses in Older Adults

Certain problems are more prevalent in older adults. The following sections discuss some of these concerns.

Confusion

Older adults are at increased risk for altered thinking patterns and confusion. Some of this change is the result of aging. Certain diseases, such as *Alzheimer's disease* (see Fading Memories in this chapter), affect the brain, resulting in impaired memory and thinking and altered behavior. Confusion that comes on suddenly, however, may be the result of medication, even a medication the person has been taking regularly. A person who has problems seeing or hearing may also become confused when injured or ill. This problem increases when the person is in an unfamiliar environment. A head injury can also result in confusion.

Confusion can be a sign of a medical emergency. An older adult with pneumonia, for example, may not run a fever, have chest pain or be coughing, but because sufficient oxygen is not reaching the brain, the person may be confused. An older adult can have a serious infection without fever, pain or nausea. An older adult having a heart attack may not have chest pain, pale or ashen skin, or other classic signs and symptoms, but may be restless, short of breath and confused.

Depression is common in older adults. A depressed older adult may seem confused at first. A depressed person may also have signs or symptoms, such as sudden shortness of breath or chest pains, without apparent cause. Whatever the reason for any confusion, do not talk down to the person or treat the person like a child.

Falls

Older adults are at increased risk for falls. In fact, falls are the leading cause of death from injury for older adults. Falls in older adults are due to slower reflexes, failing eyesight and hearing, arthritis, and problems such as unsteady balance and movement. Falls frequently result in fractures because the bones become weaker and more brittle with age.

Head Injuries

An older adult is also at greater risk for serious head injuries. As we age, the size of the brain decreases. This decrease results in more space between the surface of the brain and the inside of the skull. This space allows more movement of the brain within the skull, which can increase the likelihood of serious head injury. Occasionally, an older adult may not develop the signs and symptoms of a head injury until days after a fall. Therefore, unless you know the cause of a behavior change, you should always suspect a head injury as a possible cause of unusual behavior in an older adult, especially if the person has had a fall or a blow to the head.

Problems with Heat and Cold

An older adult is more susceptible to extremes in temperature. The person may be unable to feel temperature extremes because their body may no longer regulate temperature effectively. Body temperature may change rapidly to a dangerously high or low level.

The body of an older adult retains heat because of a decreased ability to sweat and the reduced ability of the circulatory system to adjust to heat. This can lead to heat exhaustion or heat stroke.

An older person may become chilled and suffer hypothermia simply by sitting in a draft or in front of a fan or air conditioner. Hypothermia can occur at any time of the year. People can go on for several days suffering from mild hypothermia without realizing it. The older person with mild hypothermia will want to lie down frequently; however, this will lower the body temperature even further.

See Chapter 19 for information on how to care for heat-related illnesses and cold-related emergencies.

Fading Memories

According to the Alzheimer's Association, Alzheimer's disease affects an estimated 5.4 million Americans, making it the only disease among the top 10 causes of death without prevention, a cure or a way to slow its progression. While most people with the disease are older than 65, Alzheimer's disease can strike people in their 40s and 50s. Men and women are affected almost equally. At this time, scientists are still looking for the cause.

Signs and symptoms of Alzheimer's disease develop gradually and include confusion; progressive memory loss; and changes in personality, behavior, and the ability to think and communicate. Eventually, people with Alzheimer's disease become totally unable to care for themselves. While there are no treatments to stop or reverse a person's mental decline from Alzheimer's disease, several drugs are now available to help manage some of these symptoms. In addition, because a number of disorders have signs and symptoms similar to those of Alzheimer's disease, and can be treated, it is very important for anyone who is experiencing memory loss or confusion to have a thorough medical examination.

Most people with illnesses such as Alzheimer's disease are cared for by their families for much of their illness. Giving care at home requires careful planning. The home has to be made safe, and routines must be set up for daily activities, such as mealtimes, personal care and leisure.

It is important for anyone caring for a person with Alzheimer's disease or a related problem to realize that they are not alone. There are people and organizations that can help both you and the person with Alzheimer's disease. For healthcare services, a physician—perhaps your family physician—or a specialist can give you medical advice, including help with difficult behavior and personality changes.

(Continued)

Fading Memories continued

If you are caring for a person with Alzheimer's disease living at home, you may also need help with basic services such as nutrition and transportation. A visiting nurse or nutritionist and volunteer programs such as Meals on Wheels may be helpful, and volunteer or paid transportation services may be available. Visiting nurses, home health aides and homemakers can come to your home and give help with healthcare, bathing, dressing, shopping and cooking. Many adult day care centers provide recreational activities designed for people with Alzheimer's disease. Some hospitals, nursing homes and other facilities may take in people with Alzheimer's disease for short stays.

For persons with Alzheimer's disease who can no longer live at home, group homes or foster homes may be available. Nursing homes offer more skilled nursing care, and some specialize in the care of those with Alzheimer's or similar diseases. A few hospice programs accept persons with Alzheimer's disease who are nearing the end of their lives. Search to find out which, if any, services are covered by Medicare, Medicaid, Social Security, disability or veterans' benefits in your state. A lawyer or a social worker may be able to help you.

To locate services that can help you, the person with Alzheimer's disease and other family members, search for social service organizations and state and local government listings on the Internet or in the phone book. You can also contact your local health department, area office on aging, and department of social services or senior citizens' services. Senior centers, as well as churches, synagogues and other religious institutions may also have information and programs. Another great resource is the Alzheimer's Association. To locate a chapter near you, call the association's 24-hour, toll-free number: 800-272-3900 or log onto www.alz.org.

SOURCE: Alzheimer's Association. www.alz.org. Accessed December 2016.

People with Disabilities

According to the Americans with Disabilities Act (ADA), a person with a ***disability*** is someone who has a physical or mental ***impairment*** that substantially limits one or more major life activity such as walking, talking, seeing, hearing or learning. This includes, for example, a blind person who cannot read information posted on a bulletin board or a deaf person who may need a sign language interpreter.

The Centers for Disease Control and Prevention (CDC) estimates that over 33 million people in the United States have disabilities. When giving care to people with disabilities, communicating with them can be a challenge. It may be difficult to find out what has happened and what might be wrong in an emergency situation.

Physical Disabilities

A person is considered to have a physical disability if their ability to move (also called ***motor function***) is impaired. A person also is considered to have a physical disability if their ***sensory function*** is impaired. Sensory function includes all of the senses: sight, hearing, taste, smell and touch. A person with a physical disability may have impairments in motor function, sensory function or both.

General tips for approaching an injured or ill person whom you suspect may have a physical disability include:

- Speaking to the person before touching them.

- Asking, "How can I help?" or "Do you need help?"

- Asking for assistance and information from the person who has the disability—they have been living with the disability and best understand it. If you are not able to communicate with the person, ask family members, friends or companions who are available to help.

- Not removing any braces, canes, other physical support, eyeglasses or hearing aids. Removal of these items may take away necessary physical support for the person's body.

- Looking for a medical identification tag.

- Being aware that a service animal, such as a guide or signal dog, may be present and may be protective of the person in an emergency situation. Allow the animal to stay with the person, if possible, which will help reassure both of them.

What if... *A person has a service animal? Will that change how I give care?*

No. The presence of a service animal should not change the care given, although there are several things to consider in such a situation. For starters, you should never touch, pet or provide the animal with any food or treats without the permission of the owner. Any dog that is wearing a harness or vest is considered to be "on duty." If you are asked to take the dog, hold the dog by the leash, not the harness. If the scene becomes unsafe while caring for the person, it will be necessary to evacuate the animal with the owner; never separate them. Finally, persons with a psychiatric and/or emotional disability may also have a companion animal. Their animals are just as important to them as they are for persons with a physical disability. Be understanding of this and treat the animal as a service animal.

Deaf and Hard of Hearing

Hearing loss is a partial or total loss of hearing. Some people are born with a hearing loss. Hearing loss can also result from an injury or illness affecting the ear, the nerves leading from the brain to the ear or the brain itself. You may not initially be aware that the injured or ill person has a hearing loss. Often, the person will tell you, either in speech or by pointing to the ear and shaking the head no. Some people carry a card stating that they have hearing loss. You may see a hearing aid in a person's ear.

The biggest obstacle you must overcome in caring for a person with a hearing loss is communication. You will need to figure out how to get that person's consent to give care, and you need to find out what the problem may be.

Sometimes, the injured or ill person can read lips. To assist them, position yourself where the person can see your face clearly. Look straight at the person while you speak and speak slowly. Do not exaggerate the way you form words. Do not turn your face away while you speak. Many people with a hearing impairment, however, do not read lips. In these cases, using gestures and writing messages on paper may be the most effective way to communicate in an emergency.

If you and the person know sign language, use it (Figure 21-2, A). Some people who are hearing impaired have a machine called a telecommunications device for the deaf (TDD). You can use this device to type messages and questions to the person, and the person can type replies to you (Figure 21-2, B). Many people who have

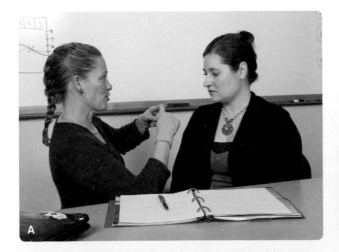 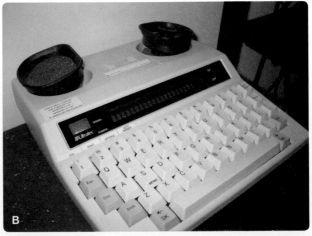

Figure 21-2, A–B. Communicate with a person with hearing loss in the best way possible. For example, **A,** use sign language or **B,** a TDD.

hearing impairments can speak, some distinctly, some not so clearly. If you have trouble understanding, ask the person to repeat what they said. Do not pretend to understand.

Blind or Visually Impaired

Vision loss is a partial or total loss of sight. Vision loss can have many causes. Some people are born with vision loss. Others lose vision as a result of disease or injury. Vision loss is not necessarily a problem with the eyes. It can result from problems with the vision centers in the brain.

It is no more difficult to communicate orally with a person who has a partial or total loss of sight than with someone who can see. You do *not* need to speak loudly or in overly simple terms. Checking a person who has a vision loss is the same as checking a person who has good vision. The person may not be able to tell you certain things about how an injury occurred, but they can usually give you a generally accurate account based on their interpretation of sound and touch.

When caring for a person with vision loss, help to reassure them by explaining what is going on and what you are doing. If you must move a visually impaired person who can walk, stand beside the person and have them hold onto your arm. Walk at a normal pace, alert the person to any obstacles in the way such as stairs and identify whether to step up or down. If the person has a service animal, try to keep them together. Ask the person to tell you how to handle the dog or ask them to do it.

> **What if...** *A person is deaf and blind and in need of care? How can I communicate?*
>
> *This type of situation is rare and can be a challenge to manage. However, there are some strategies that can help. The following communication methods are some of the options recommended by the National Federation of the Blind (www.nfb.org) based on the circumstances you find. For a person with hearing loss and low vision (or who became blind after already learning American Sign Language), try using American Sign Language—although a translator may be needed if you are not skilled in using it yourself. The person may be able to touch the hands of the person signing to communicate. For a person with hearing loss and no vision, you can also try print-in-palm, a technique in which you will "print" large block letters (not cursive) on the other person's palm using your index finger. Each letter is written in the same location on the person's palm. If you are helping someone with hearing loss and no vision at home, they may have a **Tellatouch,** a small typewriter keyboard used for communication. The person sits opposite the typist and places a finger on a small Braille "screen." As a letter is typed it appears briefly under the person's finger, allowing them to know what is being communicated.*

Motor Impairment

A person with **motor impairment** is unable to move normally. They may be missing a body part or have a problem with the bones or muscles or the nerves controlling them. Causes of motor impairment include a stroke, **muscular dystrophy, multiple sclerosis,** paralysis, **cerebral palsy** or loss of a limb. In caring for an injured or ill person with motor impairment, be aware that the person may view accepting help as failure and may refuse your help to prove that they do not need it.

Determining which problems are pre-existing and which are the result of immediate injury or sudden illness can be difficult. Care for all problems you detect as if they are new. Be aware that checking one side of the body against the other in your check for non-life-threatening conditions may not be effective with a person with motor impairment, since body parts may not look normal as a result of a specific condition.

Mental Impairment

Mental, or **cognitive, function** includes the brain's capacity to reason and to process information. A person with mental impairment has problems performing these operations. Some types of mental impairment are genetic or are genetic alterations, such as **Down syndrome.** Others result from injuries or infections that occur during pregnancy, shortly after birth or later in life. Some causes are never determined.

You may not be able to determine if a person is mentally impaired, or it may be obvious. Approach the person as you would any other person in their age group. When you speak, try to determine the person's level of understanding. If the person appears not to understand you, rephrase what you were saying in simpler terms. Listen carefully to what the person says. People who are mentally impaired often lead very orderly and structured lives. An injury or sudden illness can disrupt the order in a person's life and cause a great deal of anxiety and fear. Take time to explain who you are and what you are going to do. Offer reassurance. Try to gain the person's trust. If a parent, guardian or caregiver is present, ask that person to help you care for the person.

People with certain types of mental illness might misinterpret your actions as being hostile. If the scene becomes unsafe, you may need to remove yourself from the immediate area. Call 9-1-1 or the designated emergency number and explain your concerns about a potential psychiatric emergency. If possible, keep track of the person's location and what they are doing. Report this information to the emergency responders.

Language Barriers

Getting consent to give care and communicate about signs and symptoms with a person with whom you have a language barrier can be a problem. Find out if any bystanders speak the person's language and can help translate. Do your best to communicate nonverbally. Use gestures and facial expressions. If the person is in pain, they will probably be anxious to let you know where that pain is. Watch their gestures and facial expressions carefully. When you speak to the person, speak slowly and in a normal tone. The person probably has no trouble hearing you.

When you call 9-1-1 or the designated emergency number, explain that you are having difficulty communicating with the person and say what language you believe the person speaks. The EMS system may have someone available who can help with communication. If the person has a life-threatening condition, such as severe, life-threatening bleeding, consent is implied. The person will most likely be willing for you to give care in such a case.

Crime Scenes and Hostile Situations

In certain situations, such as giving care to a person at a crime scene or an injured person who is hostile, you will need to use extreme caution. Although your first reaction may be to go to the aid of a person, in these situations you should call 9-1-1 or the designated emergency number and stay at a safe distance.

Do *not* enter the scene of a suicide. If you happen to be on the scene when an unarmed person threatens suicide, call 9-1-1 or the designated emergency number. Do not argue with the person. Remain at a safe distance.

Leave or avoid entering any area considered to be a crime scene, such as one where there is a weapon, or the scene of a physical or sexual assault. Call 9-1-1 or the designated emergency number and stay at a safe distance.

You may encounter a situation in which there is a hostile or angry person. A person's rage or hostility may be caused by the injury, pain or fear. Some individuals, afraid of losing control, may act resentful and suspicious. Hostile behavior also may result from the use of alcohol or other drugs, a lack of oxygen or a medical condition. If a person refuses your care or threatens you, remove yourself from the situation and stay at a safe distance. Never argue with or restrain an injured or ill person. Call 9-1-1 or the designated emergency number if someone has not already done so. Never put your own safety at risk.

Uninjured family members also may display anger. This anger may stem from panic, anxiety or guilt. Try to remain calm and explain what you plan to do for giving emergency care. If possible, find a way for family members to help, such as by comforting the person.

Summary

No two emergency situations are alike. Situations involving people with special needs, problems and characteristics require your awareness and understanding. To give effective care to a child or an infant, an older adult, a person with a disability or anyone with whom communication is a challenge, you may need to adapt your approach and your attitude. Situations may also occur in which you should not intervene. If a situation is in any way unsafe, do not approach the person, and if you have already approached, withdraw. Call 9-1-1 or the designated emergency number for help. Likewise, if the situation is a crime scene, keep your distance from the scene and call for appropriate help.

READY TO RESPOND? ▶

Think back to Grandma Mary in the opening scenario and use what you have learned to respond to these questions:

1. What factors could have been responsible for Grandma Mary's collapse?

2. What steps should you take to communicate better with Grandma Mary while helping her, given her poor hearing?

Study Questions

1. **Match each term with the correct definition.**

   a. Sensory function   c. Alzheimer's disease   e. Impairment

   b. Child abuse   d. Disability   f. Motor impairment

   ____ The absence or impairment of motor, sensory or mental function

   ____ The most common type of dementia in older people, in which thought, memory and language are impaired

   ____ The total or partial inability to move or to use a body part

   ____ Action that results in the physical or psychological harm of a child; can be physical, sexual, verbal and/or emotional

   ____ Damage or reduction in quality, quantity, value or strength of a function

   ____ The ability to see, hear, touch, taste and smell

2. **You are walking to the mailbox. A young child on a bicycle, about age 5, suddenly rolls into the street from between two parked cars. A car, moving very slowly, strikes the child, knocking them to the pavement. Three people in the vicinity run to the scene, and a woman comes running out of a house and to the child's side. She says she is the mother. The driver gets out of the car, looking shocked and stunned. The child begins to cry. Describe in order the steps you should take to find out what care the child needs.**

3. **A neighbor phones saying her grandmother has fallen and is lying on the bathroom floor. She asks you to come help. When you get there, the grandmother is awake but unable to get up. She does not recognize her granddaughter. She says her left leg and hip hurt. What steps should you take to help?**

In questions 4 through 9, circle the letter of the correct answer.

4. **In which of the following ways should you move a person with vision loss who can walk?**

   a. Grasp the person's arm or belt, and support the person as you walk.

   b. Walk in front of the person, and have them keep a hand on your shoulder.

   c. Walk behind the person with a hand on the person's back.

   d. Walk beside the person, and let them grasp your arm while you are walking.

5. **The best position you can take in talking to an injured or ill young child is—**

   a. Holding the child in your arms or on your lap.

   b. Being at eye level with the child.

   c. Standing up, looking down at the child.

   d. Behind the child, out of direct sight.

(Continued)

Study Questions continued

6. **Which should you do if an injured or ill older adult appears to be confused?**

   a. Assume the person is in a permanent state of confusion.

   b. Inquire about any medications the person is taking.

   c. Assume the person has fallen and injured their head.

   d. All of the above

7. **What should you do if you become aware that a physical assault has taken place?**

   a. Call 9-1-1 or the designated emergency number and then approach the person.

   b. Call 9-1-1 or the designated emergency number and do not enter the scene.

   c. Approach the person and have someone call 9-1-1 or the designated emergency number.

   d. Assess the person for life-threatening conditions.

8. **A small child in a car seat is in a motor-vehicle collision. How would you check the child?**

   a. Remove the child from the car seat.

   b. Ask any relative of the child who is on the scene to remove the child from the seat.

   c. Check the child while the child is in the car seat.

   d. Wait until EMS personnel arrive.

9. **A responsive person who does not appear to hear or understand what you say may—**

   a. Be confused by medication.

   b. Have hearing loss.

   c. Speak a different language.

   d. All of the above

10. **List four possible causes of confusion in an older adult.**

11. **List the steps you should take if a person you are trying to help becomes hostile or uncooperative.**

Answers are listed in the Appendix.

22 EMERGENCY CHILDBIRTH

You are enjoying a maternity yoga class with your best friend Lisa, who is expecting her first child in a few weeks. You are waiting for her at the juice bar while she changes, but when she does not arrive after a while, you head back to the locker room to check on her. As you round the corner, you see Lisa grimacing in pain as a contraction begins. As it passes she gasps, "I'm sure glad to see you! My water broke, and my phone has no reception in here. This baby is ready to come!"

Learn and Respond >

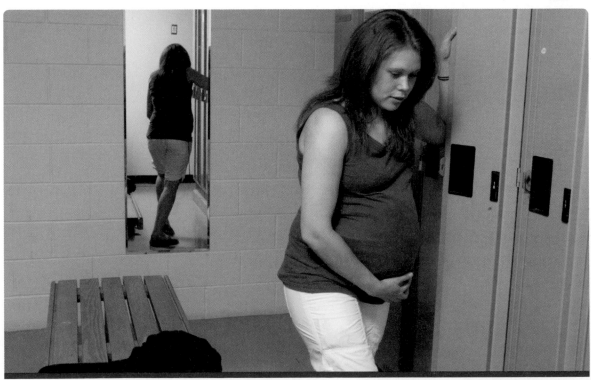

OBJECTIVES

After reading this chapter, you should be able to:

- Understand the basics of pregnancy and the birth process.

- Describe the four stages of labor.

- Identify the factors you need to know to determine the mother's condition before the birth.

- Describe techniques the expectant mother can use to cope with labor pain and discomfort.

- Identify equipment and supplies needed to assist with the delivery of a newborn.

- Describe how to assist with the delivery of a newborn.

- Identify the priorities of care for a newborn.

- Describe the steps to take in caring for the mother after delivery.

- Identify the possible complications during pregnancy and childbirth that require immediate medical care.

KEY TERMS

Amniotic sac: "Bag of waters"; sac that encloses the fetus during pregnancy and bursts during the birthing process.

Birth canal: The passageway from the uterus to the outside of the body through which a baby passes during birth.

Braxton Hicks contractions: False labor; irregular contractions of the uterus that do not intensify or become more frequent as genuine labor contractions do.

Cervix: The lower, narrow part of the uterus (womb) that forms a canal that opens into the vagina, which leads to the outside of the body; upper part of the birth canal.

Contraction: During labor, the rhythmic tightening and relaxing of muscles in the uterus.

Crowning: The phase during labor when the baby's head is visible at the opening of the vagina.

Labor: The birth process, beginning with the contraction of the uterus and dilation of the cervix and ending with the stabilization and recovery of the mother.

Placenta: An organ attached to the uterus and unborn baby through which nutrients are delivered; expelled after the baby is delivered.

Pregnancy: Begins when an egg (ovum) is fertilized by a sperm, forming an embryo.

Umbilical cord: A flexible structure that attaches the placenta to the fetus, allowing for the passage of blood, nutrients and waste.

Uterus: A pear-shaped organ in a woman's pelvis in which an embryo forms and develops into a baby; also called the womb.

Introduction

Words such as exhausting, stressful, exciting, fulfilling, painful and scary are sometimes used to describe a planned childbirth: one that occurs in the hospital or at home under the supervision of a qualified healthcare provider. However, if you find yourself assisting with the delivery of a newborn, it is probably not happening in a planned situation. Therefore, your thoughts and feelings, as well as those of the expectant mother, may be intensified by fear of the unexpected or the possibility that something might go wrong.

When presented with a possibility of delivering a child outside of a hospital, first and foremost remain calm and take control of the scene. Take comfort in knowing that things rarely go wrong during childbirth. Childbirth is a natural process. Thousands of children all over the world are born each day, without complications, in areas where no medical care is available.

By following a few simple steps, you can effectively assist in the birth process. This chapter will help you better understand the birth process and includes instruction on how to assist with the delivery of a newborn, how to give care for both the mother and newborn after the delivery, and how to recognize and care for complications until emergency medical services (EMS) personnel arrive.

Pregnancy and the Birth Process

Pregnancy begins when an egg (**ovum**) is fertilized by a sperm, forming an **embryo.** The embryo implants itself within the lining of the mother's **uterus,** a pear-shaped organ that lies at the top center of the pelvis and enlarges significantly during pregnancy. The embryo is surrounded by the **amniotic sac.** This fluid-filled sac is also called the "bag of waters." The fluid helps protect the newborn from injury and infection.

As the embryo grows, its organs and body develop. After about 8 weeks, the embryo is called a **fetus.** To continue to develop properly, the fetus must receive oxygen and nutrients. The fetus receives these items from the mother through a specialized organ called the **placenta,** which also removes carbon dioxide and waste products. The placenta is attached to the lining of the uterus and is rich in blood vessels. The placenta is attached to the fetus by a flexible structure called the **umbilical cord.** The fetus will continue to develop for approximately 40 weeks (calculated by counting back from the woman's last menstrual cycle), at which time the birth process normally will begin (Figure 22-1).

Pregnancy is broken down into three trimesters, each lasting approximately 3 months.

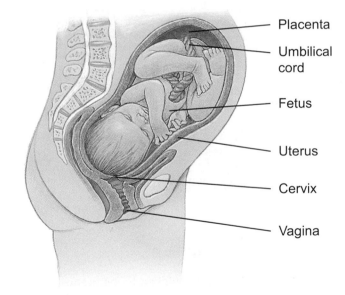

- Placenta
- Umbilical cord
- Fetus
- Uterus
- Cervix
- Vagina

Figure 22-1. Mother and fetus at 40 weeks.

Labor

Pregnancy culminates in **labor** (also called the birth process), during which the baby is delivered. Labor begins with rhythmic contractions of the uterus. This may follow or be accompanied by the rupture of the amniotic sac (often referred to as the "water breaking") and a gush or a trickle of clear fluid. As contractions continue, they dilate the cervix. When the **cervix** is sufficiently dilated, it allows the baby to travel from the uterus through the **birth canal** and into the outside world. For first-time mothers, this process normally takes between 12 and 24 hours. Subsequent deliveries usually require less time. The labor process has four distinct stages. The length and intensity of each stage varies.

Stage One—Dilation

In the first stage of labor, the mother's body prepares for the birth. This stage covers the period of time from the first contraction until the cervix is fully dilated (although dilation can begin weeks before labor and delivery). A **contraction** is a rhythmic tightening of the muscles in the uterus to allow the mother's cervix to dilate, or expand, enough for the baby to pass through the canal during the birth. Like a wave, it begins gently, rises to a peak of intensity and then subsides. A break occurs between contractions, and a contraction normally lasts about 30 to 60 seconds.

As the time for delivery approaches, the contractions occur closer together, last longer and feel stronger. Normally, when contractions are less than 3 minutes apart, delivery is near. The woman may be in considerable discomfort at this time.

Stage Two—Expulsion

The second stage of labor begins when the cervix is completely dilated and includes the baby's movement through the birth canal and delivery. During this stage of labor, the mother will experience enormous pressure, similar to the feeling she has during a bowel movement. This sensation is an indication that it is time for her to push, or "bear down," to help ease the baby through the birth canal. Considerable blood may come from the vagina at this time. Contractions are more frequent during this stage (less than 2 minutes apart) and may last between 45 and 90 seconds each. In a normal delivery, the baby's head becomes visible as it emerges from the vagina. The moment during labor when the top of the head begins to emerge is called **crowning** (Figure 22-2). When crowning occurs, birth is imminent and you must be prepared to receive the newborn. Stage two ends with the birth of the baby.

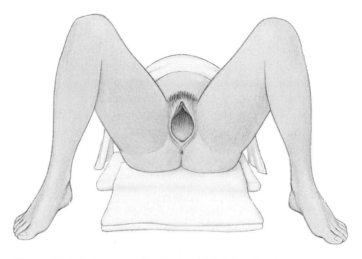

Figure 22-2. When crowning begins, birth is imminent.

Stage Three—Placental Delivery

The third stage of labor begins after the newborn's body emerges. During this stage, the placenta usually separates from the wall of the uterus and is expelled from the birth canal. This process normally occurs within 30 minutes of the delivery of the newborn.

Stage Four—Stabilization

The final stage of labor involves the initial recovery and stabilization of the mother after childbirth. Normally, this stage lasts approximately 1 hour. During this time, the uterus contracts to help control bleeding, and the mother begins to recover from the physical and emotional stress that occurred during childbirth.

Assessing Labor

If you must care for a pregnant woman, you will want to determine whether she is actually in labor and if birth is imminent. If she is in labor, you should determine what stage of labor she may be in and whether she expects any complications. You can determine these and other factors by asking a few key questions and making some observations.

Calm the mother and make her feel comfortable and confident that you are there to keep her and the baby safe. Ask the following questions:

- If 9-1-1 or the designated emergency number has been called, how long ago were they reached and what was the response?

- Is this a first pregnancy? The first stage of labor normally takes longer with first pregnancies than with subsequent ones. This may allow more time to reach the hospital or have EMS arrive.

- Does the mother expect any complications? Is there a chance of multiple births? Labor does not usually last as long in a multiple birth situation. Also, if you know there are multiples, you can prepare what you need to care for more than one newborn.

- Is there a bloody discharge? This pink or light red, thick discharge from the vagina is the **mucous plug** that falls from the cervix as it begins to dilate, also signaling the onset of labor. This discharge is also known as the "bloody show."

- Has the amniotic sac ruptured (or water broken)? When the sac ruptures, fluid flows from the vagina in a sudden gush or a trickle. Some women think they have lost control of their bladder. The breaking of the sac usually signals the beginning of labor, but not always. People often describe the rupture of the sac as "water breaking."

- What are the contractions like? Are they very close together? Are they strong? The length and intensity of the contractions will give you valuable information about the progress of labor.

  - When the contractions are 5 minutes apart or longer, there is still time to transport the woman to a medical facility if possible.

  - If the contractions are 2 minutes apart, you will not have time to transport the woman, because the birth is imminent. If no one has called 9-1-1 or the designated emergency number yet, immediately call.

- Does she have the urge to bear down, or push? If the expectant mother expresses a strong urge to push, this signals that labor is far along.

- Is the baby crowning (i.e., is the newborn's head visible)? If so, begin preparing for the delivery—the baby is about to be born.

False Labor

Be aware that the woman may be experiencing **Braxton Hicks contractions,** or false labor contractions. During false labor, the contractions do not get closer together, do not increase in how long they last and do not feel stronger as time goes on—as they would with true labor. Also, false labor contractions tend to be sporadic while true labor has regular intervals of contractions. False labor is also not accompanied by the water breaking. Because there is no real, safe way to determine whether the labor is false, however, ensuring that the woman is seen by advanced medical personnel is a prudent decision.

Assisting with Delivery

If it becomes evident that the mother is about to give birth, you will need to help the mother through the birth process, at least until EMS personnel arrive. Although childbirth can be exciting, it can also be frightening to witness. Remember that you are only assisting in the process; the expectant mother is doing all the work. Therefore, it is important that you remain calm and confident. Try not to be alarmed by the loss of blood and bodily fluid. It is a normal part of the birth process. Take a deep breath and try to relax. By following a few simple steps, you can effectively assist in the birth process.

Preparing the Mother

Explain to the expectant mother that her baby is about to be born. Be calm and reassuring. A woman having her first child often feels fear and apprehension about the pain and the condition of the newborn. Labor pain ranges from discomfort, similar to menstrual cramps, to intense pressure or pain. Many women experience something in between. Factors that can increase pain and discomfort during the first stage of labor include:

- Irregular breathing.

- Tensing up because of fear.

- Not knowing what to expect.

- Feeling alone and unsupported.

You can help the expectant mother cope with the discomfort and pain of labor. Begin by reassuring her that you are there to help. If necessary and possible, explain what to expect as labor progresses. Suggest specific physical activities that she can do to relax, such as regulating her breathing. Ask her to breathe in slowly and deeply through the nose and out through the mouth. Ask her to try to focus on one object in the room while regulating her breathing. By staying calm, firm and confident, and offering encouragement, you can help reduce fear and apprehension. Reducing fear will help relieve pain and discomfort.

Breathing slowly and deeply in through the nose and out through the mouth during labor can help the expectant mother in several ways:

- It aids muscle relaxation.

- It offers a distraction from the pain of strong contractions as labor progresses.

- It ensures adequate oxygen to both the mother and the newborn during labor.

Many expectant mothers participate in childbirth classes, such as those offered at local hospitals, that help them become more competent in techniques used to relax during the birth process. If this is the case with the mother you are helping, this could greatly simplify your role while assisting with the birth process.

Expect delivery to be imminent when you observe the following signs and symptoms:

- Intense contractions are 2 minutes apart or less and last 60 to 90 seconds.

- The woman's abdomen is very tight and hard.

- The woman reports feeling the newborn's head moving down the birth canal or has a sensation like an urge to defecate.

- Crowning occurs.

- The mother reports a strong urge to push.

Delivering the Newborn

Assisting with the delivery of the newborn is often a simple process. The expectant mother is doing all the work. She will be pushing down, using certain muscles. Your job is to create a clean environment and to help guide the newborn from the birth canal, minimizing injury to the mother and newborn.

Follow these steps:

- Position the mother so that she is lying on her back with her head and upper back raised, knees bent, feet flat and legs spread wide apart (Figure 22-3). Be sure to control the scene so that the woman will have privacy.

- Establish a clean environment for delivery. Because it is unlikely that you will have sterile supplies, use items such as clean sheets, blankets, towels or even clothes. Newspapers, which are very absorbent, can be used if nothing else is available. Place these items over the mother's abdomen and under her buttocks and legs. Also keep a clean, warm towel or blanket handy to wrap the newborn.

- Because you will be coming in contact with the mother's and newborn's body fluids, be sure to wear disposable latex-free gloves. If gloves are not available, try to find some other item to use as a barrier. For example, a plastic bag or plastic wrap may be secured around your hands. Wear protective eyewear and a mask or face shield, if available, and put something on over your clothing, if possible, to protect yourself from splashing fluids.

- If available, other helpful items to gather include a bulb syringe to suction secretions from the infant's nose and mouth immediately after birth, gauze pads or sanitary pads to help absorb secretions and vaginal bleeding, and a large plastic bag or towel to hold the placenta in after delivery.

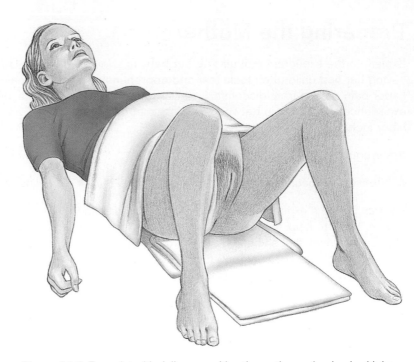

Figure 22-3. To assist with delivery, position the mother on her back with her head and upper back raised, knees bent, feet flat and legs spread wide apart in a clean environment.

- As crowning begins, place a hand on the top of the newborn's head and apply light pressure with your palm. In this way, you allow the head to emerge slowly, not forcefully. This will help prevent tearing of the vagina and avoid injury to the newborn.

- At this point, the expectant mother should stop pushing. Instruct the mother to concentrate on her breathing techniques. Ask her to pant. This technique will help her stop pushing and help prevent a forceful birth.

Once the head is out, the newborn will turn to one side. Support the head (Figure 22-4). The rotation to one side will enable the shoulders and the rest of the body to pass through the birth canal.

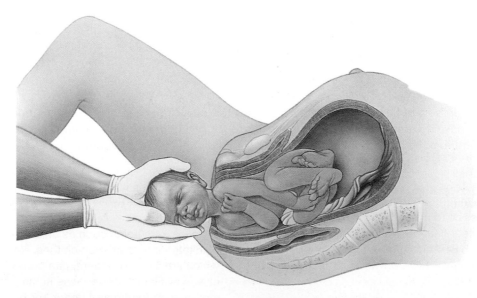

Figure 22-4. As the infant emerges and turns, be sure to support the head.

Slide your forefinger along the newborn's neck to see if the umbilical cord is looped around it. If the umbilical cord is around the neck, gently slip it over the newborn's head. If this cannot be done, slip it over the newborn's shoulders as they emerge. The newborn can slide through the loop.

- Guide one shoulder out at a time. Do *not* pull the newborn. As the newborn emerges, they will be wet and slippery. Use a clean towel to grasp the newborn.

- Place the newborn on their side, between the mother and you so that you can give care without fear of dropping the newborn.

- If possible, note the time of birth.

While assisting with delivery, also remember there are a few things you should *not* do. These include:

- Do *not* let the woman get up or leave to find a bathroom (most women will want to use the restroom).

- Do *not* hold the woman's knees together to try to slow the birth process; this will not work and may complicate the birth or harm the baby.

- Do *not* place your fingers in the vagina for any reason.

- Do *not* pull on the baby.

What if... *The expectant mother insists on getting up to go to the bathroom during delivery? What should I do?*

An expectant mother who is about to deliver should not be allowed to go to the bathroom during active labor. The pressure most women feel during labor to defecate is normally the baby putting pressure on the rectum. In fact, passing some stool during labor is common. Allowing a woman to go to the bathroom for a bowel movement, however, could damage the cervix or result in sudden delivery in the bathroom.

Caring for the Newborn and Mother

Your first priority after delivery of the newborn is to take some initial steps of care for them. Once these steps are accomplished, you can care for the mother.

Caring for the Newborn

The first few minutes of the newborn's life are a difficult transition from life inside the mother's uterus to life outside. Always be sure to support the newborn's head. You have two priorities at this point.

Your first is to see that the newborn's airway is open and clear. Because a newborn breathes primarily through the nose, it is important to immediately clear the mouth and nasal passages thoroughly. You can do this by using a bulb syringe, or your finger or a gauze pad if a bulb syringe is not available. When using a bulb syringe, clean the mouth first, and then each nostril. Also, make sure you compress the bulb *before* you place it in the newborn's mouth or nostril. The tip of the syringe should not be placed more than 1 to 1½ inches into the newborn's mouth and no more than ½ inch into the newborn's nostril.

Most babies begin crying and breathing spontaneously. If the newborn does not make any sound, stimulate the newborn to elicit the crying response by tapping your fingers on the soles of the newborn's feet or rubbing the lower back.

Crying helps clear the newborn's airway of fluids and promotes breathing. If the newborn does not begin breathing on their own within the first minute after birth, and stimulating the newborn as describe above does not work, begin CPR. You can review this technique in Chapter 6. Remember, the newborn's lungs are very small and they need very small puffs of air.

Your second responsibility to the newborn is to maintain normal body temperature. Newborns lose heat quickly; therefore, it is important to keep them warm. Dry the newborn and wrap them in a clean, warm towel or blanket. Continue to monitor breathing and skin color. You may place the baby on the mother's abdomen.

What if... I suction a newborn's nose first and then the mouth, rather than the mouth first, then the nose? Does it make a difference?

Yes, it does matter. When caring for a newborn, you should always suction the mouth (or oral airway) first using a bulb syringe (inserted 1 to 1½ inches; two or three times), followed by the nose (or nasal airway) (½ inch into the nostrils). Suctioning the nose before the mouth may stimulate the newborn to take a breath, causing them to inhale and aspirate any fluids or secretions still in the mouth.

What if... An expectant mother delivers a newborn before EMS arrives? Should I cut the umbilical cord?

No, you should never cut the umbilical cord and, in fact, there is no rush to cut the cord. Instead, keep the baby close to the mother so the cord is not pulled tight. The umbilical cord will stop pulsating approximately 10 minutes after the baby is born. When it does stop pulsating, the cord can be tied in two places very securely with gauze between the mother and child. Secure the first tie approximately 6 to 9 inches from the baby. Secure the second tie 3 inches from the first tie. However, do not delay emergency care to the newborn or mother if needed to do this.

Caring for the Mother

You can continue to meet the needs of the newborn while caring for the mother. Help the mother to begin nursing the newborn if possible. This will stimulate the uterus to contract and help slow bleeding. The placenta will still be in the uterus, attached to the newborn by the umbilical cord. Contractions of the uterus will usually expel the placenta within 30 minutes. Do not pull on the umbilical cord. Catch the placenta in a clean towel or container. It is not necessary to separate the placenta from the newborn. In the extreme event that you or another trained lay responder must transport the mother and child to the hospital under instruction by an EMS dispatcher or healthcare professional, leave the placenta attached to the newborn and place the placenta in a plastic bag or wrap it in a towel.

Expect some additional vaginal bleeding when the placenta is delivered. Gently clean the mother using gauze pads or clean towels. Place a sanitary pad or a towel over the vagina. Do *not* insert anything inside the vagina. Have the mother place her legs together. Feel for a grapefruit-sized mass in the lower abdomen. This is the uterus. Gently massage the lower portion of the mother's abdomen. Massage will cause the uterus to contract and slow bleeding.

Many new mothers experience shock-like signs and symptoms, such as cool, pale, moist skin; shivering; and slight dizziness. Keep the mother positioned on her back. Keep her from getting chilled or overheated, and continue to monitor her condition.

Special Considerations

Complications During Pregnancy

Complications during pregnancy are rare; however, they do occur. Because the nature and extent of most complications can only be determined by medical professionals during or following a more complete examination, you should not be concerned with trying to diagnose a particular problem. Instead, concern yourself with recognizing signs and symptoms that suggest a serious complication during pregnancy.

Two important signs or symptoms you should be concerned about are vaginal bleeding and abdominal pain. Any persistent or profuse vaginal bleeding, or bleeding in which tissue passes through the vagina during pregnancy, is abnormal, as is any abdominal pain other than labor contractions.

An expectant mother showing these signs or symptoms needs to receive advanced medical care quickly. Call 9-1-1 or the designated emergency number. While waiting for EMS personnel, place a pad or other absorbent material between the mother's legs. Also, take steps to minimize shock. These include:

- Helping the mother into a left lateral side-lying position if possible.
- Keeping the mother from becoming chilled or overheated.

Complications During Childbirth

The vast majority of all births occur without complication. However, this fact is reassuring only if the birth you are assisting with is not complicated. For the few that do have complications, delivery can be stressful and even life threatening for the expectant mother and the newborn. More common complications include persistent vaginal bleeding, prolapsed umbilical cord, breech birth and multiple births. If you recognize the signs of any of these complications, call 9-1-1 or the designated emergency number immediately if you have not already done so. All of these conditions require the help of more advanced medical care.

Persistent Vaginal Bleeding

The most common complication of childbirth is persistent vaginal bleeding following delivery. Persistent bleeding occurs when the uterus fails to contract after delivery, as this contraction facilitates the closing of blood vessels that were opened during the detachment of the placenta. It can also occur if the uterus was stretched too much during pregnancy or if a piece of the placenta remains inside the uterus following delivery. Abnormally long labors and multiple births also increase the risk for bleeding. While waiting for the ambulance to arrive, you should take steps to absorb the blood with sanitary napkins or towels. Do *not* pack the vagina with dressings. Try to keep the mother calm and take steps to minimize shock, as explained in Chapter 9. In addition, remember that having the mother begin to nurse her newborn and gently massaging the lower portion of the mother's abdomen will stimulate the uterus to contract and slow bleeding.

Prolapsed Umbilical Cord

A **prolapsed umbilical cord** occurs when a loop of the umbilical cord protrudes from the vagina while the unborn baby is still in the birth canal (Figure 22-5). This condition can threaten the unborn baby's life. As the unborn baby moves through the birth canal, the cord will be compressed between the unborn baby and the birth canal, and blood flow to the unborn baby will stop. Without this blood flow, the unborn baby will die within a few minutes because of lack of oxygen. If you notice a prolapsed cord, have the expectant mother assume a knee-chest position (Figure 22-6). This will help take pressure off the cord. Cover any exposed cord with a moist, sterile dressing. Never attempt to push the cord back into the vagina. Call 9-1-1 or the designated emergency number if they have not already been contacted.

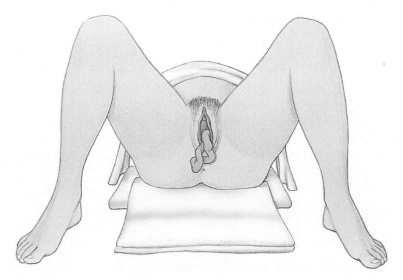

Figure 22-5. A prolapsed umbilical cord.

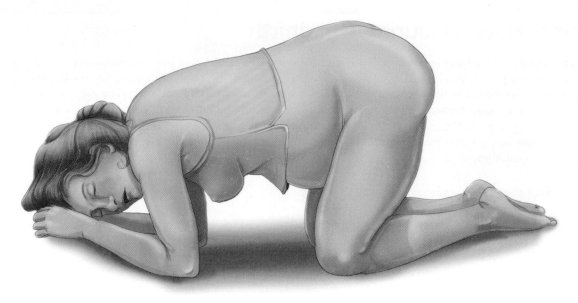

Figure 22-6. If you notice a prolapsed cord, the knee-chest position will take pressure off the cord.

Breech Birth

Most babies are born headfirst. However, on rare occasions, the newborn is delivered feet- or buttocks-first. This condition is commonly called a **breech birth.** If you encounter a breech delivery, support the newborn's body as it leaves the birth canal while you are waiting for the head to deliver. Do not pull on the newborn's body. Pulling will not help deliver the head. Do *not* attempt to push a protruding foot back up into the birth canal. If a single limb is presenting, you cannot successfully deliver the baby and the mother must be transported to a hospital as quickly as possible. Call 9-1-1 or the designated emergency number if they have not already been contacted. Place the mother in a head-down, hips-elevated position, and cover the presenting limb with a sterile towel. Do not attempt to push or pull on the protruding limb.

Because the weight of the unborn baby's head lodged in the birth canal will reduce or stop blood flow by compressing the umbilical cord, the unborn baby will be unable to get any oxygen. If the unborn baby tries to take a spontaneous breath, they will also be unable to breathe because the face is pressed against the wall of the birth canal. If the unborn baby's head is delivered, check the infant for breathing. Be prepared to give rescue breaths and perform CPR as necessary.

Multiple Births

Although most births involve only a single newborn, a few will involve delivery of more than one newborn. If the mother has had proper prenatal care, she will probably be aware that she is going to have more than one newborn. Multiple births should be handled in the same manner as single births. The mother will have a separate set of contractions for each baby being born. There may also be a separate placenta for each baby, although this is not always the case. Remember that the risk for persistent bleeding increases with multiple births.

Summary

Ideally, childbirth should occur in a controlled environment under the guidance of healthcare professionals trained in labor and delivery. In this way, the necessary medical care is immediately available for mother and newborn should any problem arise. However, unexpected deliveries may occur outside the controlled environment and may require your assistance. To assess the mother's condition before delivery and to assist in the delivery, be familiar with the four stages of labor and understand the birth process. By knowing how to prepare the expectant mother for delivery, assist with the delivery and give proper care for the mother and newborn, you can help the mother bring a new child into the world.

READY TO RESPOND? ❯

Think back to Lisa in the opening scenario, and use what you have learned to respond to these questions:

1. Which stage of labor is Lisa in? Why do you think so?

2. What information can Lisa give that will help you to assist with the delivery?

Study Questions

1. **Match each term with the correct definition.**

   a. Amniotic sac   c. Placenta   e. Crowning   g. Contraction

   b. Birth canal   d. Umbilical cord   f. Cervix   h. Uterus

   ____ A pear-shaped organ in a woman's pelvis in which a fertilized egg develops into a baby

   ____ The rhythmic tightening and relaxing of muscles in the uterus

   ____ An organ attached to the uterus and unborn baby through which nutrients are delivered

   ____ The phase during labor when the baby's head is visible at the opening of the vagina

   ____ The upper part of the birth canal

   ____ Sac that encloses the fetus during pregnancy and bursts during the birthing process

   ____ A flexible structure that attaches the placenta to the fetus, allowing for the passage of blood, nutrients and waste

   ____ The passageway from the uterus to the outside of the body through which the newborn passes during birth

2. **Name and briefly describe the four stages of labor.**

3. **List the two priorities of care for a newborn.**

Base your answers for questions 4 through 9 on the scenario below.

You happen upon a small gathering of people only to discover that a woman has gone into labor. The woman is lying on the floor in pain. She says this is her second child. She tells you that her labor pains started about an hour ago, but her contractions are already less than 3 minutes apart.

4. **The fact that this is the woman's second child, and her contractions are less than 3 minutes apart, means—**

   a. There should still be time to get this woman to the hospital to give birth.

   b. The woman may be about to give birth—when contractions are less than 3 minutes apart, delivery is near; and labor often moves more quickly in second pregnancies.

   c. The answer depends on whether her water has broken yet.

   d. The answer depends on whether she has had a bloody discharge.

(Continued)

Study Questions continued

5. **The woman now reports an urge to push. To assist with delivery of the newborn, which seems imminent now, what preparations should you take?**

   a. Ask a bystander to call 9-1-1 or the designated emergency number and help control the crowd to give the woman privacy.

   b. Place clean sheets, blankets or towels under the mother's buttocks and on her abdomen.

   c. Have the mother lie on her back with her knees bent, feet flat and legs spread wide apart.

   d. All of the above

6. **What can the woman do to help cope with the pain and discomfort of labor?**

   a. Focus on an object in the room while regulating her breathing.

   b. Assume a knee-chest position.

   c. Hold her breath then suddenly release it.

   d. Alternately tense and relax all muscles in her body.

7. **When the newborn's head is crowning at the vaginal opening, you should—**

   a. Maintain firm finger pressure against the center of the newborn's head.

   b. Place your hand lightly on the top of the newborn's head.

   c. Place the palm of your hand firmly against the newborn's head.

   d. Place one hand on either side of the newborn's head.

8. **If the mother has a breech delivery, what part of the newborn will be seen first?**

   a. Head

   b. Knee

   c. Foot (feet) or buttocks

   d. Shoulder

9. **If the newborn is not crying or does not appear to be breathing after you have cleared their airway with a bulb syringe, you should first—**

   a. Hold the newborn up by its ankles and spank its buttocks.

   b. Suction the newborn's throat with the bulb syringe.

   c. Flick the soles of the newborn's feet with your fingers or rub the lower back.

   d. Begin rescue breathing.

Answers are listed in the Appendix.

23 DISASTER, REMOTE AND WILDERNESS EMERGENCIES

You and a large group of friends are having fun along the river on a day-long kayaking outing when the unexpected happens. One of the kayaks flips over near the shore line, and Pete receives a long gash across his arm and abdomen. As he struggles to stand up in the shallow water, you can see that both wounds are bleeding profusely. You are still 2 miles away from the pickup point arranged with the rental company, and there is no mobile phone reception in the location where the incident occurred.

Learn and Respond ▶

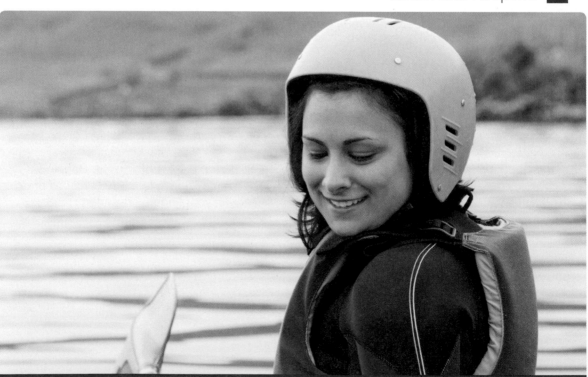

Introduction

Depending on things such as the region where you live and how active a lifestyle you enjoy, particularly with regard to outdoor pursuits, you might encounter a situation that requires extra consideration and efforts in giving first aid care. For example, you may encounter a *disaster* involving widespread destruction or large numbers of injured or ill people, or you may be faced with an emergency that occurs in a *remote* area far from resources. Even if you do not live in an area prone to natural disasters or you prefer to stay in more populated areas, you never know when extraordinary circumstances might lead to a sudden need for emergency care on a large-scale basis or with limited resources.

Consider these statistics: in the year 2016, some 103 federal disasters were declared in the United States, requiring resources from all levels of the government and private sector in order to protect, support and help citizens. These disasters included floods, wildfires, tornadoes, earthquakes and blizzards that affected practically every region of the country. While emergency medical services (EMS) networks serve reliably in the United States, even the best system can be overwhelmed in a disaster, such as during Hurricane Matthew in the Southeastern United States in October 2016 that caused disastrous flooding in North and South Carolina; the Joplin, Missouri, F5 tornado in 2011, where an entire hospital was destroyed; or the terrorist attacks of September 11, 2001.

EMS already relies on trained lay responders like you to activate the EMS system in an emergency, usually by calling 9-1-1 or the designated emergency number. But particularly in a disaster, remote or **wilderness** first aid situation, there are opportunities for trained lay responders to make life-preserving differences before advanced medical assistance becomes available by stabilizing injuries and illnesses or preventing further harm. This chapter connects what you already know about these two functions with additional considerations, helping you prepare and respond in disaster, remote or wilderness settings when advanced medical care is delayed by minutes, hours or days.

Disaster, Remote and Wilderness Emergencies

When EMS personnel are not readily available, trained lay responders can enact a number of interventions and scene management principles once someone recognizes that an emergency is developing, or one has occurred in which professional medical care will not be available within 30 minutes. You probably do not think about being away from advanced care very often, but imagine an emergency in a situation that cuts you off from communication.

Examples of such emergency situations include those that occur:

- On a boat or plane in transit.

- On a remote highway or isolated road.

- On a farm.

- While camping or hiking.

- With the occurrence of a tornado, earthquake or other natural disaster (Figure 23-1, A–C).

- Due to winter hazard conditions.

- Due to human mistakes, criminal activity or terrorism.

- As a result of a pandemic flu outbreak.

Each of these situations creates the potential for advanced care to be delayed. Factors you will need to consider along with your current first aid skills include:

- Time and/or distance that prevents access to swift advanced medical help.

- Hazards created by the environment, weather, location or time of day.

- Unavailability of EMS due to overwhelming need.

- Unavailability of EMS due to lack of workers or damaged equipment.

- Scene safety issues that demand special skills and resources.

- Lack of adequate first aid equipment.

- Issues related to managing resources, people and your own well-being for an extended amount of time.

The stress of these additional factors in first aid situations requires further mental and physical effort on your part. Additional skills and equipment to safely access, assess, care and transport injured or ill persons may be needed or improvised. Furthermore, there may be a need to manage group dynamics in an emergency with multiple injured or ill persons or multiple bystanders.

Leadership and Followership

Based on each individual's experience, the leader who emerges in one emergency may not be the same leader in another type of emergency. A designated leader may also change if that person is the one who becomes injured or ill. For example, someone who was a leader when caring for an ankle injury may later experience a heat-related illness that requires another individual to take charge. Also keep in mind that the leader in an emergency may not be the person with the highest rank, position or age in the group, but rather the person with the best training for the particular situation.

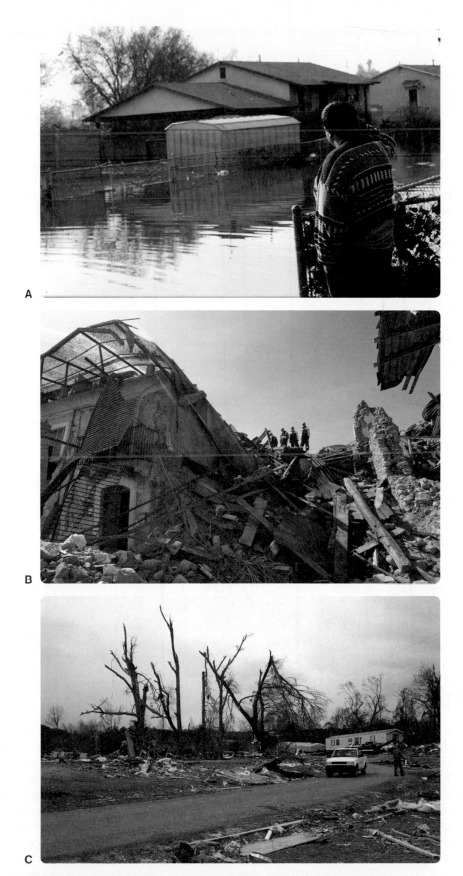

Figure 23-1, A–C. Natural disasters, such as **A,** a flood; **B,** an earthquake; or **C,** a tornado, can leave entire communities incapacitated and large numbers of people seriously injured. *Photos courtesy of:* **A,** *Robert Baker;* **B,** *Chris Helgren; and* **C,** *Joseph Songer*

With the primary goal to do the greatest good for the greatest number of people in the shortest time, and as safely as possible, leaders work to:

- Manage scene safety.

- Take a big-picture view of the scene.

- Care for life-threatening and non-life-threatening conditions (directly or indirectly).

- Provide evacuation direction for the group.

As much as a good leader depends on their own knowledge, skill and experience, a good leader also depends on the cooperation and assistance of other people in the group. If someone else takes leadership, or you are in a situation in which you are assisting EMS personnel with a major disaster response, you can be a good follower by assuming responsibility for tasks given to you. Asking pertinent questions and providing the leader with information to make informed decisions contributes to better decisions and actions by the group. Likewise, if you are the leader, you need to listen to the followers and their information because of the complexity of these situations. Providing feedback to followers maintains this relationship and keeps everyone on the same page with regard to priorities. It is good to remember your own limitations as well as the limitations of others, and realize that cases of dehydration, fatigue or environmental stress affect the judgment of everyone in a situation.

Taking Action Using Modified CHECK—CALL—CARE

In disaster, remote or wilderness emergencies, the basics of giving care that you learned in earlier chapters still apply. In Chapter 2, you learned about the emergency action steps: **CHECK—CALL—CARE.** In this chapter, you will learn to apply these same steps in a modified fashion to meet the special needs of a disaster, remote or wilderness emergency. In general, these modifications include:

- Breaking up the **CHECK** action step into three separate components that give you the information to act appropriately:

  ○ Check scene safety as part of your scene size-up.

  ○ Check the person or persons.

  ○ Check for resources.

- Recognizing that the **CALL** step will be more difficult and will require more information to be shared about the entire situation, not just the injured or ill person(s).

- Giving **CARE** for a longer term that will also require additional skills.

Each of these action steps needs a plan, based on what you see, hear and feel, along with what you anticipate. Good judgment is imperative.

Check Scene Safety

During the scene size-up, check the entire scene to get a general impression of what happened. Look for dangers that could threaten your safety or the safety of others. In a natural or human-caused disaster, this could include things such as downed wires, unstable structures, the potential presence of toxic fumes and similar hazards (Figure 23-2). In a remote or wilderness situation, dangers might include such things as falling rocks or tree limbs, difficult terrain, wild animals and the like on-site (Figure 23-3). If you see any dangers, do not approach the person(s) until you have carefully planned how you will avoid or eliminate the danger to yourself and others. Also note any impending problems, such as a threatening storm or darkness. Make the scene safe if needed or remove the person(s) with an emergency move if you can do so without putting yourself or others in jeopardy. Moving a person in a disaster, remote or wilderness area will be covered more in-depth later in this chapter. This check will also give you clues to mechanisms of injury before you start checking the person.

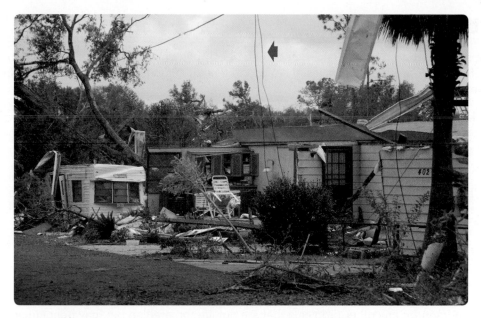

Figure 23-2. Check the scene for dangers that could threaten your safety or the safety of others, such as downed wires and unstable structures.

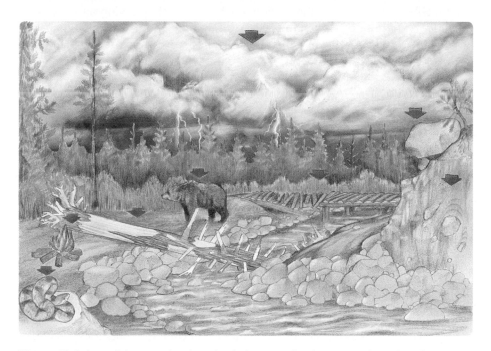

Figure 23-3. In a wilderness situation, check the scene for dangers such as changing weather conditions, wild animals, fire hazards, difficult terrain and falling rocks.

What if… *There are more injured or ill persons than I can handle?*

By their nature, disasters often create situations with multiple injured or ill persons—and limited resources for responding to their needs. When things seem overwhelming, you can help by maintaining your composure and knowing your limitations. If you are the only one with training at the scene, direct bystanders in ways to help, and encourage persons to help themselves and each other if able. You will also need to apply some basic triage principles, including quickly assessing each person, then helping the person who needs care the most and who can be saved (i.e., caring for life-threatening emergencies quickly) before helping those with less serious injuries or illnesses. Finally, offering reassurance to others can help reduce chaos at the scene until the emergency is under control.

Check the Person(s)

When you are sure it is safe, approach the person(s) carefully and check for life-threatening conditions. In disaster, remote or wilderness emergencies, the steps to identify priorities are slightly different from those taught in Chapter 5.

- First check for responsiveness and breathing as well as for severe, life-threatening bleeding. Then check the person systematically from head to toe and underneath clothing.

- Follow with checking for disability of the extremities by checking circulation, ability to move, and ability to sense in each hand or foot. The absence of any of the three could be a sign of a life-threatening head, neck or spinal injury.

If the person has fallen or if you do not know how the injury occurred, assume that they have a head, neck or spinal injury.

- Finally, consider the environment and protect the person from further harm. For example, if a disaster caused a loss of power or you are in a remote area and it is getting cold, you need to take steps to protect the person from hypothermia, which can be lethal.

Give care for any life-threatening conditions as you find them.

Next, check the person for any other problems that are not life threatening but may become so over time, using a second systematic and detailed assessment. In delayed-help situations, this check may need to occur before getting help and may also need to be repeated until help arrives. Ask the person or bystanders questions beyond the SAMPLE questions that describe what is now happening and any history that may have caused the situation but not be obvious to you (e.g., a person who fell is also a diabetic). Whenever possible, perform a head-to-toe check even if the person is unresponsive or being treated for life-threatening conditions. Write down the information that you gather so that you remember it. If you do not have anything to write with, you'll have to take mental notes of the most important or unusual observations. This subjective and objective information about the person's condition and history will help in making a care and evacuation plan.

Check for Resources

Check the scene for resources. Resources include people available to help, communication or signaling devices available, food and water, shelter, first aid supplies and means of transportation. While checking bystanders, make sure everyone else nearby is okay (e.g., if one person is hypothermic, then other bystanders may also be cold). Check the surrounding environment for conditions or developing conditions that could endanger you or the person(s) during the time it will take to get help. Note any conditions that would make it difficult for you to go get help. Also, consider whether you need to move the person(s) to prevent further harm.

As a leader, you should consider having other people do these checks, if they are able, so you can maintain control over the scene. Checking will be an ongoing step, so that you stay alert to developing dangers and deal with them in the context of the entire situation. Consider assigning a specific person as a "safety officer" to constantly check for safety-related issues, such as changes in weather conditions, unstable terrain or new threats.

Call

Once you realize help is needed, the **CALL** step is divided into two phases: making a plan for getting help and executing the plan. Proper planning based on the needs of the injured or ill person(s), changing environmental conditions and the resources available will help guide you in what to do and in which order to do it. This includes everything from the first aid needs of the person(s), to the roles of other group members, to the evacuation plan. Be sure you have all the necessary information before calling for help, as you may only have one chance depending on the situation (e.g., if you have to send someone for help or phone lines are overwhelmed with callers).

Making a Plan

In a delayed-help situation, you have four options for getting help:

- Stay where you are and call, radio or signal for help.

- Send someone to go get help or leave the person alone so you can get help.

- Transport the person to help.

- Care for the person where you are until the person has recovered enough to move on their own.

Consider all of the information you have gathered during the **CHECK** step about the conditions at the scene, the condition of the injured or ill person(s), and the resources available or needed before making the plan. Discuss your options with others, including the person(s), if appropriate. To help decide on the best approach, ask yourself and others these questions:

- Is advanced medical care needed; if so, how soon? If you discovered any conditions for which you would normally call 9-1-1 or the designated emergency number, or if these conditions seem likely to develop, you should plan to get help immediately.

- Is there a way to call from the scene for help or advice? If communication is possible, call 9-1-1 or the designated emergency number as soon as you have enough information about the condition of the person(s) and they are safe from dangers at the scene. Emergency medical personnel can tell you how to give care and advise you about getting help.

- If phone or radio communication is not possible, is there a way to signal for help? The advantages of signaling are that it is faster and safer than going for help. The disadvantages include not knowing if your signal has been received and not being able to communicate with the receiver exactly the type of help you need.

- If there is no way to call for help, is it possible to go get help yourself? Consider whether you can get help safely while not jeopardizing the safety of the person(s) or yourself as well as how long it might take. Carefully weigh the decision if going to get help means leaving a person alone, and determine what to do before leaving to keep them safe.

- Is there a way to transport the person(s) to help? Consider whether you have a safe and practical way to transport the person(s), and whether any injuries allow for safe transport. If a person cannot walk, it will be extremely difficult to carry them any distance, even if you have a large number of people to assist. Unless a vehicle or other means of transportation is available, you probably will not be able to transport the person to help without great difficulty or risk to others.

- Is it possible to give care where you are until the person(s) can travel? Think about the risks of caring for the person(s) without medical assistance and the possibility that serious complications may develop. On the other hand, consider how quickly the person(s) may be able to recover, allowing you to safely transport them to medical care.

- Is it safe to wait for help where you are? Environmental hazards, such as a threatening storm or falling temperatures, may make it unsafe to wait for help.

You will discover that there is no "best" plan for getting help in a disaster, remote or wilderness emergency. You may have to compromise, reducing overall risk by accepting certain risks. For example, if you are hiking in a remote area late in the afternoon on a cold, sunny day and one of your companions injures an ankle, generally, the safest thing to do for the person would be to immobilize the ankle in place, send someone for help and wait with the person until emergency transportation arrives. However, if you know that it will take until nightfall for someone to summon help and no one in your party is dressed to survive the low temperatures overnight, you may decide to immobilize the ankle and help the person walk to a shelter, even though following this plan could cause further injury to the ankle.

Calling for Help

If you have some means of quickly calling for help, such as a mobile phone or two-way radio, make sure you have gathered all the necessary information about the condition of the person(s) and your location so that EMS or rescue personnel will be able to plan their response. Having essential information when you call reduces confusion and improves the likelihood that the right type of help will be sent to the right location. In addition, if you include all essential information in your first communication call, emergency personnel will be able to respond even if later communication attempts fail.

Make sure you give the dispatcher specific information about your location. Identifying prominent landmarks and marking your area can help responders find your location. Consider that some landmarks are clearly visible during the day but are not visible at night, or may have been destroyed by a disaster. Flares are one way of marking your location, although you should not use flares in dry or heavily wooded areas that could ignite and start a fire. You may need to send someone to meet EMS personnel at a main road or easy-to-identify location and have them guide EMS personnel to the person(s). Do not give mileage approximations to the EMS dispatcher unless you are sure of the distance.

Improvised Distress Signals

If you have no way to call for help and it is dangerous or impractical to use flares or send someone for help, you may have to improvise. Two of the most widely used general distress signals are:

- Signals in threes. A series or set of three signals alert others to your call for "Help!" (Figure 23-4). Three shots, three flashes of light, three shouts, three whistles or three smoky fires are all examples. Use extreme caution when building fires. Always remain near the fire and have water or dirt close by to extinguish sparks. Do not use fires in dry areas. A small fire can easily get out of control. Build your fires in a triangle at least 50 yards (46 meters) apart so that they are visible as separate fires.

- Ground-to-air signals. To signal an aircraft, use either signals in threes (three fires or three flashes of light) or else mark a large "X" on the ground. The X ground-to-air signal is a general distress signal meaning "unable to proceed" or "need immediate help." If constructing an X signal, make sure that you choose a large open area and that the X you construct stands out against its background. The X signal should be at least 20 feet (6 meters) across.

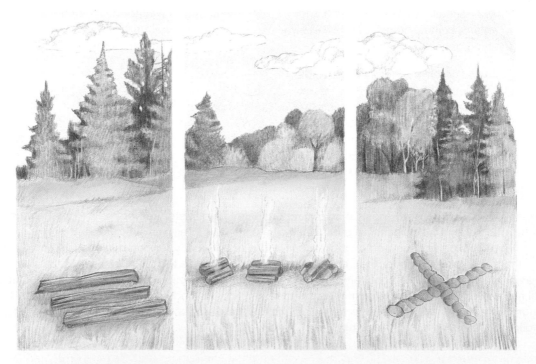

Figure 23-4. A series or set of three signals or a ground-to-air signal can be used to signal "Help!"

In addition, smoke, mirrors, flare guns and whistles create visual or auditory signals to attract responders. Smoke signals can be effective because they can be seen for many miles. If you are on a boat, making an urgent call over marine radio indicates that you have an emergency. You should be familiar with various ways of signaling that are appropriate for your location and environment.

Sending for Help

If calling or signaling is not an option, such as in an area where no mobile service is available, consider sending two or three people to get help. Ideally, they should have the following information:

- A note indicating the condition of the injured or ill person(s)

- A map indicating the location of the person(s)

- A list of other members in the group

- A list of available resources

- A description of the weather, terrain and access routes if known

- A list of immediate and long-term plans, as well as contingency plans if needed

This information will help emergency personnel determine their needs for the rescue. The information should be carried in writing in the event that the individuals seeking help become lost or something happens to them.

The safety of the messengers seeking help is extremely important. Make sure you send enough people to ensure safety and success in delivering the message. If going for help involves hazards or challenges, do not send individuals who are not prepared to overcome these problems. Taking personal safety equipment, food, water and shelter is essential. Also, if the plan involves accessing a vehicle, for example at a trail head, be sure to send the keys with the individuals seeking help.

Another consideration in going for help is making sure those sent can lead responders back to the person. Whenever you find yourself in a large urban disaster, or a remote location such as on a boat or in the wilderness, the most accurate way to describe your location is to use maps, perhaps in coordination with a Global Positioning System (GPS), compass or other instrument. You should be trained in map and chart reading and know how to use your GPS or compass if you travel or work in delayed-help environments. Of course, today many people rely solely on GPS devices. While these can be helpful and often provide accurate information, they do have limitations, including the fact that they can run out of batteries or break.

If going for help, another important step is to always mark the way so that you can return more easily with responders. Regularly look back at the area you just traveled, which can assist you on your return trip. What you see behind you will look different from the area you are facing.

Finally, before sending anyone for help, consider whether tasks at the scene require everyone's help. For instance, moving an injured or ill person a short distance to a shelter or gathering firewood is easier to do when everyone helps. When sending someone for help, make sure you also leave behind enough trained individuals to care for the injured or ill person(s) while waiting for help. Those remaining with the person should be equipped to care for the person and themselves.

Leaving a Person Alone

Generally, it is not a good idea to leave an injured or ill person alone. However, if you are alone with the person, have no way to call or signal for help, and are reasonably sure that no one will happen by, then you may decide that it is best to leave the person and go get help.

Follow the guidance above for having a plan and executing it. Write down the route, the time you are leaving and when you expect to arrive, and then leave this information with the person. Be sure to provide for the injured or ill person's needs while you are gone. Ensure that the person has food, water and a container to use as a urinal or bedpan. If the person cannot move, make sure that these things are within reach.

Also make certain that the person has adequate clothing and shelter and that they are protected from the ground. See Protection from the Environment later in this chapter for more information. Recheck any splints or bandages, and adjust them if necessary so that they are not too tight. If the person is awake, make sure they understand that you are going to get help. Give the person an idea of when to expect a response. Be as reassuring and positive as the situation allows.

If the person is unresponsive or completely unable to move, place them in a recovery position, lying on one side with their face angled toward the ground, to maintain an open and clear airway and prevent aspiration in case the person vomits. To put them in the recovery position, extend the person's arm that is closest to you above their head. Then roll the person toward yourself onto their side so that their head rests on their extended arm. Once on their side, bend both of their knees to stabilize the body. Be careful to keep the head and spine as straight as possible if you suspect an injury in those areas. For instructions on how to place an adult, child or infant in a recovery position, refer to Chapter 5.

Transporting a Person to Help

In situations involving injury or sudden illness, it is usually best to have help come to you. Consider transporting a person to help only if a vehicle or other means of transportation is available rather than simply carrying the person. Carrying a person is very difficult and can be hazardous, especially if the terrain is not smooth and flat.

Factors to consider when deciding to move a person include the extent of the injuries, distance to be traveled and available help at the scene. Remember that excessive movement may aggravate or worsen the person's condition. You should not attempt to move or transport a person with a suspected head, neck or spinal injury unless a potential for greater danger exists.

If you decide to transport a person to help, plan the route you will follow. Remember that you may need to travel more slowly to avoid further injury to the person or responders. Once you get to your vehicle, remember it is better to have someone come along in addition to the driver who will care for the person during transport. If possible, inform someone else of your route and alternate plans.

Being Prepared . . . In Your Vehicle

If you plan to travel by car through remote areas, or live in an area prone to winter storms, making sure to stock your vehicle with some minimal survival supplies can make the difference between life and death should you find yourself stranded. In addition to the items listed below, you should also always be prepared by ensuring your vehicle is in proper working order, keeping the gas tank full and avoiding traveling when you know the weather could be severe.

At a minimum, your vehicle survival kit should include:

- Battery-powered radio and extra batteries.
- Flashlight and extra batteries.
- Blankets or sleeping bags.
- Jumper cables.

- Bottled water.
- Nonperishable snacks.
- Compass and road map.
- First aid kit.

Also consider including:

- A fire extinguisher (5 lb, A-B-C).
- A small shovel.
- A tire repair kit and pump.

- Flares or reflective triangles.
- A sack of sand or cat litter (for traction).

Care

In a delayed-help situation, your plan for caring for each person in need extends from the initial stabilization of an injury or illness to long-term care of those issues and personal care. The best care possible, whether for a few minutes or a few hours, will come if you remain calm, use the information in all of the checks to create a sound plan, and demonstrate good leadership or followership. This provides you a focus and will support and reassure the person and bystanders until EMS personnel take over.

Monitoring the Person

After you complete your initial check of the person and give care for the conditions found, continue to monitor the person's condition. Monitoring provides you with ongoing information so you can modify your plan as needed and gives you reference points with regard to the person's improvement (or lack of improvement).

Continuously monitor the breathing of a person who is unresponsive or has an altered level of consciousness. Listen to and watch the person's breathing. If the person stops breathing, you will need to perform CPR. If the person vomits, you will need to put them in a side-lying recovery position and clear their mouth. Otherwise, recheck the person about every 15 minutes until they are stable.

If the person can answer questions, ask the person if their condition has changed. You should also watch for changes in skin appearance and temperature and level of consciousness. Changes in these conditions may indicate developing problems, such as heat-related illnesses or cold-related emergencies and shock. Recheck any splints or bandages, and adjust them if they are too tight or loose. If minutes turn into hours, you will also have to provide a safe means for the person to eat as well as urinate and defecate. If hours turn into days, you will need to assess and care for wounds that may become infected.

Keep a written record, noting any changes you find and the time the changes occur, and describe the care you give.

Fractures, Dislocations, Sprains and Strains

In Chapters 11 and 12, you learned how to recognize and give care for musculoskeletal injuries and not to attempt to move a person with a serious musculoskeletal injury unless it is absolutely necessary. However, in delayed-help situations where advanced medical personnel will not arrive quickly to help, splinting may reduce pain and will allow you to more safely move a person with a musculoskeletal injury. First splint the injured part using the techniques learned earlier. It is more likely that you will need to improvise a splint in a disaster, remote or wilderness situation (Figure 23-5). Be sure to continue to check the splinted area for

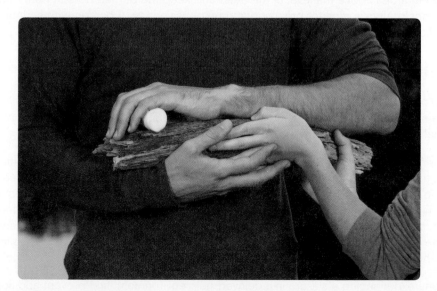

Figure 23-5. You may need to improvise a splint in a disaster, remote or wilderness situation.

feeling, warmth and color about every 15 minutes, and adjust the splint if necessary. Using the principles of RICE (rest, immobilize, cold and elevate) for this type of injury may help speed healing time, where a person could walk out versus being carried out, and will address pain issues. Refer to Chapter 11 for specifics about these care steps. For long-term care and faster healing, repeat RICE three to four times a day, until pain and swelling subside.

Bleeding

In delayed-help situations, use the same principles that you learned to control severe bleeding in Chapter 8. Direct pressure controls most external bleeding and should be maintained for at least 10 minutes to allow a blood clot to form. Long-term management of small and large wounds includes cleaning the wound with large amounts of clean water and protecting the wound from infection with ointments and dressings. The wound should be checked periodically for infection, cleaned and redressed as needed.

Also as taught in Chapter 8, if direct pressure fails to control severe, life-threatening external bleeding on an extremity or is not possible, application of a manufactured (commercial) tourniquet may be necessary. However, because of the concerns about prolonged use of a tourniquet, and additional factors complicating delayed-help situations, it is recommended that any individual planning to be in a possible delayed-help situation get full training on the use of tourniquets and hemostatic dressings to control bleeding, such as that offered in a specific wilderness first aid course.

Burns

General steps for caring for a burn in a delayed-help environment are the same as in any other situation. Refer back to Chapter 10 for details.

Keep in mind that using cold water on large or serious burns increases the possibility of hypothermia and shock, especially in a cold environment. Be careful not to use more water than necessary and focus on cooling only the burned area. In areas with limited water, you may need to reuse water, so plan ahead.

Since the danger of infection is greater in delayed-help environments, keep a dressing over the cooled burn. Apply a thin layer of wound gel to the dressing first if available. If an emergency facility is more than a day away, you must redress the burn daily. Redressing includes taking old dressings off, cleaning the burned area with sterile water and mild soap, reapplying a thin layer of wound gel and covering with a clean dressing. If none of these materials are available, leave the burn alone; it will form a scab.

Partial- and full-thickness burns, or burns covering more than one body part, can cause serious loss of body fluids. Elevate burned areas above the level of the heart and keep the burned person from becoming chilled while treating for shock. Always monitor breathing and responsiveness. A person with serious burns requires transport to a medical facility as soon as possible.

Sudden Illness

When caring for a person with sudden illness, such as someone experiencing a diabetic emergency or a seizure, follow the same procedures as if you were not in a delayed-help situation (see Chapter 15). However, there are additional factors to consider when you are far from help or transportation.

A person recovering from a diabetic emergency due to low blood sugar should rest after eating or drinking something sweet. If the person does not show improvement within 10 to 15 minutes, you need to give the person water in the amounts described in the following section on shock. Consider a fast evacuation. Some wilderness first aid experts recommend rubbing small amounts of a sugar and water mixture (or some other sweet liquid, such as fruit juice or a sports drink) on the gums of an unresponsive person. Remember, however, that while a person having a diabetic emergency needs to get a sugary substance into their system immediately, you should never attempt to give an unresponsive person anything to eat or drink.

To care for someone experiencing a seizure in a delayed-help environment, first prevent additional harm, for example, by clearing the area around the person. During the seizure, place the person in a side-lying recovery position if it is safe to do so. Complete a detailed check for injuries after the seizure ceases. Maintain the person's body temperature and help prevent shock by placing some form of insulation between the person and the ground. Cover the person with a blanket or coat if necessary. If you are on a recreational outing, such as a camping trip or hike, consider ending the trip if you suspect any injuries or possible recurrence of the seizure.

Shock

With all injuries and illnesses in a delayed-help situation, it is likely that you will have to give care for shock to minimize or delay its onset while waiting for advanced medical care. If untreated, shock will worsen and lead to death.

Remember that shock does not always occur right away; it may develop while you are waiting for help because of a hidden injury or illness. Check for signs and symptoms of shock (see Chapter 9) every time you check the person's condition. Be alert for conditions that may cause shock to develop slowly, such as internal bleeding, vomiting, diarrhea or heat loss.

For those in shock, if medical care is more than 2 hours away, you should consider providing the responsive and awake person with cool water or clear juices. This fluid will help the body compensate for fluid loss in an injury or illness. You can give an adult about 4 ounces (½ cup) or more of water to sip slowly over a 20-minute period if it is tolerated. For a child, give 2 ounces (¼ cup), and for an infant, 1 ounce (⅛ cup), over the same 20-minute period. Giving frequent, small amounts of fluid, rather than fewer large amounts, reduces the chance of vomiting. If no injuries are present or suspected, you may also consider placing them in the supine position (i.e., lying face-up on their back) and raising their feet 6 to 12 inches to maintain more blood volume to their vital organs.

Even in a delayed-help situation, do not give fluids if the person is unresponsive, having seizures, has a serious head or abdominal injury, or if vomiting is frequent and sustained. If you give fluids and the person then starts to vomit, wait before giving the person any more to drink. Remember to keep the person from becoming chilled or overheated.

If you or someone you are with is susceptible to anaphylaxis or anaphylactic shock as a result of an allergy, bite or sting, be sure someone knows the location of necessary medication, such as oral antihistamines or injectable epinephrine (see Chapters 16 and 17), and knows how to use it. Anaphylactic shock is life threatening if the person does not receive care immediately. Advanced medical support for a person who shows signs and symptoms of anaphylactic shock, such as swelling and trouble breathing, is needed as quickly as possible, as the condition is often reversible with specific drugs, but life threatening without them.

Head, Neck and Spinal Injuries

If you suspect a head, neck or spinal injury based either on the cause or your assessment of a person, the goal and the care are the same as in any other emergency: prevent further injury by having the person remain still.

Caring for a person with a head, neck or spinal injury who will be exposed to the elements for an extended period is more difficult, as the person will not be able to maintain normal body temperature without your help. The person will need help drinking, eating, urinating and defecating. Help the person maintain normal body temperature by placing insulation underneath them or providing shelter from the weather. If two or more people are available, roll the person onto one side to place insulation underneath the body, being careful not to twist the head, neck or spine.

Difficult Decisions

Dealing with a life-threatening condition when advanced medical care is not easily obtainable is one of the most emotionally charged and stressful situations you can face as a trained lay responder. The most difficult question of all in a delayed-help situation may be how long to continue resuscitation efforts if the condition of a person in cardiac arrest does not improve and advanced medical help is hours away. While there is no simple answer, following are some general principles that can help you decide.

As you learned in Chapter 6, the purpose of CPR is to partially and temporarily substitute the functions of the respiratory and circulatory systems. However, CPR is not designed for and is not capable of sustaining a person's life indefinitely. Usually, the longer CPR is continued, the less likely it is that the person will survive. Prolonged CPR efforts may be unsafe for you or the group due to exhaustion or environmental changes.

The person's survival depends largely on what caused the heart to stop in the first place. If the cause was a direct injury to the heart, such as from a heart attack or from crushing or penetrating trauma to the chest, little chance exists that the person will survive in a delayed-help environment, regardless of whether CPR is performed. On the other hand, if the heart is not injured but stops as a result of hypothermia, suffocation (e.g., from an avalanche), a lightning strike or drowning (especially in cold water), the person's heart has a better chance of restarting. CPR can limit brain damage in case the heart starts and may even improve the chance that the heart will start. In such a case, CPR should be continued until one of the following occurs:

- You find an obvious sign of life such as normal breathing.

- You are relieved by another trained responder.

- EMS personnel arrive and take over.

- You are too exhausted to continue.

- The scene becomes unsafe.

If a person dies or is found dead, you will then need to manage the physical and emotional needs of yourself and the group. Try yourself, and encourage others, to begin functioning normally (e.g., sleeping, eating), and take steps to decrease the intensity of the emotional experience (e.g., by covering the body or performing a service). You will also need to notify authorities and protect the body. Document and do not disturb the area as best as possible.

Protection from the Environment

When caring for a person in a disaster, remote or wilderness emergency where help will be delayed, it is critical to protect the person from environmental conditions, such as heat, cold, wind, rain, sleet or snow, while waiting. You may need to construct a shelter using whatever materials you have on hand.

Protecting the Person

An injured or ill person who is not able to move may develop a heat-related illness or cold-related emergency that is life threatening. To keep the person from getting chilled or overheated, you will need to provide some type of insulation to protect the person. If the ground is dry, you can use cloth items such as towels, blankets, clothing or sleeping bags to insulate the person from the ground; also, dry leaves or grass may serve as natural insulators. If the ground is wet, you will also need a moisture barrier, such as a waterproof tarp, raincoat or poncho, between the insulating material and the ground.

Constructing a Shelter

A person exposed to hot sun, rain, snow or chilling wind needs appropriate shelter (Figure 23-6, A–D). Remember that you may need to protect bystanders as well, and they may also be a good resource for constructing or finding shelter. The following are four basic types of shelters:

- Natural shelters

- Artificial shelters

- Snow shelters

- Tents and bivouac bags

A car can also be an effective shelter. If stranded, your car generally offers more visibility and protection, so consider staying in it. If you need heat, running the heater for 15 to 20 minutes each hour should sustain you. Make sure nothing, such as snow, blocks the exhaust pipe and causes carbon monoxide fumes to back up into the car. Leave the window opened a little to prevent carbon monoxide poisoning. You can also use candles as a source of heat. It is important, especially in the winter months, that you keep your car in good working condition, filled with gasoline, and carry a vehicle survival kit.

Whether a shelter is natural or artificial, it should be well ventilated to prevent buildup of condensation or toxic fumes.

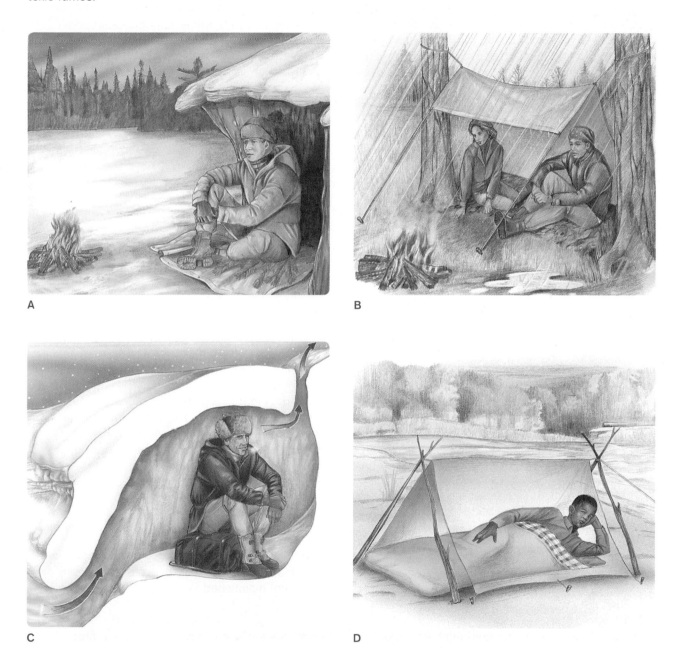

Figure 23-6, A–D. Types of shelters include: **A,** natural shelters; **B,** artificial shelters; **C,** snow shelters and **D,** a pole tent.

Being Prepared . . . On the Farm

To many, a farm or ranch may seem peaceful and idyllic. Yet historically, farming has been one of the most hazardous occupations in the United States. The very nature of farming puts workers—as well as the many children who live and help on family farms—at risk for injuries, illness and death.

Farms are often far from neighbors or towns, many roads in rural communities have no identifying signs and emergencies may occur in isolated areas of the farm where vehicle access is problematic. In addition, EMS is generally more limited than in urban areas, with responders who are often volunteers who have other duties and may be far from the scene of the emergency. As a result, the first person on the scene of a farm emergency, often a family member, is generally the person who gives the initial care and whose actions often determine whether a person who is injured or ill lives or dies.

Fortunately, there are many resources to help prepare those who live and work in agricultural settings for an emergency. One such organization is Farm Safety For Just Kids, which works to prevent farm-related childhood injuries, health risks and fatalities. It puts out a variety of resource materials and activity ideas, including a catalogue of items to teach farm safety. To learn more about this organization, visit *www.farmsafetyforjustkids.org.*

Another resource is the National Ag Safety Database, developed with funding from the National Institute of Occupational Safety and Health (NIOSH) to provide comprehensive access to prevention, safety and training information. To learn more about what is available, visit *www.nasdonline.org.*

Preparing for Emergencies

If you live or work in a disaster-prone area or delayed-help environment or plan to be in one, develop a plan for how you will prepare and respond to emergencies that may arise. Ideally, everyone in the situation should know how to react, whether you are a part of a remote survey team, family farm or youth group outing.

As you have read, there are risks in everyday life and even more risks in delayed-help situations. Mitigating or preventing emergencies makes the most sense for enjoying and profiting from wilderness and remote locations. And while disasters are generally thought of as unpredictable, you can mitigate many issues through preparedness activities and early detection of risk factors. Minor incidents can lead to major ones quickly and occur for a variety of reasons:

- Bad judgment, such as traveling unprepared, without water or other essentials; using inadequate equipment, such as an improper helmet or clothing; practicing poor sleep, hydration and hygiene habits; engaging in activities that exceed the abilities of one or more members of the group; and getting separated or stranded from the group

- Environmental conditions, such as bad weather, darkness or falling debris, perhaps caused by disasters, such as earthquakes or hurricanes

- Equipment failure, such as farm vehicles, deer stands or bicycles that do not work properly or are not maintained

Although not all factors that contribute to incidents or accidents are avoidable, many can be prevented through preparation.

Being Prepared . . . Remote and Wilderness Activities

Planning for emergencies is an important part of preparation for any trip or activity. Adequate preparation will not only reduce the risk of certain problems, but will also help make your trip more enjoyable. When planning a trip, several major considerations will help you determine special safety needs. These include:

- Knowledge level of first aid training among group members.

- Distance you will be from medical help.

- Duration of the trip or activity.

- Level of risk associated with the activity and environment.

- Group-related factors, such as pre-existing medical or physical conditions.

- Requirements for special equipment and supplies for high-risk or other specific activities.

- Group size. It is best to travel in a group larger than two so that at least one person is always available to stay with an injured or ill person.

In addition, when you are traveling in a wilderness or back-country area, the Boy Scouts of America recommend having the following with you at all times:

- A map, preferably a topographical map, of the area in which you will be traveling

- A compass—and know how to use it before you leave

- Matches in a waterproof container

- 24 hours of *extra* high-energy food

- Water (1 to 2 liters [1 to 2 quarts])

- Extra clothes, such as socks and a sweater

- Rain gear

- A pocket knife and whistle

- Sun protection, such as a wide-brimmed hat, sunglasses and sunscreen

- A first aid kit with an emergency blanket

Types of Preparation

There are three general types of preparation—knowledge, skills and equipment.

Knowledge

Knowledge includes learning about the emergency care resources available and how to access them, as well as educating yourself on how to react in an emergency that may be common in the region where you live or travel. It also includes familiarizing yourself with local geography, including landmarks and hazards. For instance, if you are going on a hiking trip, talk with park rangers or others who know the environment. Plan your route and write it down. Decide when and where you will check in, and let others know about your timing, routes, destination and companions. Letting others know your destination and estimated time of arrival may lessen the response time in the event of an emergency.

If you are planning a boating expedition, consult the Coast Guard about possible weather hazards for that time of year. If you will be boating on inland waters, also consult the local authority with control over dam water releases. People in rural areas should meet with local EMS personnel and ask what to do if an emergency occurs and the estimated response time to their particular location.

Additionally, you should know the people in the group you are living, working or traveling with, both to find out who has relevant training and to learn who might have special health concerns that put them at greater risk for an injury or illness. Youth programs, such as Girl Scouts of the USA, require individuals to have health forms that prepare leaders and individuals to understand health risks beforehand and provide important information to care providers if something happens. Ideally, group members know what resources (i.e., skills and equipment) lay in the group or location you may be in; this will keep confusion down and efficiency up.

Skills

Skills preparation includes having proficiency in implementing disaster plans, and wilderness or survival techniques, along with having the technical skills necessary to safely engage in certain activities, such as scuba diving or rock climbing. In addition, if you plan to use a two-way radio, you need to know how to operate it and how to call for help. Rural inhabitants should know how to safely handle the hazards they encounter on a regular basis, such as pesticides or farm machinery. Courses are available that address specific situations, such as wilderness first aid and farming emergencies.

Equipment

Equipment preparation includes having the essentials of water, food and shelter prepared and available to help keep people alive during long-term events. Equipment includes appropriate clothing for your location and activities, first aid supplies suitable for your activities and expected hazards, and devices for signaling and communication.

First aid kits are also important as not all first aid materials can be improvised (e.g., sterile bandages). Chapter 1 lists supplies for a basic first aid kit, but you should modify the contents of a first aid kit to suit your particular needs. For example, boaters should waterproof their kits by placing the contents in a waterproof container. People driving on long trips may want to add flares, a blanket and a flashlight to their kits.

Here are some factors to help you adjust the contents of your basic first aid kit:

- The environment (e.g., bring prescription medications for high altitudes or anti-itch topical agents for lower altitudes with biting insects)

- The setting (e.g., if you are going to a wilderness area with few trees, pack splints; if you anticipate humidity, bring fragrance-free powder to prevent chafing)

- The season (e.g., if you expect cold or hot weather, include a high-sugar drink solution or ample amounts of sunscreen)

- The terrain (e.g., if paddling or hiking long distances, bring blister supplies)

The number of people in your location, or the number of days you will be in a remote area, will also affect the kit you bring. For example, if you are preparing a disaster-readiness kit, you should have a 3-day minimum supply. You will also want to know what other group members have in their kits as this will help you add to or reduce the size of a group kit. This becomes more important particularly in activities where you expect to travel a long distance from definitive medical care. To keep kits manageable, know what things could be improvised from personal equipment (e.g., a t-shirt for a sling). Evaluate and repack your first aid kit before every trip.

Medications

In standard first aid, there is no recommended routine use of medication, except for aspirin in suspected heart attack cases, epinephrine auto-injectors for anaphylaxis, and antibiotic ointment or wound gel for some soft tissue injuries. When preparing for disasters or extended trips, you should have an adequate supply of medicine for routine issues in your disaster or first aid kit. For anticipated trips, healthcare professionals may be able to provide instructions or medications specific to the conditions you expect to be encountering (e.g., prescribing a medicine for altitude sickness or nausea and vomiting). As a trained first aid provider, you are *not* licensed to give medications; a person you are helping needs to be able to decide to take over-the-counter medications (i.e., they are competent and of age, or you have permission from their guardian). The person should only take oral medication if they can swallow and have no known contraindications. You can assist or have the person read and follow all label or healthcare provider instructions. Check state and local regulations regarding the use of prescription and over-the-counter medications.

For the long term, renew medications that have reached expiration dates and replace items that have been damaged by heat, cold or moisture on a regular basis. Do not fill your kit with items you do not know how to use. You—and all members of your group—must maintain a high level of familiarity with the proper uses of all the items in your disaster, remote or wilderness first aid kit. Remember that knowledge and skill are more valuable in an emergency than the contents of a kit.

Being Prepared . . . Homeland Security

Terrorism has been around for many years, yet the threat of terrorism is something that has been increasingly on the minds of Americans after the events of the past decade and the uncertainty about what lies in the future. As with any type of disaster, however, being informed about what is happening in the areas in which you live or travel, and having an emergency plan in place, are steps you can take now to prepare for and respond to future threats.

In response to public concerns after the attacks of September 11, 2001, the U.S. government launched the website *www.ready.gov* in order to educate and empower Americans to prepare for a wide spectrum of emergencies, whether human-made, such as terrorist acts, or natural. Go there to learn how you can best "prepare, plan and stay informed" both at home and in the work setting. In addition, *redcross.org* provides tips and information on how to prepare for, and respond to, a terrorist attack or other disaster situation.

Ensuring Adequate Preparation

Get trained. Take courses and talk to people with experience. Disaster professionals in your local health department, adventure guides, park rangers and Coast Guard personnel, as well as enthusiasts of the activity you will be engaged in, are good sources of information and training. You may find experienced people in clubs or in stores that sell equipment for the intended activity. Ask what preparations they recommend to make your experience safe and enjoyable. If possible, talk to more than one person to get a range of viewpoints.

Look for books, magazines and websites that include information on how to be prepared for common weather or natural events in your intended destination and risks associated with any activity. Find more than one source of written information so that you get more than one author's point of view. Also, find out about local emergency resources, including whether the emergency number is 9-1-1, and if not, what the designated emergency number is. Get other important phone numbers, such as for hospitals, clinics and law enforcement agencies. If traveling to a foreign country, find out whatever details you can about the medical care that is available.

As you work to be prepared individually and as a group, incorporate practice to assess knowledge, skills and behaviors. This practice should include skills for successful experiences, physical fitness and dealing with emergency scenarios. Scenario-based learning can be both fun and meaningful in developing skills and knowing limitations. The Wilderness and Remote First Aid program of the American Red Cross is one option for more in-depth training.

Being Prepared . . . For Every Type of Disaster

Since 2012, the American Red Cross has been actively developing and improving many disaster mobile apps for smart phones and tablets. To date, our selection of apps includes: First Aid, Emergency, Tornado, Earthquake, Hurricane, Wildfire and Flood, plus other non-disaster-related apps. The apps provide extensive just-in-time information on how to be prepared for a disaster before, during and after it occurs. This just-in-time information can even be accessible without mobile phone connectivity. When connectivity is available, these apps have storm tracker and alerting capability, as well as shelter locations in your community and real-time National Oceanic and Atmospheric Administration (NOAA) alerts/warnings.

Summary

Emergencies do not always happen where there is quick and easy access to advanced medical care. In delayed-help situations, such as those that may occur with disaster, remote and wilderness emergencies, you will need to be prepared to give care for a much longer time than usual.

As with all other emergencies, use the emergency action steps: **CHECK—CALL—CARE.** However, in a delayed-help situation, you will need to check the scene, the person and resources in detail before calling for help. You will also need to develop a more detailed plan for getting help and caring for the person for the long term. Getting help may involve calling for help, sending for help, leaving the person alone while you go for help, transporting the person to help or allowing the person to recover sufficiently so that they can walk to help.

In general, the care you give a person in a delayed-help situation is the same as what you have learned in previous chapters. However, you will spend more time caring for the person and assisting with their personal needs. Regularly checking the person's condition while waiting for help and writing down any changes that you find are important in a delayed-help situation. You may also need to protect the person from heat and cold by constructing a shelter if help is delayed for an extended period.

If you live in a region that is prone to natural disasters, or if you live in, work in or are planning to venture into a delayed-help environment, think about how you can reduce the risk of emergencies. Adequately preparing yourself for a delayed-help environment includes early planning, talking to people with experience, researching your location, finding out about local weather conditions and emergency resources, planning your route and constructing plans to deal with emergencies should they arise.

READY TO RESPOND?

Think back to Pete in the opening scenario, and use what you have learned to respond to these questions:

1. Is this a delayed-help situation? If so, what factors make it a delayed-help situation?

2. What dangers should you look for at the scene of Pete's injury?

3. What life-threatening conditions might Pete have, and what conditions might shortly become life threatening?

4. What do you think would be the best method for getting help in this situation? Why?

Study Questions

1. List five factors that contribute to a delayed-help situation, requiring trained lay responders to act differently.

2. List the four primary roles of a leader in a disaster, remote or wilderness emergency.

3. List four options for getting help in a delayed-help situation.

In questions 4 through 7, circle the letter of the correct answer.

4. During the emergency action steps, your priorities should include checking—

   a. The scene.   b. The person.   c. The resources.   d. All of the above

5. Periodically rechecking the person's condition while giving care until help arrives is necessary because—

   a. It helps you remember changes in their condition.
   b. The person may become hungry.
   c. It provides information for planning and action.
   d. The person needs to be comfortable.

6. A series or set of _____ signals can be used to signal "Help!"

   a. One   b. Three   c. Five   d. Ten

7. Which would you do if you would have to leave the person alone for an extended period?

   a. Write down the route you are going to take and the time you are leaving.
   b. Make sure the person has a shelter, food and water.
   c. Adjust any splints or bandages to ensure they are not too tight.
   d. All of the above

(Continued)

Study Questions continued

8. In the following scenario, circle the information you should consider before making a plan to get help.

You are trekking with your hiking club in Greenleaf National Forest and are now on a trail about 5 miles from the main road. As you are crossing a stream, a group member slips and falls into the icy water. You all help the member out and sit the person on the bank. The person is shivering violently in the cool breeze. They say their right knee is very painful and feels as if it is swelling. You notice overcast skies and estimate the temperature to be about 50° F (10° C). The sun will begin to set in about 4 hours. A group member gives you a sweater, which you substitute for the person's soaked jacket. Other group members provide clothing.

9. In the above scenario, what information would you share if you sent a small group to get help?

10. What are the three general types of preparation?

Answers are listed in the Appendix.

APPENDIX

Chapter 1

Answers to Ready to Respond? Questions

1. One person can call 9-1-1 or the designated emergency number on a mobile phone, or find a phone nearby; another can begin helping the person in the car if trained, or find a trained lay responder. Someone can keep the area free of onlookers and traffic. Someone could go find supplies, blankets or a first aid kit if needed.

2. Although you may feel ill and be incapacitated by the sight of blood or cries of pain, you can still help. If possible, turn away for a moment, take a few deep breaths and try to control your feelings. If you are still unable to proceed, make sure EMS personnel have been called. Then find other ways to help, such as asking bystanders to assist you or helping to keep the area safe.

Answers to Study Questions

1. a. I was fixing sandwiches and talking with my next-door neighbor, Mrs. Roberts, who had come by to borrow a book. My 3-year-old, Jenny, was in her room playing with some puzzles. As Mrs. Roberts got up to leave, **I heard a loud thump and a shriek from upstairs**.

   b. I was on the bus headed for work. A man from the back of the bus came down the aisle, and I noticed that **he was moving unsteadily**. It was cold in the bus, but **I noticed he was sweating and looked very pale. "I don't know where I am," I heard him mumble to himself**.

   c. On my way into the grocery store from the parking lot, **I heard the loud screech of tires and the crash of metal. I saw that a car had struck a telephone pole, causing the telephone pole to lean at an odd angle. Wires were hanging down from the pole onto the street**. It was very frightening.

2. Being uncertain than an emergency actually exists; being afraid of giving the wrong care or inadvertently causing the person more harm; assuming that the situation is already under control; squeamishness related to unpleasant sights, sounds or smells; fear of catching a disease; and fear of being sued.

3. A trained lay responder can overcome these fears or concerns by mentally preparing themselves to face these challenges ahead of time.

4. c, e, a, d, b, f

5. Calling, meeting and directing the ambulance; keeping the area free of unnecessary traffic; or giving first aid. Bystanders can go for additional supplies or give comfort to others on the scene. Finally, bystanders may be able to give you important information about the person or what happened.

Chapter 2

Answers to Ready to Respond? Questions

1. The main danger in the garage could be the presence of carbon monoxide. Another danger could be fumes from a spilled toxic substance or an electrical hazard.

2. The presence of poisonous fumes would be the major factor that could make you decide to move your friend immediately. Avoid breathing in poisonous fumes as you execute the move.

3. You would call 9-1-1 or the designated emergency number. Since you are alone, and your friend is unresponsive, it is a *call first* situation.

Answers to Study Questions

1. **CHECK—CALL—CARE**

2. Downed power lines; traffic; fire; dangerous fumes; freezing rain; broken glass; metal shards; spilled fuel.

3. Do not approach the person. Make sure you are a safe distance away and call 9-1-1 or the designated emergency number.

4. The exact location of the emergency (in this case, mile marker posts or landmarks can be helpful); what happened; the number of people involved; the person's condition; and the care being given. Tell the bystander to report back to you after making the call and tell you what the EMS call taker said.

5. *Call first;* that is, call 9-1-1 or the designated emergency number before giving care since the driver is unresponsive.

Chapter 3

Answers to Ready to Respond? Questions

1. After checking the scene to make sure it is safe, and obtaining consent to give care, you should take steps to prevent disease transmission, such as wearing disposable latex-free gloves to avoid contact with the boy's blood before checking him.

2. You should immediately wash your hands with soap and water after giving care.

Answers to Study Questions

1. a

2. d

3. b

4. a

5. c

6. When you must move the person to protect them from immediate danger. When you have to get to another person who may have a more serious problem. When it is necessary to give proper care.

7. Any dangerous conditions at the scene. The size of the person. The distance the person must be moved. Your physical ability. Whether others (bystanders) can help you. The person's condition. Any aids or equipment to facilitate moving the person at the scene.

8. Use your legs, not your back, when you bend. Bend at the knees and hips, and avoid twisting your body. Maintain a firm grip on the person. Walk forward when possible, taking small steps and watching where you are going to maintain a firm footing. Avoid twisting or bending anyone with a possible head, neck or spinal injury. Do not move a person who is too large to move comfortably. Use good posture.

9. Walking assist. Two-person seat carry. Clothes drag. Blanket drag. Ankle drag.

Chapter 4

Answers to Ready to Respond? Questions

1. The impact of an injury or a disease is rarely restricted to one body system. An injury to the head could affect the brain and nervous system, which could in turn affect breathing.

2. Nervous—he is unresponsive. Integumentary—he has a cut on his head.

Answers to Study Questions

1. (a) Respiratory (b) airway, lungs (c) circulatory (d) transports oxygen and other nutrients to cells and removes wastes (e) skin, hair, nails (f) part of the body's communication network, helps prevent infection and dehydration, assists with temperature regulation, aids in production of certain vitamins (g) bones, ligaments, muscles, tendons (h) supports body, allows movement, protects internal organs and structures, produces blood cells, stores minerals, produces heat (i) nervous (j) brain, spinal cord, nerves.

2. g, e, f, c, d, a, b

3. a

4. c

5. c

6. c

7. b

8. b

9. d

Chapter 5

Answers to Ready to Respond? Questions

1. Because of the person's location on the bike trail, you should try to guard against the possibility that another biker might round the curve and hit you or the person.

2. Interview the person using the SAMPLE questions and check the person from head to toe.

3. You or the other cyclist would need to call 9-1-1 or the designated emergency number. If neither of you have a mobile phone with you, one of you will need to leave the person to call 9-1-1 or the designated emergency number and then return to the person as soon as possible. You may be asked to meet EMS personnel and take them to the person.

Answers to Study Questions

1. Unresponsiveness; trouble breathing or breathing that is not normal (agonal breathing); absence of breathing; severe, life-threatening bleeding.

2. There's a stopped car on the road and a mangled bicycle that could cause another crash. There are also dangers from being in the middle of the street. You can use bystanders to direct traffic.

3. If the person is awake and has no life-threatening conditions, you can begin to check for other conditions that may need care. Checking a responsive person who is awake with no immediate life-threatening conditions involves two basic steps: interview the person and bystanders using the SAMPLE questions and check the person from head to toe.

4. 2, 1, 3, 5, 4

5. b

6. c

7. b

8. a

9. b

Chapter 6

Answers to Ready to Respond? Questions

1. Yes. The exertion of mowing grass in the heat can add an extra burden on the body, increasing its demand for oxygen. The heart works harder to keep up with the body's demand for oxygen, increasing its own oxygen needs. If the arteries are narrowed as a result of atherosclerosis, the delivery of oxygen-rich blood to the heart is severely restricted or completely cut off, causing the heart to beat irregularly or stop beating.

2. Resting eases the heart's need for oxygen.

3. If Mr. Getz is suffering cardiac arrest, his greatest chance of survival occurs when you follow the Cardiac Chain of Survival, starting with recognition of cardiac arrest and activation of the EMS system, followed by early CPR, early defibrillation, early advanced life support and integrated post-cardiac arrest care.

4. CPR—the combination of chest compressions and rescue breaths—helps maintain a low level of circulation in the body, but if Mr. Getz also has an abnormal heart rhythm (such as V-fib or V-tach), it needs to be corrected by defibrillation. Prompt CPR, early defibrillation and other advanced cardiac life support measures in combination are needed to sustain life.

Answers to Study Questions

1. c, f, d, b, a, e

2. The person will be unresponsive and not breathing, or only gasping.

3. You notice an obvious sign of life, such as normal breathing. An AED becomes available and is ready to use. Another trained responder or EMS personnel arrive and take over. You are too exhausted to continue. The scene becomes unsafe.

4. Breathing problems (such as airway obstruction, smoke inhalation, asthma attack and severe epiglottitis) and trauma (such as a motor-vehicle crash or a hard blow to the chest, drowning, electrocution, poisoning, firearm injuries and falls).

5. b

6. d

7. d

8. c

9. d

10. c

11. c

12. b

13. Her chest and shoulder hurt; she is sweating heavily; she is breathing fast; she looks ill.

14. 3, 2, 1, 4, 5

15. c

16. a

17. d

Chapter 7

Answers to Ready to Respond? Questions

1. If James could cough forcefully, cry or speak at all, you would know his airway was only partially blocked.

2. If James's airway was only partially blocked, you would encourage James to keep coughing to try to dislodge the object. If James could no longer speak, cough, cry or breathe, however, that would be a sign of a complete airway obstruction. You would need to give James 5 back blows, followed by 5 abdominal thrusts in order to try to dislodge the object.

3. Carefully lower James to the ground and begin CPR, starting with chest compressions. Before giving rescue breaths, open his mouth and look for the object. If an object is seen, remove it with your finger. If no object is seen, open James's airway using the head-tilt/chin-lift maneuver and attempt 2 rescue breaths, then resume CPR with compressions. Continue this process until the obstruction is cleared or your rescue breaths go in, then continue CPR.

Answers to Study Questions

1. a, b, d, e, c

2. When Rita walked into Mr. Boyd's office, **she found him collapsed** across his desk. His eyes were closed but she could hear him breathing, **making a high whistling noise.** He was **flushed, sweating** and seemed to be **trembling uncontrollably**. When he heard Rita, he raised his head a little. **"My chest hurts,"** he gasped, **"and I feel dizzy and can't seem to catch my breath."** He looked frightened.

3. Talking or laughing with their mouth full or eating too fast. Medical conditions (such as a neurological or muscular condition that affects the person's ability to chew, swallow or both). Dental problems or poorly fitting dentures that affect the person's ability to chew food properly.

4. c, a, b

5. d

6. b

7. a

8. b

9. c

10. a

11. 1, 3, 2, 5, 4

Chapter 8

Answers to Ready to Respond? Questions

1. The bleeding from Joe's wound is probably from a vein. The blood is flowing rather than spurting. Spurting would indicate that the bleeding is from an artery.

2. If not controlled, severe bleeding can reduce the blood volume in the body and become life threatening. An adequate amount of blood is needed to maintain the flow of oxygen-rich blood to the body, particularly to the vital organs.

3. You should use PPE, such as disposable latex-free gloves. If gloves are not available, you can also use plastic wrap, a clean folded cloth or have Joe use his hand to control the bleeding. You should also wash your hands after giving care even if you wore gloves.

Answers to Study Questions

1. b, a, d, g, f, e, c

2. Blood spurting or pouring from the wound; bleeding that fails to stop after direct pressure is applied.

3. Put on disposable latex-free gloves. If blood has the potential to splatter, you may need to wear eye and face protection. Cover the wound with a dressing and press firmly against the wound with a gloved hand. Apply a pressure bandage over the dressing to maintain pressure on the wound and to hold the dressing in place. If blood soaks through the dressing or bandage, reapply or redirect pressure to the wound. Consider alternative techniques to control bleeding, such as applying a tourniquet or a hemostatic dressing. Continue to monitor the person's condition. Observe the person closely for signs that may indicate that the person is developing shock. Take steps to minimize shock, such as helping the person to lie down and preventing them from getting chilled or overheated. Have the person rest comfortably and reassure them while waiting for EMS personnel to arrive. Wash your hands with soap and water immediately after giving care, even if you wore gloves.

4. Tender, swollen, bruised or rigid areas of the body, such as the abdomen; rapid breathing; skin that feels cool or moist or looks pale or bluish; vomiting blood or coughing up blood; excessive thirst; an injured extremity that is blue or extremely pale, swollen and rigid; an altered level of consciousness, such as the person becoming confused, faint, drowsy or unresponsive.

5. Internal bleeding.

6. a

Chapter 9

Answers to Ready to Respond? Questions

1. Her body could not compensate for her significant injuries, which probably involved severe bleeding.

2. You could care for shock by controlling any external bleeding as possible in the situation; having her lie flat on her back (supine); helping maintain her normal body temperature (e.g., covering her if she was getting chilled); offering reassurance and helping her rest comfortably; and monitoring her condition and watching for changes in her level of consciousness.

Answers to Study Questions

1. False. Shock can result from severe blood loss, as well as the loss of other body fluids; failure of the heart to pump enough oxygenated blood (resulting from trauma, disease, poisoning, respiratory distress); abnormal dilation of the blood vessels (resulting from spinal cord or brain trauma, infection, anaphylaxis); or injury to the chest, obstruction of the airway or any respiratory problem that decreases the amount of oxygen in the lungs.

2. Apprehension, anxiety, restlessness or irritability; altered level of consciousness; nausea or vomiting; pale, ashen or grayish, cool, moist skin; rapid breathing; rapid, weak heartbeat; excessive thirst.

3. Severe vomiting or diarrhea.

4. Take steps to control any external bleeding and prevent further blood loss. Immobilize his leg (using the ground for support) to prevent movement that could cause more bleeding and damage. Have him lie down flat on his back. Help maintain normal body temperature by covering him with a blanket. Do not give him anything to eat or drink, even though he is likely to be thirsty and may ask for a drink. Talk to him in a calm and reassuring manner to reduce the harmful effects of emotional stress and help him rest comfortably. Continue to monitor his breathing and for any changes in his condition.

5. d

6. b

7. d

8. b

Chapter 10

Answers to Ready to Respond? Questions

1. Jeremy has sustained a partial-thickness heat (thermal) burn, evidenced by his red skin and the formation of blisters caused by exposure to the heat.

2. Jeremy's burns will require medical attention as the burn is to his hands and blistered.

3. Call 9-1-1 or the designated emergency number. Stop the burning by removing Jeremy from the source of the burn. Check for life-threatening conditions. As soon as possible, cool the burn with large amounts of cold running water for at least 10 minutes or until pain is relieved. Cover the burn loosely with a dry, sterile dressing. Take steps to minimize shock. Have Jeremy lie down flat on his back, and keep him from getting chilled or overheated. Comfort and reassure Jeremy.

Answers to Study Questions

1. c, f, a, d, e, b

2. c, d, a, b

3. a, b, d, c

4. The area around the wound becomes swollen and red; the area may feel warm or throb with pain; there may be a pus discharge; more serious infections may cause a person to develop a fever and feel ill; red streaks may develop that progress from the wound.

5. Bandages are used to hold dressings in place, to apply pressure to control bleeding, to protect a wound from dirt and infection, and to provide support to an injured limb or body part.

6. Abrasion (skin that is rubbed or scraped away); laceration (cut with jagged or smooth edges); avulsion (a portion of the skin and sometimes other soft tissue is partially or completely torn away); amputation (a body part is severed); puncture/penetration (skin is pierced with a pointed object; sometimes results in an embedded objected); crush injury (a body part, usually an extremity, is subjected to a high degree of pressure).

7. Heat (thermal), electricity, chemicals, radiation.

8. a. Involves only the top layer of the skin (superficial). Skin is red and dry, and the burn is usually painful. The area may swell. Usually heals within a week without permanent scarring.

    b. Involves the top layers of the skin (partial thickness). May look red and have blisters. Blisters may open and weep clear fluid. Burned skin may look mottled. Burns are painful and often swell. Usually heals in 3 or 4 weeks. May scar.

    c. May destroy all layers of the skin and some or all of underlying structures (full thickness). Skin may look brown or charred (black). Tissues underneath may appear white. Burns can be extremely painful or relatively painless if the burn destroyed nerve endings. Healing requires medical assistance. Scarring is likely.

9. a

10. d

11. d

12. b

13. a

14. b

15. d

16. b

17. d

18. b

19. b

20. d

21. d

22. c

Chapter 11

Answers to Ready to Respond? Questions

1. Kelly likely sprained or strained her ankle or foot. A fracture is also a possibility.

2. A snapping sound at the time of the injury. The injured area is very painful to touch or move. There is significant bruising and swelling. There is significant deformity. She is unable to use the affected part normally. There are bone fragments sticking out of a wound. She feels bones grating. The injured area is cold, numb and tingly. The cause of the injury suggests that it may be severe.

3. Help Kelly rest in the most comfortable position; immobilize her foot, using the ground to support it; apply cold to the injured area for periods of 20 minutes on, 20 minutes off (if 20 minutes of cold cannot be tolerated, apply a cold pack for periods of 10 minutes); and elevate the injury above the level of the heart, only if it does not cause more pain.

Answers to Study Questions

1. h, b, f, c, a, i, k, d, j, g, e

2. There is obvious deformity; there is moderate or severe swelling and discoloration; bones sound or feel like they are rubbing together; a snap or pop was heard or felt at the time of the injury; there is a fracture with an open wound at, or bone piercing through, the injury site; the injured person cannot move or use the affected part normally; the injured area is cold and numb; the injury involves the head, neck or spine; the injured person has trouble breathing; the cause of the injury suggests that the injury may be severe; it is not possible to safely or comfortably move the person to a vehicle for transport to a hospital.

3. Splint only if you have to move the injured person and you can do so without causing more pain and discomfort to the person. Splint an injury in the position in which you find it; do not move, straighten or bend angulated bones or joints. Splint the injured area and the joints or bones above and below the injury site. Check for proper circulation (feeling, warmth and color) before and after splinting. If circulation has changed with splinting, loosen the splint slightly and reassess circulation.

4. c

5. b

6. b

7. a

8. b

Chapter 12

Answers to Ready to Respond? Questions

1. Yes. Sue's leg is bleeding and she cannot move her ankle without pain.

2. You should call 9-1-1 or the designated emergency number since there are signs and symptoms of a possible open fracture; stabilize the injury in the position found (do not use a splint as you cannot transport Sue yourself without a vehicle); control external bleeding (do not use direct pressure on an open fracture; instead apply pressure around the wound); apply a cold pack if available; and take steps to minimize shock. If shock is suspected, assess for other injuries and have Sue lie down flat on her back if possible. You should also help reassure Sue until EMS personnel arrive.

Answers to Study Questions

1. c, b, d, a

2. Falling on the hand of an outstretched arm.

3. A dislocation or fracture of the shoulder and a fractured leg.

4. Left arm looks deformed at the shoulder. No sensation in the fingers of that arm, arm is beginning to look bruised and is painful. Unable to move the leg, which is beginning to swell.

5. Call 9-1-1 or the designated emergency number; immobilize the injured parts in the position found; apply a cold pack, placing gauze or cloth between the cold pack and the skin; help the person rest in the most comfortable position; prevent them from becoming chilled or overheated; reassure the person. Continue to monitor the person's level of consciousness, breathing, skin color and temperature. Be alert for any signs, such as changes in breathing rate, skin color or level of consciousness that may indicate the person's condition is worsening. If needed, take steps to minimize shock.

6. Injured leg is noticeably shorter than the other leg; injured leg may be turned outward. Additional signs and symptoms include severe pain and inability to move the lower extremity.

7. Soft, rigid and anatomic.

8. b

9. c

10. Do not move or straighten the injured area. Stabilize the injury in the position found. If the person's lower extremity is supported by the ground, do not move it. Use rolled towels or blankets to support the leg in the position in which you found it. Control any external bleeding with direct pressure, unless the bleeding is located directly over a suspected fracture. With a fracture, apply pressure around the area. If you must transport or move the person, and it does not cause more pain, create an anatomic splint by securing the injured lower extremity to the uninjured lower extremity with several wide cravats placed above and below the site of the injury. Place a pillow or rolled blanket between the lower extremities, and bind them together above and below the site of the injury. Apply a cold pack. Take steps to minimize shock.

Chapter 13

Answers to Ready to Respond? Questions

1. No. Signs or symptoms could develop later. He did strike his head and could have a concussion or have injured his neck or back in doing so.

2. Since the person cannot move his arms, you should suspect a serious head, neck or spinal injury. Have the person remain still and keep their head in the position it is in until EMS personnel arrive. Check for life-threatening conditions, monitor responsiveness and breathing, and take steps to minimize shock.

Answers to Study Questions

1. d, b, a, c

2. A person is unresponsive; was involved in a motor-vehicle crash or subjected to another significant force; was injured as a result of a fall from greater than the person's standing height; is wearing a safety helmet that is broken; complains of neck or back pain; has tingling or weakness in the extremities; is not fully awake; appears to be intoxicated; appears to be frail or older than 65 years; is a child younger than 3 years with evidence of a head or neck injury.

3. Changes in the level of consciousness; severe pain or pressure in the head, neck or spine; tingling or loss of sensation in the extremities; partial or complete loss of movement of any body part; observable, unusual bumps or depressions on the head or neck; sudden loss of memory; blood or other fluids in the ears or nose; profuse external bleeding of the head, neck or back; seizures in a person who does not have a seizure disorder; impaired breathing or impaired vision as a result of injury; nausea or vomiting; persistent headache; loss of balance; bruising of the head, especially around the eyes or behind the ears.

4. Place the person in a face-up position and enlist someone to help stabilize the person's head. Do not attempt to remove any object embedded in the eye. Stabilize the object by encircling the eye with a gauze dressing or soft sterile cloth, being careful not to apply any pressure to the area. Position bulky dressings, such as roller gauze, around the impaled object and then cover it with a shield such as a paper cup. Do not use Styrofoam®-type materials, as small particles can break off and get into the eye. The shield should not touch the object. Bandage the shield and dressing in place with a self-adhering bandage and roller bandage covering the person's injured eye, as well as the uninjured eye, to keep the object stable and minimize movement. Comfort and reassure the person. Do not leave the person unattended.

5. d

6. d

7. c

8. c

9. a

10. b

11. d

12. Do not put direct pressure on the wound; attempt to control bleeding with pressure on the area around the wound; secure the dressings with a roller bandage or triangular bandage; call 9-1-1 or the designated emergency number.

Chapter 14

Answers to Ready to Respond? Questions

1. The person is holding his chest and his breathing sounds shallow as if it is painful to breathe. Both are common signs and symptoms of a rib fracture.

2. You should have the man rest in a position that will make breathing easier and encourage him to breathe normally if tolerated. You should also give him a blanket, pillow or other similar available object to hold against his ribs to support and immobilize the area. If supplies are available, you could also use a sling and binder to hold the person's arm against the injured side of the body. In addition, you should monitor breathing and take steps to minimize shock.

Answers to Study Questions

1. c, a, b, e, d

2. Call 9-1-1 or the designated emergency number; limit movement; monitor breathing and signs of life; control bleeding; take steps to minimize shock.

3. Trouble breathing or no breathing; severe pain at the site of the injury; flushed, pale, ashen or bluish skin; obvious deformity, such as that caused by a fracture; coughing up blood (may be bright red or dark like coffee grounds); bruising at the site of a blunt injury, such as that caused by a seat belt; a "sucking" noise or distinct sound when the person breathes.

4. Severe abdominal pain; bruising; external bleeding; nausea; vomiting (sometimes vomit containing blood); pale, or ashen, cool, moist skin; weakness; thirst; pain, tenderness or a tight feeling in the abdomen; organs protruding from the abdomen; rigid abdominal muscles; signs and symptoms of shock.

5. a

6. A sucking chest wound (an open chest wound).

7. Trouble breathing; considerable pain at the site of the injury; a sucking sound from the chest when the person breathes.

8. Call 9-1-1 or the designated emergency number; control any major bleeding, but do not allow the wound to become occluded by a dressing or bandage; do *not* cover or seal the wound; monitor the person's breathing; take steps to minimize shock.

Chapter 15

Answers to Ready to Respond? Questions

1. Paul is likely having a diabetic emergency based on the information given by the receptionist that he has diabetes and skipped lunch after exercising vigorously on his break—risk factors for hypoglycemia. A change in level of consciousness is also a sign of a diabetic emergency.

2. Check Paul for responsiveness and normal breathing. If he is not responding but breathing normally, you should ask the receptionist to call 9-1-1 or the designated emergency number, and then care for Paul as you would any unresponsive person who is breathing normally. This includes interviewing any bystanders using the SAMPLE questions; conducting a head-to-toe check and placing him in a recovery position if no injuries are found; making sure his airway is clear of any vomit; monitoring his breathing and giving care until advanced medical personnel take over.

3. If a person is unresponsive or responsive but not fully awake, you should not give the person anything by mouth—including a form of sugar for a diabetic emergency.

Answers to Study Questions

1. f, c, h, g, e, d, b, i, a

2. A person with a sudden illness may have any of these signs or symptoms: changes in level of consciousness such as drowsiness, confusion, or unresponsiveness; numbness, tingling, light-headedness, dizziness or giddiness; breathing problems (i.e., trouble breathing or no breathing); signs and symptoms of a possible heart attack, including persistent chest pain, discomfort or pressure lasting more than a few minutes that goes away and comes back or that spreads to the shoulder, arm, neck, jaw, stomach or back; signs and symptoms of a stroke, including sudden weakness on one side of the face (facial droop); sudden weakness, often on one side of the body; sudden slurred speech or trouble forming words; a sudden, severe headache; loss of vision or blurred vision; signs and symptoms of shock, including rapid breathing, changes in skin appearance and cool, pale or ashen (grayish) skin; sweating; persistent abdominal pain or pressure; nausea or vomiting; diarrhea and abdominal cramping; seizures.

3. Do no further harm; monitor the person's level of consciousness and breathing; help the person rest in the most comfortable position or the position recommended for a specific condition; keep the person from getting chilled or overheated; comfort and reassure the person, but do not provide false hope; give any specific care as needed.

4. After the seizure passes, position the person on their side in a recovery position so that fluids (saliva, blood, vomit) can drain from the mouth. Check to see if the person was injured during the seizure. Offer comfort and reassurance, especially if the seizure occurred in public, as the person may feel embarrassed and self-conscious. If this is the case, keep bystanders well back to provide maximum privacy, and stay with the person until they are fully awake and aware of their surroundings. If this is the person's first seizure, or if the cause of the seizure is unknown, call 9-1-1 or the designated emergency number if you have not already done so as part of the scene size-up.

5. a

6. c

7. c

8. a

9. b

10. a

11. c

12. a

Chapter 16

Answers to Ready to Respond? Questions

1. Your cousin is wiping something from Sophia's mouth and looking distressed. Sophia is seated next to cleaning supplies that were on the floor.

2. Although Sophia is young, you could try to have her tell you what bottles she might have touched or tasted. You should also call the national Poison Help line for advice and information, and watch for any signs and symptoms that might develop if Sophia ingested or absorbed a poison. You'll need to tell the national Poison Help line what substances she potentially had contact with.

Answers to Study Questions

1. e, b, f, c, a, d

2. Remove the person from the source of poison if the scene is dangerous. Do this only if you are able to without endangering yourself or bystanders. Check the person's level of consciousness and breathing. For life-threatening conditions, such as if the person is unresponsive or is not breathing, or if a change in the level of consciousness occurs, call 9-1-1 or the designated emergency number immediately and care for any life-threatening conditions. If the person is awake, ask questions to get more information. Look for any containers and/or packaging and take them with you to the telephone. Call the national Poison Help line at 800-222-1222 and follow any directions given.

3. The type and amount of the substance; the time that has elapsed since the poison entered the body; and the person's age, size (build), weight and medical conditions.

4. Follow standard precautions and then immediately rinse the affected area thoroughly with water. In the case of poison ivy, using soap cannot hurt, but soap may not do much to remove the poisonous plant oil that causes the allergic reaction. Before washing the affected area, you may need to have the person remove any jewelry. This is only necessary if the jewelry is contaminated or if it constricts circulation due to swelling. Rinse the affected areas for at least 20 minutes, using a shower or garden hose if possible. If a rash or weeping lesion (an oozing sore) develops, advise the person to seek additional advice from a pharmacist or healthcare provider.

5. If a person is unresponsive, confused or seems to be losing responsiveness; has trouble breathing; has persistent chest pain or pressure; has pressure or pain in the abdomen that does not go away; is vomiting blood or passing blood in the stool or urine; exhibits signs of shock such as pale, ashen or grayish, cool, moist skin; has a seizure, severe headache or slurred speech; acts aggressively or violently.

6. Itching and burning hands; swollen fingers; red bumps all over her forearm.

7. Wear gloves to protect her hands when gardening.

8. d

9. c

10. a

Chapter 17

Answers to Ready to Respond? Questions

1. Given Sara's report that she was bitten by a tick last week, and now has a rash appearing in various spots on her body, Sara could potentially have Rocky Mountain Spotted Fever.

2. While you cannot provide first aid for Rocky Mountain Spotted Fever, you can help Sara by following general care guidelines for an unknown sudden illness. These steps include: do no further harm; monitor Sara's level of consciousness and breathing; help Sara rest in the most comfortable position or the position recommended for a specific condition; keep Sara from getting chilled or overheated; comfort and reassure Sara, but do not provide false hope; and give any specific care as needed. In addition, you should advise Sara's parents that you observed signs and symptoms that could indicate a tickborne illness and recommend that she visit her healthcare provider for follow-up.

Answers to Study Questions

1. a, b, d, c

2. With a gloved hand, grasp the tick with fine-tipped, pointed, non-etched, non-rasped tweezers as close to the skin as possible and pull slowly, steadily and firmly upward. If you do not have tweezers, use a glove, plastic wrap, a piece of paper or a leaf to protect your fingers. Wash the bite area with soap and warm water. Apply antiseptic or antibiotic ointment to help prevent infection. Wash your hands thoroughly. If a rash, flu-like signs and symptoms or joint pain develop, seek medical attention.

3. Presence of a stinger; pain; swelling; redness; signs and symptoms of an allergic reaction.

4. Call 9-1-1 or the designated emergency number. Wash the site with soap and water. Keep the injured area still and lower than the heart. The person should walk only if absolutely necessary.

5. a

6. d

7. b

8. d

9. a

10. d

Chapter 18

Answers to Ready to Respond? Questions

1. The signs and symptoms exhibited by Tom are talkativeness, then a sudden mood change and becoming unresponsive.

2. The signs and symptoms of Tom's condition, along with the fact that he has been drinking, seem to indicate a case of alcohol poisoning. There could, however, be some other type of emergency that caused the same signs and symptoms.

3. Yes, you should call 9-1-1 or the designated emergency number because EMS personnel should be called in cases when someone becomes unresponsive.

Answers to Study Questions

1. f, c, d, e, a, h, b, g

2. Behavioral changes not otherwise explained; sudden mood changes; restlessness, talkativeness or irritability; changes in level of consciousness, including becoming unresponsive; slurred speech or poor coordination; moist or flushed skin; chills, nausea or vomiting; dizziness or confusion; abnormal breathing.

3. Stimulants; hallucinogens; depressants; opioid narcotics; inhalants; cannabis products.

4. Read the product information and use products only as directed. Ask your physician or pharmacist about the intended use and side effects of prescription and over-the-counter medication. If you are taking more than one medication, check for possible interaction effects. Never use another person's prescribed medications. Always keep medications in their appropriate, marked containers. Destroy all out-of-date medications by dropping them off at local medication disposal sites. Always keep medications out of the reach of children.

5. Check the scene to be sure it is safe to help the person. Do not approach the person if they are behaving in a threatening manner. Call 9-1-1 or the designated emergency number immediately if the person is unresponsive, confused or responsive but not fully awake; has trouble breathing or is breathing irregularly; has persistent chest pain or pressure; has pain or pressure in the abdomen that does not go away; is vomiting blood or passing blood; has a seizure, a severe headache or slurred speech; or acts violently. If none of the above conditions are present, and you have good reason to suspect a substance was taken, call the national Poison Help line at 800-222-1222 and follow the call taker's directions. Try to learn from the person or others what substances may have been taken. Calm and reassure the person. Keep the person from getting chilled or overheated.

6. b, c, a, d, e, f

7. c

8. b

Chapter 19

Answers to Ready to Respond? Questions

1. Kelly is showing signs and symptoms of hypothermia, including shivering and impaired judgment (wanting to just stop walking despite the fact she is cold and the conditions are unpleasant).

2. The wind and rain; the fact that Kelly does not have enough layers to put on to keep her warm and dry in the conditions.

3. Your priority should be getting Kelly to a warmer place.

Answers to Study Questions

1. c, e, d, a, b

2. Air temperature; humidity; wind.

3. Exercise-associated muscle cramps; exertional heat exhaustion; heat stroke.

4. Cool, pale, clammy or slightly flushed skin; fatigue; nausea and/or vomiting; loss of appetite; dehydration; dizziness with possible fainting; elevated heart and respiratory rate; muscle cramps.

5. The person's condition does not improve; the person refuses fluids; there is a change in the person's level of consciousness; the person vomits.

6. Rapidly cool the body by immersing the person up to the neck in cold water (preferred); douse the person with ice-water-soaked towels over the entire body, frequently rotating the cold, wet towels, spraying with cold water, fanning the person, or covering the person with ice towels or bags of ice placed over the body.

7. Frostbite; hypothermia.

8. Avoid being outdoors in the hottest or coldest part of the day. Dress appropriately for the environment and your activity level. Change your activity level according to the temperature. Take frequent breaks by removing yourself from the environment. Drink large amounts of nonalcoholic or non-caffeinated fluids before, during and after activity.

9. a

10. d

11. Lack of feeling in fingers; fingers look waxy and white and feel cold.

12. Keep your friend inside where it is warm. Handle the area gently. Because there is no reason to believe the part will refreeze, rapidly rewarm the affected part using skin-to-skin contact such as with a warm hand. Loosely bandage the area with dry, sterile dressings. Place dry, sterile gauze between the fingers to keep them separated. Avoid breaking any blisters. Take precautions to prevent hypothermia. Monitor the person and care for shock. Do not give any ibuprofen or other nonsteroidal anti-inflammatory drugs. Seek emergency medical care as soon as possible.

13. No response to your questions; glassy eyes; seems weak and exhausted; does not seem to feel your touch.

14. Call 9-1-1 or the designated emergency number. Move the person into a warmer environment if possible. Make the person comfortable. Remove any wet clothing and dry the person if needed. Put on dry clothing if available. Warm the body gradually by wrapping the woman in blankets and plastic sheeting to hold in body heat. Also, keep her head covered to further retain body heat. Keep the woman positioned near a heat source or apply heating pads or other heat sources to the body, such as containers filled with warm water. Carefully monitor any heat source to avoid burning the person. If the person is alert and can swallow, give warm liquids that do not contain alcohol or caffeine. Check breathing, monitor for any changes in the person's condition and care for shock.

Chapter 20

Answers to Ready to Respond? Questions

1. You can make a reaching assist by firmly bracing yourself on the pool deck and using an object that you find near the pool (e.g., pole, oar, towel) to extend your reach. You may also attempt a reach by lying down on the pool deck and extending your arm or leg for the child to grab. Another option is to throw an item that floats, such as a picnic jug, an air mattress or an inflatable toy, out to the child with a line attached. Try to throw it over the child's shoulder, with the line resting on the shoulder. The child can grasp the object and then be pulled to safety. Remember that your first priority is to stay safe. By rushing into the water to help a person, you could become a drowning victim, too.

Answers to Study Questions

1. Reaching assist; throwing assist; wading assist.

2. A drowning victim—active could be at the surface or sinking. They could be positioned vertically in the water and leaning back slightly. This person may not have a supporting kick or the ability to move forward. The person's arms could be at the side pressing down in an instinctive attempt to keep the head above water to breathe. All energy is going into the struggle to breathe, and the person may not be able to call out for help.

3. d

4. c

5. If it is safe to do so and you are trained, make sure the person is face-up in the water. Open the person's airway and check for breathing for no more than 10 seconds. If they are breathing normally, hold the person steady in the water until advanced help arrives. If the person is not breathing, remove the person from the water immediately and begin CPR, starting with chest compressions.

Chapter 21

Answers to Ready to Respond? Questions

1. Falls in older adults are due to slower reflexes, failing eyesight and hearing, arthritis, and problems such as unsteady balance and movement. However, Grandma Mary should be fully checked to ensure that another condition did not lead to her fall, such as a sudden illness or musculoskeletal injury.

2. You should get at Grandma Mary's eye level so that she can see and hear you more clearly. If she seems confused at first, the confusion may be the result of her impaired hearing. Speak slowly and clearly, and look at her face while you talk. Notice if she has her hearing aid in. If not, it may be helpful to have your friend find it so she can put it in. If Grandma Mary seems truly confused, try to find out if the confusion is the result of the injury, sudden illness or a condition she already has. Information from your friend may be helpful.

Answers to Study Questions

1. d, c, f, b, e, a

2. Check the scene for safety. Have a bystander call 9-1-1 or the designated emergency number. Introduce yourself as someone who knows first aid and ask permission from the parent to give care. Observe the child before actually touching them. Look for signs and symptoms that indicate changes in the level of consciousness, any trouble breathing, and any apparent injuries and conditions. Realize that the situation may change as soon as you touch the child because they may become more anxious and upset. Allow the child's mother to stay with the child to help comfort the child, and reassure both the parent and child. Ask the child simple questions to find out what is wrong. Whenever necessary (e.g., when the child is agitated), begin your check of the child who is awake at their toes and work your way to their head if no life-threatening conditions have been found.

3. Introduce yourself and explain that you are there to help. Get consent to give care. Ask the woman her name and use it when you speak to her. Tell her to lie still; as part of your SAMPLE questions, try to find out from the neighbor if the woman is generally confused or is taking any medication. Have the neighbor call 9-1-1 or the designated emergency number if you have not done so already. Reassure and comfort the person. Support and immobilize the injured area, probably using blankets and pillows.

4. d

5. b

6. b

7. b

8. c

9. d

10. Diseases such as Alzheimer's disease; medication; vision or hearing loss; head injury; medical emergency such as illness or infection; depression.

11. If a hostile person refuses your care or threatens you, remove yourself from the situation and stay at a safe distance. Never argue with or restrain an injured or ill person. Call 9-1-1 or the designated emergency number if someone has not already done so. Never put your own safety at risk.

Chapter 22

Answers to Ready to Respond? Questions

1. Because this is Lisa's first pregnancy, she is probably still in stage one of labor, but getting close to stage two. The fact that her water has broken is often a sign that labor is beginning.

2. Lisa can tell you if this is a first pregnancy; if she expects any complications; if there has been a bloody discharge; how close together and strong the contractions are, and when she began to have them; and if she has the urge to bear down or push.

Answers to Study Questions

1. h, g, c, e, f, a, d, b

2. Stage one: dilation—the mother's body prepares for birth; from the first contraction until the cervix is completely dilated. Stage two: expulsion—begins when the cervix is completely dilated and includes the baby's movement through the birth canal and delivery. Stage three: placental delivery—the placenta separates from the wall of the uterus and is expelled from the birth canal. Stage four: stabilization—the initial recovery and stabilization of the mother after childbirth.

3. See that the airway is open and clear; maintain normal body temperature.

4. b

5. d

6. a

7. b

8. c

9. c

Chapter 23

Answers to Ready to Respond? Questions

1. The fact that you are traveling by kayak on a river, at least 2 miles from help without a vehicle or way to call, all make this a delayed-help situation as it will very likely take more than 30 minutes for you to get help for Pete.

2. When checking the scene, you should check for dangerous conditions due to the water, such as loose or slippery rocks where he is trying to stand up near the shore. You should be sure there are no environmental hazards, such as wild animals or impending severe weather.

3. Pete is bleeding profusely from two wounds, including one in his abdomen. If left uncontrolled, bleeding can be life threatening. An injury to the abdomen could also cause internal injuries if the force was enough, and this could also be life threatening. Because Pete is also wet, he could be prone to hypothermia as well, and is at increased risk for shock.

4. Because you have no means of calling for help, but know that there is a scheduled pick-up point 2 miles down the river, and there are enough people available with the proper equipment to go safely, you should send a kayak ahead for help in this situation. Ideally, you should send them with a note explaining Pete's condition; a map indicating the location of the emergency; a list of other members in the group; a list of available resources; a description of the weather, terrain and access routes if known; and the group's list of immediate and long-term plans, with possible contingency plans if needed.

Answers to Study Questions

1. Time and/or distance that prevents access to swift advanced medical help. Hazards created by the environment, weather, location or time of day. Unavailability of EMS due to overwhelming need. Unavailability of EMS due to lack of workers or damaged equipment. Scene safety issues that demand special skills and resources. Lack of adequate first aid equipment. Issues related to managing resources, people and your own well-being for an extended amount of time.

2. Manage scene safety. Take a big-picture view of the scene. Care for life-threatening conditions and non-life-threatening conditions (directly or indirectly). Provide evacuation direction for the group.

3. Stay where you are and call, radio or signal for help. Send someone to go get help or leave the person alone to get help. Transport the person to help. Care for the person where you are until the person has recovered enough to travel on their own.

4. d

5. c

6. b

7. d

8. You are trekking with your hiking club in Greenleaf National Forest and are now on a trail **about 5 miles from the main road**. As you are crossing **a stream**, a **group member slips and falls into the icy water**. You all help the member out and sit the person on the bank. **The person is shivering violently** in the **cool breeze**. They say their **right knee is very painful and feels as if it is swelling**. You notice **overcast skies** and **estimate the temperature to be about 50° F** (10° C). The **sun will begin to set in about 4 hours**. **A group member gives you a sweater, which you substitute for the person's soaked jacket. Other group members provide clothing**.

9. Information you would share includes the person's name and condition; care given; names and contact information of all people in the group; resources available; a map indicating the location of the person; a description of the weather, terrain and access routes if known; and a list of immediate and long-term plans, as well as contingency plans.

10. Knowledge, skills and equipment.

GLOSSARY

Abandonment: Ending the care of an injured or ill person without obtaining that person's consent or without ensuring that someone with equal or greater training will continue care.

Abdomen: The middle part of the trunk, containing the stomach, liver, intestines and spleen.

Abdominal thrusts: Inward and upward thrusts just above the navel, used in combination with back blows to force the object out of the airway when a person is choking.

Abrasion: The most common type of open wound; characterized by skin that has been rubbed or scraped away.

Absence seizure: A type of generalized seizure in which there are minimal or no movements; the person may appear to have a blank stare; also known as a petit mal or nonconvulsive seizure.

Absorbed poison: A poison that enters the body through the skin.

Acute: Having a rapid and severe onset, then quickly subsiding.

Addiction: The compulsive need to use a substance; stopping use would cause the user to suffer mental, physical and emotional distress.

Adhesive compress: A small pad of nonstick gauze on a strip of adhesive tape, applied directly to minor wounds.

Advanced cardiac life support (ACLS): Techniques and treatments designed for use by EMS personnel with victims of cardiac emergencies.

Advanced emergency medical technician (AEMT): A person trained to give basic and limited advanced emergency medical care and transportation for critical and emergent patients who access the emergency medical services (EMS) system.

Agonal breathing: Irregular or gasping breaths. In an unresponsive person, isolated or infrequent gasping in the absence of normal breathing; can occur even after the heart has stopped beating. Agonal breaths are a sign of cardiac arrest.

Airway obstruction: Complete or partial blockage of the airway, which prevents air from reaching a person's lungs; a common cause of respiratory emergencies.

Allergens: Substances that induce allergies.

Alzheimer's disease: The most common type of dementia in older people, in which thought, memory and language are impaired.

Amniotic sac: "Bag of waters"; sac that encloses the fetus during pregnancy and bursts during the birthing process.

Amputation: The complete removal or severing of an external body part.

Anaphylaxis: A severe, life-threatening allergic reaction. A form of distributive shock caused by an often sudden severe allergic reaction, in which air passages may swell and restrict breathing; also referred to as anaphylactic shock.

Anatomical airway obstruction: Complete or partial blockage of the airway by the tongue or swollen tissues of the mouth, throat or other airway structures.

Anatomy: The study of structures, including gross anatomy (structures that can be seen with the naked eye) and microscopic anatomy (structures seen under the microscope).

Aneurysm: An abnormal bulging of an artery due to weakness in the blood vessel; may occur in the aorta (main artery of the heart), brain, leg or other location.

Angina pectoris: Pain in the chest that comes and goes at different times; caused by a lack of oxygen reaching the heart.

Anorexia nervosa: An eating disorder characterized by a long-term refusal to eat food with sufficient nutrients and calories.

Antihistamine: A medication that counteracts the effects of histamine, a chemical released by the body during an allergic reaction.

Antitoxins: Antibodies capable of neutralizing specific disease-producing poisonous substances.

Antivenom: A substance used to counteract the poisonous effects of venom.

Arteries: Large blood vessels that carry oxygen-rich blood from the heart to all parts of the body, except for the pulmonary arteries, which carry oxygen-poor blood from the heart to the lungs.

Aspiration: Inhalation of blood, vomit, saliva or other foreign material into the lungs.

Asthma: An ongoing condition in which the airways swell; the air passages can become constricted or blocked when affected by various triggers.

Asthma action plan: A written plan that the person develops with their healthcare provider that details daily management of the condition as well as how to handle an asthma attack.

Asystole: A condition in which the heart has stopped generating electrical activity.

Atherosclerosis: A condition in which deposits of plaque, including cholesterol (a fatty substance made by the liver and found in foods containing animal or animal products) build up on the inner walls of the arteries, causing them to harden and narrow, reducing the amount of blood that can flow through; develops gradually and can go undetected for many years.

Aura: An unusual sensation or feeling that may signal the onset of a seizure in some people. An aura can include a strange sound, taste or smell, or an urgent need to get to safety.

Aura phase: The first stage of a generalized seizure, during which the person experiences perceptual disturbances, often visual or olfactory in nature.

Automated external defibrillator (AED): A portable electronic device that analyzes the heart's electrical rhythm and, if necessary, can deliver an electric shock to a person in cardiac arrest.

Avulsion: An injury in which a portion of the skin, and sometimes other soft tissue, is partially or completely torn away.

Back blows: Blows between the shoulder blades, used in combination with abdominal thrusts to force the object out of the airway when a person is choking.

Bacteria: One-celled organisms that can cause infection; a common type of pathogen.

Bandage: Material used to wrap or cover a part of the body; commonly used to hold a dressing or splint in place.

Bandage compress: A thick gauze dressing attached to a bandage.

Binder: A cloth wrapped around a person to securely hold the arm against the person's chest to add stability; also called a *swathe*.

Birth canal: The passageway from the uterus to the outside of the body through which a baby passes during birth.

Blood volume: The total amount of blood circulating within the body.

Blunt trauma: Injury caused by impact with a flat object or surface; a common cause of internal bleeding.

Body system: A group of organs and other structures that work together to carry out specific functions.

Bone: A dense, hard tissue that forms the skeleton.

Braxton Hicks contractions: False labor; irregular contractions of the uterus that do not intensify or become more frequent as genuine labor contractions do.

Breathing emergency: An emergency in which breathing is impaired; can become life threatening; also called a respiratory emergency.

Breech birth: The delivery of a baby's feet or buttocks first.

Bronchitis: A disease resulting in inflammation of the lining of the trachea, bronchi and bronchioles.

Bulimia: An eating disorder characterized by eating excessively then purging unwanted calories by vomiting or using laxatives.

Burn: An injury to the skin or to other body tissues caused by heat, chemicals, electricity or radiation.

Cannabis products: Substances such as marijuana and hashish that are derived from the *Cannabis sativa* plant; can produce feelings of elation, distorted perceptions of time and space, and impaired motor coordination and judgment.

Capillaries: Tiny blood vessels linking arteries and veins; they transfer oxygen and other nutrients from the blood to all body cells and remove waste products.

Cardiac arrest: A condition in which the heart has stopped beating or beats too irregularly or weakly to pump blood effectively.

Cardiac Chain of Survival: Five actions that, when performed in rapid succession, increase the person's likelihood of surviving cardiac arrest.

Cardiopulmonary resuscitation (CPR): A technique that combines chest compressions and rescue breaths to circulate blood containing oxygen to the brain and other vital organs for a person whose heart and normal breathing have stopped.

Carpals: The bones of the wrist.

Cells: The basic units that combine to form all living tissue.

Cerebral palsy: A dysfunction of the central nervous system in which a person has little or no control of the muscles.

Certification: Credentialing at the local level; usually entails completing a probationary period and updating and/or recertification to cover changing knowledge and skills.

Cervix: The lower, narrow part of the uterus (womb) that forms a canal that opens into the vagina, which leads to the outside of the body; upper part of the birth canal.

Chest: The upper part of the trunk, containing the heart, major blood vessels and lungs.

Chest thrusts: Thrusts to the chest to force the object out of the airway when a person is choking.

Child abuse: Action that results in the physical or psychological harm of a child; can be physical, sexual, verbal and/or emotional.

Child neglect: The most frequently reported type of child abuse in which a parent or guardian fails to provide the necessary, age-appropriate care to a child; insufficient medical or emotional attention or respect given to a child.

Cholesterol: A fatty substance made by the liver and found in foods containing animal or animal products; diets high in cholesterol contribute to the risk of heart disease.

Chronic: Persistent over a long period of time.

Chronic obstructive pulmonary disease (COPD): A progressive lung disease in which the person has difficulty breathing because of damage to the lungs; the airways become obstructed and air sacs lose their ability to fill with air.

Circulatory system: A group of organs and other structures that carry blood and other nutrients throughout the body and remove waste.

Circumferential burn: A burn that encircles an extremity; considered a critical burn requiring immediate medical attention.

Clavicle: The collarbone; the slender, curved bone that extends from the sternum to the scapula (shoulder blade).

Clonic phase: The third phase of a generalized seizure, during which the person experiences the seizure itself.

Closed fracture: A type of fracture in which the skin over the broken bone is intact.

Closed wound: A wound in which soft tissue damage occurs beneath the skin and the skin is not broken.

Clotting: The process by which blood thickens at a wound site to seal an opening in a blood vessel and stop bleeding.

Compartment syndrome: Condition in which there is swelling and an increase in pressure within a limited space that presses on and compromises blood vessels, nerves and tendons that run through that limited space; usually involves the leg, forearm, arm, thigh, shoulder or buttock.

Competence: The injured or ill person's ability to understand the responder's questions and the implications of the decisions made.

Complex partial seizure: A type of partial seizure in which the person may experience an altered mental status or be unresponsive.

Compression-only CPR: A CPR technique that involves giving continuous chest compressions, with no rescue breaths.

Concussion: A temporary loss of brain function caused by a blow to the head.

Consent: Permission to receive emergency care granted by a competent adult either verbally or nonverbally.

Contraction: During labor, the rhythmic tightening and relaxing of muscles in the uterus.

Contusion: An injury to the soft tissues that results in blood vessel damage (usually to capillaries) and leakage of blood into the surrounding tissues; caused when blood vessels are damaged or broken as the result of a blow to the skin, resulting in swelling and a reddish-purple discoloration on the skin; commonly referred to as a bruise.

Coronary arteries: Blood vessels that supply the heart muscle with oxygen-rich blood.

Coronary heart disease (CHD): A disease in which cholesterol and plaque build up on the inner walls of the arteries that supply blood to the heart; also called *coronary artery disease* (CAD).

Critical burn: Any burn that is potentially life threatening, disabling or disfiguring; a burn requiring advanced medical care.

Croup: A common upper airway virus that affects children under the age of 5; marked by a harsh, repetitive cough.

Crowning: The phase during labor when the baby's head is visible at the opening of the vagina.

Crush injury: An injury to a body part, often an extremity, caused by a high degree of pressure; may result in serious damage to underlying tissues and cause bleeding, bruising, fracture, laceration and compartment syndrome.

Crush syndrome: Common in people who are trapped in collapsed structures. The injury does not happen at the time that the tissue is crushed, but once the crushed muscle is released from compression and the tissue is reperfused with blood. At that point, multiple adverse processes occur, as the products of muscle breakdown are released into the blood. The person may suffer major shock and renal failure, and death may occur.

Cyanotic: Bluish discoloration of the skin around the mouth or the fingertips resulting from a lack of oxygen in the blood.

Defibrillation: An electric shock that disrupts the electrical activity of the heart long enough to allow the heart to spontaneously develop an effective rhythm on its own.

Dependency: The desire or need to continually use a substance.

Depressant: A substance that affects the central nervous system and slows down physical and mental activity; can be used to treat anxiety, tension and high blood pressure.

Dermis: The deeper layer of skin; contains the nerves, sweat glands, oil glands and blood vessels.

Designer drugs: Potent and illegal street drugs formed from a medicinal substance whose drug composition has been modified (designed).

Diabetes: A disease in which there are high levels of blood glucose due to defects in insulin production, insulin action or both.

Diabetic coma: A life-threatening complication of diabetes in which very high blood sugar causes the person to become unresponsive.

Diabetic emergency: A situation in which a person becomes ill because of an imbalance of insulin and sugar (glucose) in the bloodstream.

Diabetic ketoacidosis (DKA): An accumulation of organic acids and ketones (waste products) in the blood; occurs when there is inadequate insulin and high blood sugar levels.

Digestive system: A group of organs and other structures that digest food and eliminate waste.

Direct contact transmission: Mode of transmission of pathogens that occurs through directly touching infected blood or other potentially infectious materials (OPIM), or other agents such as chemicals, drugs or toxins.

Direct pressure: Pressure applied on a wound to control bleeding.

Disability: The absence or impairment of motor, sensory or mental function.

Disaster: An event that causes widespread destruction, including possible large numbers of casualties; can be natural or man-made.

Disease transmission: The passage of a disease from one person to another.

Dislocation: The displacement of a bone from its normal position at a joint.

Distressed swimmer: A swimmer showing anxiety or panic; often identified as a swimmer who has gone beyond their swimming abilities.

Down syndrome: A condition caused by a genetic accident and characterized by varying degrees of mental retardation and physical defects.

Dressing: A pad placed directly over a wound to absorb blood and other body fluids and to prevent infection.

Drowning: An event in which a person experiences respiratory impairment due to submersion in water. Drowning may or may not result in death.

Drug: Any substance, other than food, intended to affect the functions of the body.

Elastic roller bandage: A bandage designed to keep continuous pressure on a body part; also called an elastic wrap.

Embedded object: An object that remains in an open wound.

Embolus: A sudden blockage of a blood vessel by a traveling clot or other material, such as fat or air, that circulates in the bloodstream until it becomes lodged in a blood vessel.

Embryo: The term used to describe the early stage of development in the uterus from fertilization to the beginning of the third month.

Emergency: A situation requiring immediate action.

Emergency action steps: Three basic steps you should take in any emergency: **CHECK—CALL—CARE**.

Emergency medical dispatcher (EMD): A telecommunicator who has received special training to respond to a request for emergency medical services via 9-1-1 or a designated emergency number and to allocate appropriate resources to the scene of an emergency. Some EMDs are trained to provide prearrival medical instructions to a responder before emergency medical services (EMS) personnel arrive.

Emergency medical responder (EMR): A person trained in emergency care who may be called on to give such care as a routine part of their job until more advanced emergency medical services (EMS) personnel take over. EMRs often are the first trained professionals to respond to emergencies; also called "first responders."

Emergency medical services (EMS) personnel: Trained and equipped community-based personnel who give emergency care for injured or ill persons and who are often dispatched through 9-1-1 or a designated emergency number.

Emergency medical services (EMS) system: A network of professionals linked together to give the best care for people in all types of emergencies.

Emergency medical technician (EMT): A person who gives basic emergency medical care and transportation for critical and emergent patients who access the EMS system. EMTs are typically authorized to function after completing local and state certification requirements; formerly referred to as EMT-Basic.

Emphysema: A chronic, degenerative lung disease in which there is damage to the alveoli (air sacs in the lungs).

Endocrine system: A group of organs and other structures that regulate and coordinate the activities of other systems by producing chemicals (hormones) that influence tissue activity.

Epidermis: The outer layer of skin; provides a barrier against bacteria and other organisms that can cause infection.

Epiglottitis: A serious bacterial infection that causes severe swelling of the epiglottis (the flap of tissue that covers the trachea during swallowing to keep food and liquid out of the lungs), which can result in a blocked airway, causing respiratory failure in children; may be fatal.

Epilepsy: A brain disorder characterized by recurrent seizures.

Epinephrine: A drug that slows or stops the effects of anaphylaxis.

Epinephrine auto-injector: A syringe system, available by prescription only, that contains a single dose of epinephrine.

Exercise-associated muscle cramps: Formerly known as heat cramps, these muscle spasms can be intense and debilitating and occur typically in the legs, arms and abdomen; painful involuntary muscle spasms occur during or after physical exertion, particularly in high heat and humidity, possibly due to loss of electrolytes and water from perspiration; not associated with an increase in body temperature.

Exertional heat exhaustion (EHA): An inability to cope with heat and characterized by fatigue, nausea and/or vomiting, loss of appetite, dehydration, exercise-associated muscle cramps, dizziness with possible fainting, elevated heart and respiratory rate, and skin that is pale, cool and clammy or slightly flushed; if a core temperature can be obtained, it is typically higher than 104° F (40° C). The person may be weak and unable to stand but has *normal mental status;* often results from strenuous work or wearing too much clothing in a hot, humid environment, and may or may not occur with dehydration and electrolyte imbalance.

Exertional heat stroke (EHS): The most serious form of heat-related illness; life threatening and develops when the body's cooling mechanisms are overwhelmed and body systems begin to fail; people with EHS have exaggerated heat production and an inability to cool themselves.

External bleeding: Bleeding on the outside of the body; often, visible bleeding.

Extremity: A limb of the body; *upper extremity* is the arm; *lower extremity* is the leg.

Fainting: Temporary loss of consciousness; usually related to temporary insufficient blood flow to the brain; also known as syncope, "blacking out" or "passing out."

Febrile seizure: Seizure activity brought on by a rapid increase or spike in body temperature in a young child or an infant.

Femoral arteries: The arteries that supply blood to the lower extremities.

Femur: The bone of the thigh.

Fetus: The term used to describe the stage of development in the uterus after the embryo stage, beginning at the start of the third month.

Fibula: One of the two bones of the lower leg.

First aid: The helping behaviors and initial care given for an acute injury or illness.

Forearm: The part of the upper extremity from the elbow to the wrist.

Fracture: A break or disruption in bone tissue.

Frostbite: A condition in which body tissues freeze; most commonly occurs in the fingers, toes, ears and nose.

Full-thickness burn: A burn injury involving all layers of skin and underlying tissues; skin may be brown or charred, and underlying tissues may appear white; formerly referred to as a third-degree burn.

Gastric distention: A condition in which the abdomen becomes swollen with air.

Generalized tonic-clonic seizure: A seizure that affects most or all of the brain.

Genitals: The external reproductive organs.

Genitourinary system: A group of organs and other structures that eliminate waste and enable reproduction.

Glucose: A simple sugar that is the primary source of energy for the body's tissues.

Good Samaritan laws: Laws that protect people against claims of negligence when they give emergency care in good faith without accepting anything in return.

Grand mal seizure: A type of generalized seizure that involves whole-body contractions with loss of consciousness.

Hallucinogen: A substance that affects mood, sensation, thinking, emotion and self-awareness; alters perception of time and space; and produces hallucinations or delusions.

Head-tilt/chin-lift maneuver: A maneuver used to open a person's airway by pushing down on the forehead while pulling up on the bony part of the jaw.

Hearing loss: Partial or total loss of hearing.

Heart attack: A sudden illness involving the death of heart muscle tissue when it does not receive oxygen-rich blood; also known as *myocardial infarction*.

Heat stroke: The most serious form of heat-related illness; life threatening and develops when the body's cooling mechanisms are overwhelmed and body systems begin to fail.

Hemorrhage: A loss of a large amount of blood in a short time or when there is continuous bleeding.

Hemostatic dressing: A dressing treated with a substance that speeds clot formation.

Humerus: The bone of the arm from the shoulder to the elbow.

Hyperglycemia: A condition in which too much sugar (glucose) is in the bloodstream, resulting in higher than normal blood glucose levels; also known as high blood glucose.

Hyperventilation: Breathing that is faster than normal.

Hypodermis: A layer of skin located beneath the dermis and epidermis; contains fat, blood vessels and connective tissues.

Hypoglycemia: A condition in which too little sugar (glucose) is in the bloodstream, resulting in lower than normal blood glucose levels; also known as low blood glucose.

Hypothalamus: Control center of the body's temperature; located in the brain.

Hypothermia: The state of the body being colder than the usual core temperature, caused by either excessive loss of body heat and/or the body's inability to produce heat.

Immobilize: To use a splint or other method to keep an injured body part from moving.

Impairment: Damage or reduction in quality, quantity, value or strength of a function.

Impaled object: An object, such as a branch or piece of metal, that penetrates the body and remains in the body.

Implied consent: Legal concept that assumes a person would consent to receive emergency care if they were able or old enough to do so.

Indirect contact transmission: Mode of transmission of pathogens that occurs when a person touches objects that have the blood or other potentially infectious materials (OPIM) of an infected person, and that infected blood or OPIM enters the body through a correct entry site.

Infection: A condition caused by disease-producing microorganisms, called pathogens or germs, in the body.

Ingested poison: A poison that is swallowed.

Inhalant: A substance, such as a medication, that a person inhales to counteract or prevent a specific condition; also a substance inhaled to produce mood-altering effects.

Inhaled poison: A poison that is breathed into the lungs.

Injected poison: A poison that enters the body through a bite, sting or syringe.

Injury: Damage that occurs when the body is subjected to an external force, such as a blow, a fall, a collision, an electrical current or temperature extremes.

Insulin: A hormone produced by the pancreas to help glucose move into cells; in persons with diabetes, it may not be produced at all or may not be produced in sufficient amounts.

Insulin shock: A life-threatening condition in which too much insulin is in the bloodstream.

Integumentary system: A group of organs and other structures that protect the body, retain fluids and help to prevent infection.

Internal bleeding: Bleeding inside the body.

Joint: A structure where two or more bones are joined.

Kidney: An organ that filters waste from the blood to form urine.

Labor: The birth process, beginning with the contraction of the uterus and dilation of the cervix and ending with the stabilization and recovery of the mother.

Laceration: A cut, usually from a sharp object, that can have either jagged or smooth edges.

Lay responder: A layperson who is not trained to provide first aid, but who recognizes an emergency and decides to act.

Life-threatening emergency: An injury or illness that impairs a person's ability to circulate oxygenated blood to all parts of the body and will likely cause death if not cared for immediately.

Ligament: A fibrous band that holds bones together at a joint.

Long-term control medications: Medications taken regularly to help prevent asthma attacks by reducing inflammation and swelling and making the airways less sensitive to triggers.

Lower extremity: The parts of the body from the hip to the toes.

Lower leg: The part of the lower extremity from the knee to the ankle.

Lyme disease: A disease transmitted by the deer tick and black-legged tick.

Mechanical airway obstruction: Complete or partial blockage of the airway by a foreign object, such as a piece of food or a small toy, or by fluids such as vomit or blood.

Medical emergency: A sudden illness requiring immediate medical attention.

Medication: A drug given therapeutically to prevent or treat the effects of a disease or condition, or otherwise enhance mental or physical well-being.

Mental (cognitive) function: The brain's capacity to reason and to process information.

Metabolism: The process by which cells convert nutrients to energy.

Metacarpals: The bones of the hand.

Metatarsals: The bones of the foot.

Motor function: The ability to move the body or a body part.

Motor impairment: The total or partial inability to move or to use a body part.

Mucous plug: A collection of mucus that blocks the opening of the cervix and is expelled, usually toward the end of the pregnancy when the cervix begins to dilate.

Multiple sclerosis: A progressive disease characterized by nerve degeneration and patches of hardened tissue in the brain or spinal cord.

Muscle: A tissue that contracts and relaxes to create movement.

Muscular dystrophy: A hereditary disease characterized by progressive deterioration of muscles, leading to disability, deformity and loss of strength.

Musculoskeletal system: A group of tissues and other structures that support the body, protect internal organs, allow movement, store minerals, manufacture blood cells and create heat.

Narcotic: A drug derived from opium or opium-like compounds; used to reduce pain and can alter mood and behavior.

Nervous system: A group of organs and other structures that regulate all body functions.

Nitroglycerin: A prescribed medication, often in tablet or spray form, given for the prevention or relief of angina pectoris.

Non-life-threatening emergency: A situation that does not have an immediate impact on a person's ability to circulate oxygenated blood but still requires medical attention.

Occlusive dressing: A special type of dressing that does not allow air or fluid to pass through.

Open fracture: A type of fracture in which there is an open wound in the skin over the fracture.

Open wound: A wound with a break in the skin's surface.

OPIM: Other potentially infectious materials such as body fluids (other than blood).

Opioid narcotic: A drug used to dull the senses or reduce pain; often derived from opium or opium-like compounds.

Organ: A structure of similar tissues acting together to perform specific body functions.

Osteoporosis: The gradual, progressive weakening of bone.

Overdose: The use of an excessive amount of a substance, resulting in adverse reactions ranging from mania (mental and physical hyperactivity) and hysteria to coma and death.

Ovum: A female's egg; once fertilized by a sperm, it forms an embryo.

Paralysis: A loss of muscle control; a permanent loss of feeling and movement; the inability to move.

Paramedic: An allied health professional whose primary focus is to give advanced emergency medical care for critical and emergency patients who access the EMS system. Paramedics may also give nonemergency, community-based care based on state and local community paramedicine or mobile integrated healthcare programs.

Partial seizure: A seizure that affects only part of the brain; may be simple or complex.

Partial-thickness burn: A burn injury involving the epidermis and dermis, characterized by red, wet skin and blisters; formerly referred to as a second-degree burn.

Patella: The kneecap.

Pathogen: A term used to describe a germ; a disease-causing agent (e.g., bacterium or virus).

Pelvis: The lower part of the trunk, containing the intestines, bladder and internal reproductive organs.

Penetrating trauma: Trauma that occurs when the body is pierced by or impaled on a sharp object.

Personal protective equipment (PPE): The equipment and supplies that help prevent the responder from directly contacting infected materials; includes disposable latex-free gloves, gowns, masks, shields and protective eyewear.

Phalanges: The bones of the fingers and toes.

Physiology: How living organisms function (e.g., movement and reproduction).

Placenta: An organ attached to the uterus and unborn baby through which nutrients are delivered; expelled after the baby is delivered.

Plasma: The liquid part of the blood.

Platelets: Disk-shaped structures in the blood that are made of cell fragments; help stop bleeding by forming blood clots at wound sites.

Poison: Any substance that can cause injury, illness or death when introduced into the body, especially by chemical means.

Poison Control Center (PCC): A specialized health center that provides information on poisons or suspected poisoning emergencies.

Post-ictal phase: The fourth and final phase of a generalized seizure, during which the person becomes extremely fatigued.

Pregnancy: Begins when an egg (ovum) is fertilized by a sperm, forming an embryo.

Prehospital care: Emergency medical care given before a person arrives at a hospital or medical facility.

Pressure bandage: A bandage applied snugly to create pressure on a wound to aid in controlling bleeding.

Prolapsed umbilical cord: A complication of childbirth in which a loop of umbilical cord protrudes through the vagina before delivery of the baby.

Puncture/penetration wound: A type of wound that results when the skin is pierced with a pointed object.

Quick-relief (rescue) medications: Medications taken when a person is experiencing an acute asthma attack to open the airways right away.

Rabies: An infectious viral disease that affects the nervous system of humans and other mammals; has a high fatality rate if left untreated.

Radius: One of the two bones of the forearm.

Reaching assist: A method of rescuing someone in the water by using an object to extend the responder's reach or reaching with an arm or leg.

Refusal of care: The declining of care by a competent person; a person has the right to refuse the care of anyone who responds to an emergency scene.

Remote: Far away from populated areas or resources.

Reproductive system: A group of organs and other structures that enables sexual reproduction.

Respiratory arrest: A condition in which breathing has stopped but the heart is still beating.

Respiratory distress: A condition in which a person is having trouble breathing or requires extra effort to breathe.

Respiratory system: A group of organs and other structures that bring air into the body and remove waste through a process called breathing, or respiration.

Retroperitoneal space: The space posterior to the abdominal cavity that contains the kidneys, pancreas, blood vessels and other structures.

Reye's syndrome: An illness brought on by high fever that affects the brain and other internal organs; can be caused by the use of aspirin in children and infants.

Rib cage: The cage of bones formed by the 12 pairs of ribs, the sternum and the spine.

Risk factors: Conditions or behaviors that increase the chance that a person will develop a disease.

Rocky Mountain Spotted Fever: A disease caused by the transmission of microscopic bacteria from the wood tick or dog tick host.

Roller bandage: A bandage made of gauze or gauze-like material that is wrapped around a body part, over a dressing, using overlapping turns until the dressing is covered.

Saturated fat: The fat in animal tissue and products.

Scapula: The shoulder blade.

Scene size-up: A brief survey done prior to entering the scene of an emergency to ensure safety, form an initial impression about what happened and the nature of the person's illness or injury, identify any life-threatening conditions and determine necessary resources.

Sensory function: The ability to see, hear, touch, taste and smell.

Severe, life-threatening bleeding: Profuse bleeding from a wound that is a potential threat to life.

Shock: A life-threatening condition that occurs when the circulatory system fails to provide adequate oxygenated blood to all parts of the body.

Simple partial seizure: A seizure in which a specific body part experiences muscle contractions; does not affect memory or awareness.

Skeletal muscles: Muscles that attach to the bones.

Soft tissues: Body structures that include the layers of skin, fat and muscles.

Spinal column: See *spine*.

Spinal cord: A cylindrical structure extending from the base of the skull to the lower back, consisting mainly of nerve cells and protected by the spinal column.

Spine: The series of vertebrae extending from the base of the skull to the tip of the tailbone (coccyx); also referred to as the spinal column or the vertebral column.

Spleen: Located behind the stomach and protected somewhat by the lower left ribs, the spleen is the most commonly injured intra-abdominal organ.

Splint: A device used to immobilize body parts.

Sprain: The partial or complete tearing or stretching of ligaments and other soft tissue structures at a joint.

Standard precautions: Safety measures taken to prevent exposure to blood and OPIM when giving care to injured or ill persons; assumes that all body fluids, secretions and excretions (except sweat) are potentially infective.

Status epilepticus: An epileptic seizure (or repeated seizures) that lasts longer than 5 minutes without any sign of slowing down; should be considered life threatening and requires prompt advanced medical care.

Sternum: The long, flat bone in the middle of the front of the rib cage; also called the breastbone.

Stimulant: A substance that affects the central nervous system and speeds up physical and mental activity.

Stoma: See *tracheostomy*.

Strain: The excessive stretching and tearing of muscles or tendons; a pulled or torn muscle.

Stroke: A disruption of blood flow to part of the brain that may cause permanent damage to brain tissue. The disruption can be caused by an obstruction (a clot) or by bleeding in the brain.

Substance abuse: The deliberate, persistent, excessive use of a substance without regard to health concerns or accepted medical practices.

Substance misuse: The use of a substance for unintended purposes or for intended purposes but in improper amounts or doses.

Sudden cardiac arrest: Cardiac arrest that happens suddenly and without any warning signs. Sudden cardiac arrest can happen in people who appear healthy and have no known heart disease or other risk factors for the condition. A person who experiences sudden cardiac arrest is at very high risk for dying and needs immediate care.

Sudden illness: A physical condition requiring immediate medical attention.

Sudden infant death syndrome (SIDS): The sudden death of an infant younger than 1 year that remains unexplained after the performance of a complete postmortem investigation (autopsy).

Superficial burn: A burn injury involving only the top layer of skin, the epidermis, characterized by red, dry skin; formerly referred to as a first-degree burn.

Supraventricular tachycardia (SVT): An abnormal heart rhythm resulting in a very rapid heartbeat. People with SVT often feel palpitations in their chest or their heart racing.

Syncope: A term used to describe the temporary loss of consciousness; also known as fainting or "passing out."

Synergistic effect: The outcome created when two or more drugs are combined; the effects of each may enhance those of the other.

Tarsals: The bones of the ankle.

Tellatouch: A small typewriter keyboard used for communication by a person with hearing and/or vision loss.

Tendon: A fibrous band that attaches muscle to bone.

Tetanus: An acute infectious disease caused by a bacterium that produces a powerful poison; can occur in puncture wounds, such as human and animal bites; also called lockjaw.

Thigh: The part of the lower extremity from the pelvis to the knee.

Thrombus: A blood clot that forms in a blood vessel and remains there, slowing the flow of blood and depriving tissues of normal blood flow and oxygen.

Throwing assist: A method of rescuing someone in the water by throwing the person a floating object, with or without a line attached.

Tibia: One of the two bones of the lower leg.

Tissue: A collection of similar cells acting together to perform specific body functions.

Tolerance: The condition in which the effects of a substance on the body decrease as the result of continued use.

Tonic phase: The second phase of a generalized seizure, during which a person becomes unresponsive and muscles become rigid.

Tourniquet: A wide band placed tightly enough around an arm or a leg to constrict blood vessels in order to stop blood flow to a wound.

Tracheostomy: A surgical opening created in the front of the neck following surgery on the trachea to allow the person to breathe; also called a stoma.

Trained lay responder: A layperson who is trained in basic emergency care (i.e., trained to give first aid), but who does not have special or advanced medical training, and is willing to act in an emergency.

Transient ischemic attack (TIA): A condition that produces stroke-like symptoms but causes no permanent damage; may be a precursor to a stroke; sometimes called a mini-stroke.

Traumatic brain injury (TBI): An injury to the brain resulting from an external force such as a blow to the head or a penetrating injury to the brain. TBIs are associated with temporary and/or permanent impairment to brain function, including physical, emotional and cognitive functioning. A concussion is a common type of TBI.

Triggers: Substances or conditions that initiate an asthma attack when the person is exposed to them.

Ulna: One of the two bones of the forearm.

Umbilical cord: A flexible structure that attaches the placenta to the fetus, allowing for the passage of blood, nutrients and waste.

Upper arm: The part of the upper extremity from the shoulder to the elbow.

Upper extremity: The parts of the body from the shoulder to the fingers.

Urinary system: A group of organs and other structures that eliminates waste products from the blood.

Uterus: A pear-shaped organ in a woman's pelvis in which an embryo forms and develops into a baby; also called the womb.

Veins: Blood vessels that carry oxygen-poor blood from all parts of the body to the heart, except for the pulmonary veins, which carry oxygen-rich blood to the heart from the lungs.

Ventricular fibrillation (V-fib): A life-threatening heart rhythm in which the heart is in a state of totally disorganized electrical activity, and does not pump blood effectively.

Ventricular tachycardia (V-tach): A life-threatening heart rhythm in which there is very rapid contraction of the ventricles (the lower chambers of the heart), causing the heart to pump blood ineffectively or not at all.

Vertebrae: The 33 bones of the spine.

Vertebral column: See *spine*.

Virus: A common type of pathogen that depends on other organisms to live and reproduce; can be difficult to kill.

Vision loss: Partial or total loss of sight.

Vital organs: Those organs whose functions are essential to life, including the brain, heart and lungs.

Wading assist: A method of rescuing someone in the water by wading out to the person in distress and using a reaching assist to help pull them to safety; use this assist only in water no deeper than the responder's chest.

Wheezing: A high-pitched whistling sound heard during inhalation but heard most loudly on exhalation; an abnormal breath sound that can often be heard without a stethoscope.

Wilderness: An area that is uninhabited by human beings, is uncultivated and has been left in its natural condition.

Withdrawal: The condition of mental and physical discomfort produced when a person stops using or abusing a substance to which they are addicted.

Wound: An injury to the soft tissues.

SOURCES

American Academy of Allergy, Asthma and Immunology: *Food allergy.* http://www.aaaai.org/patients/gallery/foodallergy.asp. Accessed October 2015.

American Academy of Orthopaedic Surgeons: *Growth plate fractures.* http://orthoinfo.aaos.org/topic.cfm?topic=A00040. Accessed December 2016.

American Academy of Pediatrics: *Ear infection information.* https://healthychildren.org/English/health-issues/conditions/ear-nose-throat/Pages/Ear-Infection-Information.aspx. Accessed December 2016.

American Association of Poison Control Centers: *2014 annual report of the American Association of Poison Control Centers' National Poison Data System (NPDS): 32nd annual report.* http://dx.doi.org/10.3109/15563650.2015.1102927. Accessed December 2016.

American Diabetes Association: *Living with diabetes: Hyperglycemia (high blood glucose).* http://www.diabetes.org/living-with-diabetes/treatment-and-care/blood-glucose-control/hyperglycemia.html. Accessed October 2015.

American Diabetes Association: *Living with diabetes: Hypoglycemia (low blood glucose).* http://www.diabetes.org/living-with-diabetes/treatment-and-care/blood-glucose-control/hypoglycemia-low-blood.html. Accessed October 2015.

American Diabetes Association: *Statistics about diabetes.* http://www.diabetes.org/diabetes-basics/statistics/. Accessed January 2017.

American Heart Association: *CPR facts and stats.* http://cpr.heart.org/AHAECC/CPRAndECC/AboutCPRFirstAid/CPRFactsAndStats/UCM_475748_CPR-Facts-and-Stats.jsp. Accessed October 2015.

American Lung Association: *Asthma.* http://www.lung.org/lung-health-and-diseases/lung-disease-lookup/asthma/. Accessed October 2015.

American Stroke Association: *About stroke: Understanding risk.* http://www.strokeassociation.org/STROKEORG/AboutStroke/About-Stroke_UCM_308529_SubHomePage.jsp. Accessed December 2016.

Armstrong LE, Crago AE, Adams R, Roberts WO, Maresh CM: Whole-body cooling of hyperthermic runners: comparison to two field therapies, *American Journal of Emergency Medicine* 14:355–358, 1996.

Armstrong LE, Maresh CM, Crago AE, Adams R, Roberts RO: Interpretation of aural temperatures during exercise, hyperthermia, and cooling therapy, *Medicine, Exercise, Nutrition and Health* 3:9–16, 1994.

Armstrong LE, Szlyk PC, DeLuca JP, Sils IV, Hubbard RW: Fluid-electrolyte losses in uniforms during prolonged exercise at 30 degrees C, *Aviation, Space, and Environmental Medicine* 63:351–355, 1992.

Asthma and Allergy Foundation of America: *Asthma overview.* http://www.aafa.org/display.cfm?id=8&cont=8. Accessed October 2015.

Binkley HM, Beckett J, Casa DJ, Kleiner DM, Plummer PE: National Athletic Trainers' Association position statement: Exertional heat illnesses, *Journal of Athletic Training* 37(3):329–343, 2002.

Brodeur VB, Dennett SR, Griffin LS: Exertional hyperthermia, ice baths, and emergency care at the Falmouth Road Race, *Journal of Emergency Nursing* 15:304–312, 1989.

Casa DJ, Armstrong LE, Ganio MS, et al: Exertional heat stroke in competitive athletes, *Current Sports Medicine Reports* 4:309–317, 2005.

Casa DJ, Armstrong LE, Hillman SK, Montain SJ, Reiff RV, Rich B, Roberts WO, Stone JA: National Athletic Trainers' Association position statement: Fluid replacement for athletes, *Journal of Athletic Training* 35(2):212–224, 2000.

Centers for Disease Control and Prevention: *Deaths and mortality*. http://www.cdc.gov/nchs/fastats/ deaths.htm. Accessed December 2016.

Centers for Disease Control and Prevention: Increases in drug and opioid overdose deaths—United States, 2000–2014, *Morbidity and Mortality Weekly Report* 64(50):1378–1382, 2016. http://www.cdc.gov/mmwr/ preview/mmwrhtml/mm6450a3.htm?s_cid=mm6450a3_w. Accessed September 2016.

Centers for Disease Control and Prevention: *Prevent Lyme disease*. http://www.cdc.gov/Features/ LymeDisease/. Accessed October 2015.

Centers for Disease Control and Prevention: *Unintentional drowning: Get the facts*. https://www.cdc.gov/ homeandrecreationalsafety/water-safety/waterinjuries-factsheet.html. Accessed January 2017.

Centers for Disease Control and Prevention: *West Nile Virus (WNV) fact sheet*. https://www.cdc.gov/ westnile/resources/pdfs/wnvFactsheet_508.pdf. Accessed December 2016.

Centers for Disease Control and Prevention: *Winter weather frequently asked questions*. https://www.cdc. gov/disasters/winter/faq.html. Accessed December 2016.

Cianferoni A, Muraro A: Food-induced anaphylaxis, *Immunology and Allergy Clinics* 32(1):165–195, 2012.

Clements J, Casa D, Knight J, McClung J, Blake A, Meenen P, et al: Ice-water immersion and cold-water immersion provide similar cooling rates in runners with exercise-induced hyperthermia, *Journal of Athletic Training* 37(2):146–150, 2002.

Epilepsy Foundation: *Epilepsy and seizure statistics*. http://www.epilepsy.com/learn/epilepsy-statistics. Accessed December 2016.

FEMA: *Disaster declarations for 2016*. https://www.fema.gov/disasters/grid/year/2016?field_disaster_type_ term_tid_1=All. Accessed January 2017.

Foundation for Spinal Cord Injury Prevention, Care and Cure: *Spinal cord injury facts*. http://fscip.org/ facts.htm. Accessed December 2016.

Hadad E, Moran D, Epstein S: Cooling heat stroke patients by available field measures, *Intensive Care Medicine* 30(2):338, 2004.

Hayward JS, Collis M, Eckerson JD: Thermographic evaluation of relative heat loss areas of man during cold water immersion. *Aerospace Medicine* 44:708–711, 1973.

Home Safety Council: *Safety tips: Poison*. http://homesafetycouncil.org/SafetyGuide/sg_poison_w001.asp. Accessed September 2015.

Lederer W, Mair D, Rabl W, et al: Frequency of rib and sternum fractures associated with out-of-hospital cardiopulmonary resuscitation is underestimated by conventional chest X-ray, *Resuscitation* 60(2):157–162, 2004.

Maguire S, Mann M, John N, et al: Does cardiopulmonary resuscitation cause rib fractures in children? A systematic review, *Child Abuse and Neglect* 30(7):739–751, 2006.

MayoClinic.com: *Hypothermia: Risk factors*. http://www.mayoclinic.org/diseases-conditions/hypothermia/ basics/risk-factors/CON-20020453. Accessed October 2015.

MedlinePlus: *Epiglottitis*. https://www.nlm.nih.gov/medlineplus/ency/article/000605.htm. Accessed October 2015.

MedlinePlus: *Hypothermia*. http://www.nlm.nih.gov/medlineplus/hypothermia.html. Accessed October 2015.

Mizukami H, Shimizu K, Shiono H, Uezono T, Sasaki M: Forensic diagnosis of death from cold. *Legal Medicine* 1(4):204–209, 1999.

Mozaffarian D, Benjamin EJ, Go AS, Arnett DK, Blaha MJ, Cushman M, Das SR, de Ferranti S, Després J-P, Fullerton HJ, Howard VJ, Huffman MD, Isasi CR, Jiménez MC, Judd SE, Kissela BM, Lichtman JH, Lisabeth LD, Liu S, Mackey RH, Magid DJ, McGuire DK, Mohler ER III, Moy CS, Muntner P, Mussolino ME, Nasir K, Neumar RW, Nichol G, Palaniappan L, Pandey DK, Reeves MJ, Rodriguez CJ, Rosamond W, Sorlie PD, Stein J, Towfighi A, Turan TN, Virani SS, Woo D, Yeh RW, Turner MB; on behalf of the American Heart Association Statistics Committee and Stroke Statistics Subcommittee. Heart disease and stroke statistics—2016 update: a report from the American Heart Association [published online ahead of print December 16, 2015]. *Circulation.* DOI: 10.1161/CIR.0000000000000350.

National Center for Injury Prevention and Control: *10 leading causes of death, United States 2007, all races, both sexes.* http://webappa.cdc.gov/sasweb/ncipc/leadcaus10.html. Accessed December 2016.

National Highway Traffic Safety Administration: *Car seat by child's age and size.* http://www.safercar.gov/parents/CarSeats/Right-Car-Seat-Age-Size.htm. Accessed October 2015.

National Institute of Allergy and Infectious Diseases: *NIAID's food allergy research.* https://www.niaid.nih.gov/diseases-conditions/food-allergy. Accessed December 2016.

National Osteoporosis Foundation: *What is osteoporosis and what causes it?* https://www.nof.org/patients/what-is-osteoporosis/. Accessed December 2016.

National Spinal Cord Injury Statistical Center: *Spinal cord injury facts and figures at a glance, February 2013.* https://www.nscisc.uab.edu/PublicDocuments/fact_figures_docs/Facts%202013.pdf. Accessed December 2016.

Powner D, Holcombe P, Mello L: Cardiopulmonary resuscitation-related injuries, *Critical Care Medicine* 12(1):54–55, 1984.

Princeton University: *Cold stress facts.* https://ehs.princeton.edu/workplace-construction/occupational-health/heat-cold-stress/cold-stress-facts. Accessed December 2016.

REI: *Layering basics.* http://www.rei.com/expertadvice/articles/dress+layers.html. Accessed December 2016. United States Department of Health and Human Services: *The poison help line.* http://poisonhelp.hrsa.gov/the-poison-help-line/index.html. Accessed October 2015.

United States Department of Justice: *Burn injuries in child abuse.* https://www.ncjrs.gov/pdffiles/91190-6.pdf. Accessed October 2015.

United States Department of Labor: *Welcome to OSHA's campaign to prevent heat illness in outdoor workers.* https://www.osha.gov/SLTC/heatillness/index.html. Accessed October 2015.

United States Federal Communications Commission: *Guide: 911 wireless services.* https://www.fcc.gov/guides/wireless-911-services. Accessed October 2015.

United States Food and Drug Administration: *Disposal of unused medicines: What you should know.* http://www.fda.gov/Drugs/ResourcesForYou/Consumers/BuyingUsingMedicineSafely/EnsuringSafeUseofMedicine/SafeDisposalofMedicines/ucm186187.htm. Accessed December 2016.

United States National Library of Medicine: *Transient ischemic attack.* http://www.nlm.nih.gov/medlineplus/ency/article/000730.htm. Accessed October 2015.

Wedin B, Vanggaard L, Hirvonen J: Paradoxical undressing in fatal hypothermia, *Journal of Forensic Sciences* 24(3):543–553, 1979.

Williams D: Giving birth "in place": A guide to emergency preparedness for childbirth, *American College of Nurse-Midwives* 49(4):48–52, 2004.

PHOTOGRAPHY CREDITS

CHAPTER 1 Chapter Opener: ©iStockphoto.com/Willowpix

CHAPTER 2 Chapter Opener: ©iStockphoto.com/Willowpix

CHAPTER 3 Chapter Opener: ©iStockphoto.com/emesilva

CHAPTER 4 Chapter Opener ©iStockphoto.com/SimplyCreativePhotography

CHAPTER 6 Chapter Opener: ©iStockphoto.com/choja

CHAPTER 7 Chapter Opener: ©iStockphoto.com/AlbanyPictures

CHAPTER 9 Chapter Opener: ©iStockphoto.com/Wibofoto

CHAPTER 10 Chapter Opener: ©iStockphoto.com/skynesher

CHAPTER 13 Chapter Opener: ©iStockphoto.com/grandriver

CHAPTER 14 Chapter Opener: ©iStockphoto.com/miljko

CHAPTER 18 Chapter Opener: Courtesy of the Canadian Red Cross

CHAPTER 19 Chapter Opener: ©iStockphoto.com/Jim_David

CHAPTER 21 Chapter Opener: ©iStockphoto.com/Imagesbybarbara

CHAPTER 22 Chapter Opener: Courtesy of the Canadian Red Cross

CHAPTER 23 Chapter Opener: wavebreakmedia/Shutterstock.com

INDEX

Note: Page locators with *b* indicate box; *f*, figure; and *t*, table.